ask a **midwife**

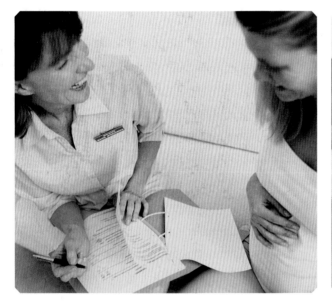
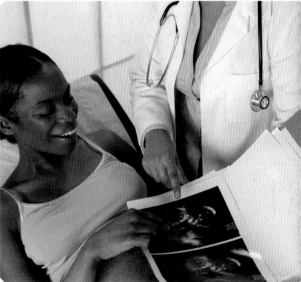

ask a midwife

All your pregnancy and birth
questions answered with wisdom,
insight, and expertise

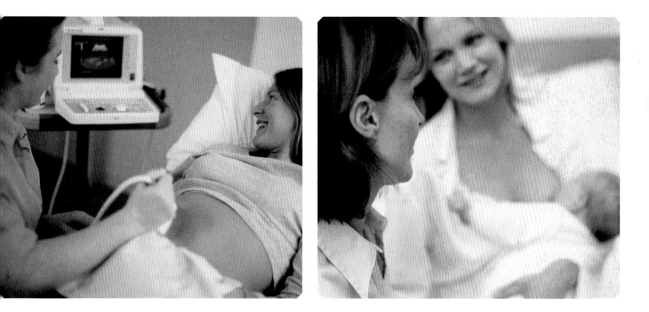

Catharine Parker-Littler
in conjunction with www.midwivesonline.com

London, New York, Munich, Melbourne, Delhi

Project Editor Claire Cross
Design Carole Ash at Project 360
Senior Editors Esther Ripley, Emma Woolf
Senior Art Editor Nicola Rodway
Production Editor Jenny Woodcock
Production Controller Bethan Blase
Creative Technical Support Sonia Charbonnier
Managing Editors Penny Warren, Esther Ripley
Managing Art Editor Marianne Markham
Publisher Peggy Vance

Contributing midwives
Diane Jones RM
Joanne Daubeney RM
Dawn Lewis RM
Julie Scott RM
Emma Whapples RM
Tamsin Oxenham RM
Sarah Fleming RM
Anne Thysse RM
Dr Mary Steen

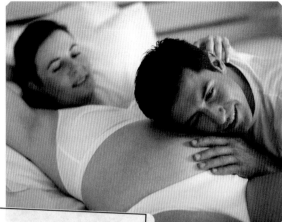

First published in Great Britain in 2008 by
Dorling Kindersley Limited
80 Strand, London WC2R ORL

Penguin Group (UK)

A CIP catalogue record for this book is available from
the British Library

ISBN: 978-1-4053-3110-4

Printed and bound in China by Sheck Wah Tong Printing Press Ltd

Discover more at
www.dk.com

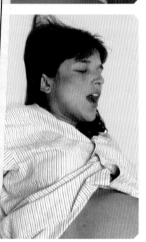

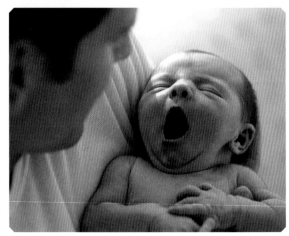

Foreword

My own career as a midwife has spanned over twenty years and covers a broad range of midwifery experience, including hospital-based midwifery, working in the local community, attending home births in the east end of our capital, working with traditional birth attendants on the west coast of Africa, and clinical research.

Since 2002, my attention has been focused on using the internet to deliver midwifery information. My initial vision was to set up a contemporary website to help my midwifery collegues to access relevant links on the web for evidence-based information to inform their clinical practice. I developed and launched a simple webpage with web-based resources and links. As a result, a growing number of midwives began using the site to access the informative quick links. I provided direct email access for my fellow midwives to communicate with me and was surprised when a growing number of users who were not midwives but were either wanting to become pregnant or were expectant mothers began to access my web page and email box, typically asking "Are you a real midwife? Can I ask you a question as my midwife is always so busy?". I began to recognize the need for a complementary online midwifery information service. I also saw that, at a time when our midwives were thin on the ground, expectant mothers wanted and needed contact with a midwife for reassurance.

In 2003, I launched www.midwivesonline.com. It has grown to be one of the most frequently accessed pregnancy information sites and is the UK's leading midwifery-led website for expectant and new parents, attracting thousands of users from across the nation, with a growing interest worldwide. There is something about writing an email that encourages expectant parents to share their concerns freely and ask questions that they perhaps wouldn't in a more formal clinical environment. At a time when there is such a shortage of midwives, our *Ask a Midwife* service provides invaluable support to many mothers- and fathers-to-be.

In this book I, and a great team of midwives, have observed the most frequently asked questions that expectant parents ask and have collated them into a user-friendly, midwifery-led resource. We hope that the wisdom contained within *Ask a Midwife* will help you to be more confident when called to make choices about antenatal care and tests, and most of all that the book will help you to have a positive birth and parenting experience.

Catharine Parker-Littler

Contents

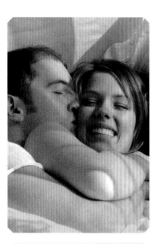

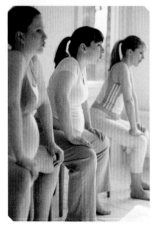

Labour and birth

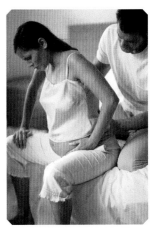

New parents

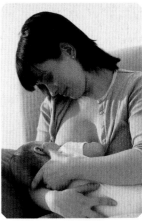

A new life

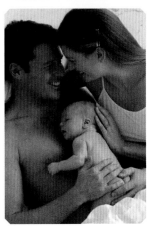

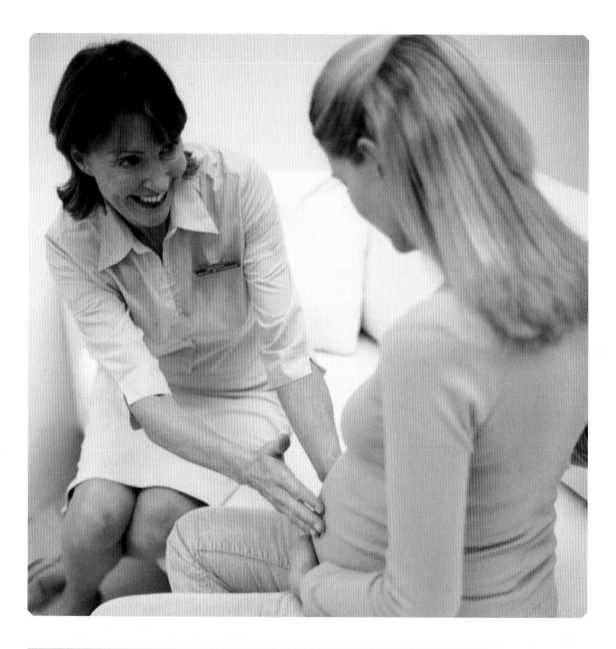

As midwives, we know that seemingly trivial questions can cause unnecessary fear if left unanswered

Introduction

I'm so thrilled about your desire for a baby and say with confidence that there are few experiences in life that top the moment when **your pregnancy is confirmed! It's always a miracle** when you consider how many couples experience difficulties when trying for a baby, so our warm congratulations – whether you are just starting a family or bringing a new addition into your current family – a baby to love and be loved by.

Tune in to every passing moment and enjoy this season in your life as much as you can. Although time passing during pregnancy can feel like an eternity as the months roll on and your pregnancy grows, believe me when I say "enjoy"! This is such a special period for expectant parents and you will probably look back and marvel at just how quickly it really passed. My advice is to slow down and enjoy this chapter in your life. Before too long you will have entered into the next season following the birth – don't wish this time away too quickly.

The word "midwife" is rooted in the concept of "wise woman" and "being with woman", which is what a good midwife aspires to be and do. Part of the midwife's role is to be your first point of contact, so as soon as you confirm your pregnancy, get in touch and arrange an early appointment. It is the desire of a midwife to remain as accessible and available to mothers and families in their care as possible, and to provide antenatal care, support during your labour, and guidance during those initial weeks following the birth. Midwives view your pregnancy as a normal occurrence rather than a medical condition; however, they are also highly skilled and trained to provide support and care along with other specialist healthcare professionals should challenges occur during your pregnancy, birth, or the post-birth period.

In almost every culture, village, town, and city throughout the world there have been and will always be midwives. It's a given that even in the most remote areas of the world a midwife will exist in some form with a passion and commitment to care for women, their babies, and their families throughout this very special time of their lives – almost like a special calling or life-work! A midwife's overall aim is to be your number one carer, advocate, and support thoughout your pregnancy and birth. For myself, it has been a privilege as a midwife to serve countless women, their partners, and their families for over twenty years. Today I remain an active midwifery practitioner and feel as passionate, if not even more so, about being a midwife as when I delivered my first baby as a student midwife many years ago! It has humbled me over the years to see how women and their partners trust their midwives so completely, opening up their hearts to them about their dreams, hopes, and fears.

When midwives are over-stretched and thin on the ground, mothers and midwives feel it deeply. Most midwives are driven by a love and passion to provide excellent care and support for "their mums" – a term of endearment often used by many midwives. Your midwife understands and often anticipates the many questions you may have over the coming months and, no matter how trivial some of these may seem to you, they are of the highest priority to her. She realizes that if those seemingly trivial questions are not answered quickly, that gap of knowledge and lack of reassurance can lead to unnecessary worry and anxiety for both you and your partner. When pressures of work make it hard for midwives to devote the time they would wish to their mothers, this can mean that both mother and midwife are compromised in receiving and in delivering that excellent care that is in the heart of most midwives' role – ultimately, expectant parents may have less contact with a midwife than they would really love and indeed need. Midwives accept that there is no substitute for having a midwife who knows you by your name and is there whenever you need her; however, this may not always be possible and we have thought long and hard about how we can offer you the next best thing.

Ask a Midwife **is more than just a book; it is your own personal midwife resource for all the family.** In this book you have access to your very own "midwife" at any time of the day or night. Arranged in an easily accessible question-and-answer format, the aim of the book is to help close the gap that may exist between the times of your antenatal appointments, allowing you to touch base and access our knowledge, expertise, and experience right at your fingertips – night and day, twenty-four hours a day – and all in the comfort of your own home, work place, or when you are out and about. Access hundreds of the most frequently asked questions that expectant mothers, fathers, grandparents, family, and friends ask when they or someone else close to them is undertaking the journey of pregnancy, birth, and caring for a newborn baby. The questions in this book are down to earth, gritty, and leave no stone unturned – often the types of questions you think about, but can't quite find the words or courage to ask, such as "Will I poo in labour?" There! We have asked the question that is asked by most women albeit often in silence! So now flick over to find the answer. All the questions in the book have been plucked from real-life scenarios and situations and span the period from couples first trying to become pregnant through to their first walk out with their baby in the buggy.

Ultimately, midwives want you to enjoy a safe and positive experience of pregnancy and birth and to give you the best preparation for the early parenting of your new baby. The desire of a midwife is to share her clinical knowledge, expertise, and experience as a practitioner to equip and empower you, your partner, and your supporters with reliable knowledge and timely and relevant information at exactly the time you need it. With this resource, you will feel more in control and reassured and supported, and hopefully less worried and anxious during what can feel like a vulnerable time in your life. In the

The access to midwifery knowledge and clinical experience within the book provides timely, relevant information to allay anxiety and put minds at rest

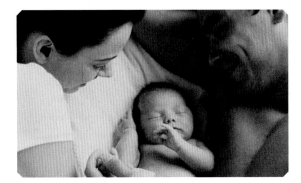

book we have taken time to provide you with answers that reflect the current best practice, and where possible we have integrated reliable scientific evidence. It's important for us to know that we are equipping you with the information you will need to make informed decisions that are right for you and your family, as it is this that will give you confidence during pregnancy and birth and help you to stay in control.

We have come to realize that fathers often voice and experience feelings of exclusion, especially during pregnancy. Throughout the book, we have tried to be sensitive to this and wish to reassure all dads-to-be that this is as much a user-friendly resource for them as it is for expectant mothers. We also realize that more and more grandparents are participating in providing support during pregnancy and ongoing childcare following the birth and this is a helpful resource for them, too.

The questions in *Ask a Midwife* have been collated by a great team of midwives working with me. The topics covered relate to all areas of pregnancy and birth, from Trying for a baby and Now you're pregnant through to Labour and birth, and A new life. Examples of the style of questions include: "I'm on the pill, but want a baby – what is the next step for me?"; "Why does pregnancy make you feel so sick?"; "What does a skin-to-skin birth mean?"; and "Should I pick my baby up every time she cries?" Plus the more difficult questions that can follow the loss of a baby, such as "I feel so angry I can't even cry – is this part of grief?" And much much more. Throughout the book, I have also included select quotes to inspire and encourage; for example, "Visualize your dream birth and work towards making this a reality – whether a home birth, or creating a calm environment in your hospital birthing room".

It is our hope that we have been able to engage with you and offer our midwifery support through what can be a confusing time. *Ask a Midwife* is indeed a partnership between expectant parents, their families, and their midwives. Most of the wisdom within these pages has been drawn from our knowledge of other women's experiences, paving the way for you to have a smooth ride. Our greatest wish is that you will have a fulfilling and safe pregnancy, will have the confidence to choose what is best for you, and will have the right information to help you achieve this. We hope that your baby has a safe passage all the way to be finally enveloped in the loving arms of her long-awaiting parents.

Enjoy your own *Ask a Midwife*.

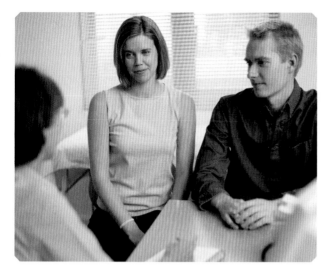

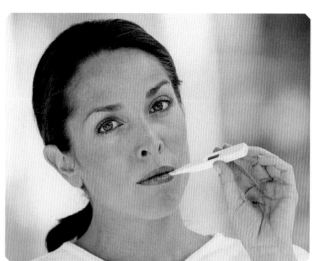

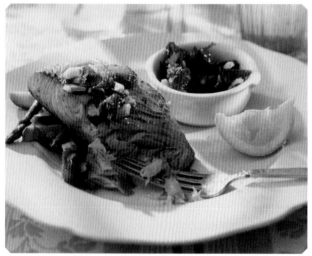

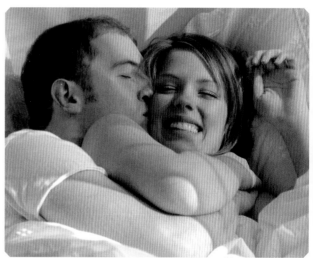

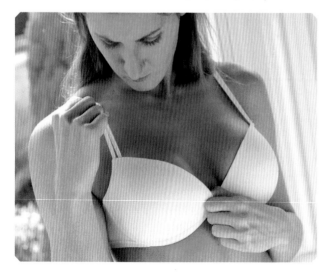

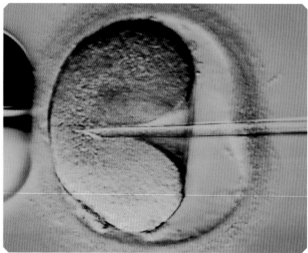

Trying for
a baby

- **We want to be parents**
  preparing for pregnancy

- **I've had a miscarriage**
  why did it happen to me?

- **We're not getting pregnant**
  what do we do now?

- **How will I know I'm pregnant?**
  confirming your pregnancy

We want to be parents
preparing for pregnancy

Q **We've been trying for a baby for months and I dread seeing my period– why isn't it happening?**

Trying to conceive can be very stressful, leading to feelings of anxiety and depression as the months pass without a positive pregnancy test. However, try not to become too disheartened; even if you don't conceive in the first few months, statistically, you have a 90 per cent chance of conceiving within a year.

It is a good idea to keep a note of the dates of your menstrual periods, as this makes it easier to calculate the fertile time of your cycle. The best time for "baby-making" sex is just before ovulation. The average length of a woman's fertility cycle is 28 days, counting the first day of your period as day one. So if you have a regular 28-day cycle, you can predict that ovulation is likely to occur mid-cycle, on around day 14. If your cycle length varies, this can make calculating the mid-point more difficult, but observing and recording your body's fertility indicators during your menstrual cycle can help you to identify your fertile time (see p.17).

Other measures you can take to maximize your reproductive health include taking pre-conceptual folic acid (see p.16), minimizing your intake of alcohol, avoiding recreational drugs, stopping smoking, and avoiding smoky environments. You should also check your rubella immunity before you become pregnant (see opposite).

Q **How long should I leave it before I go to see my doctor?**

There is no wrong or right amount of time to wait before going to see your doctor, but a lot will depend on your age and personal circumstances. If you're both under 35 and have no reason to suspect problems, for example, previous surgery or irregular periods, then the usual advice is to seek help after about a year of trying to conceive. Women over 35 are advised to seek help earlier, as fertility starts to decline more rapidly after your mid-30s. Your doctor can carry out a few basic tests straight away to rule out obvious fertility problems, such as monitoring your hormone levels, screening for sexually transmitted infections, such as chlamydia (see p.18), and semen analysis for your partner. Your doctor may then refer you to a specialist.

Q **My periods are really irregular – what are my chances of falling pregnant?**

Menstrual cycles that vary more than a few days in length from month to month are considered irregular periods. An irregular cycle can be troublesome when trying to get pregnant, but being aware of your fertility signs (see p.17) can help you to determine when you are approaching your short window of fertility. Irregular ovulation and menstruation account for around 30–40 per cent of fertility problems. Although there are many factors that determine how fertile a woman is, such as her age, whether her cervical fluid is wet enough to sustain sperm, or whether her Fallopian tubes are open, the most important factor is whether she ovulates – releases

Preparing your body for a future pregnancy will improve your chances of a healthy outcome for you and your baby

Preconception diet

A varied, balanced diet is key to good reproductive health. Certain foods in particular contain essential vitamins and minerals that are thought to benefit eggs and sperm and the health of the future embryo. These include foods rich in vitamins A, B, C, and E, folic acid, calcium, omega-3 and omega-6 essential fatty acids, zinc, and selenium.

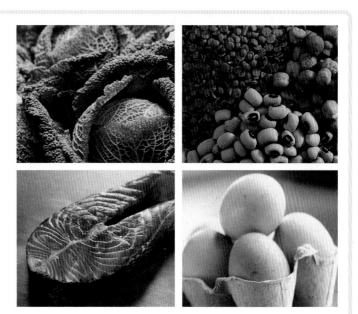

TOP LEFT: Dark green leafy vegetables contain minerals and vitamins. **TOP RIGHT:** Pulses are a source of folic acid. **BOTTOM LEFT:** Fish contains essential fatty acids. **BOTTOM RIGHT:** Eggs provide zinc, which boosts sperm production.

an egg – regularly each month. Sometimes, a condition called anovulation occurs in which there is a menstrual bleed but no ovulation. If you don't release an egg each month, you won't have as many chances to get pregnant, in which case you may be given drugs to encourage ovulation. It would be wise to talk to your doctor about your cycle.

Q I don't want to get pregnant yet but maybe next year – what can we do now to prepare?

Adopting a healthy lifestyle and improving your general wellbeing are sensible measures if you are planning a pregnancy. Start by looking at your diet (see above). Is it well balanced? Could you cut back on the amount of salt, sugar, and fast or processed food you eat? You should also increase your intake of fruit and vegetables, particularly green leafy vegetables, which are a good source of folic acid. Exercise is important too. If you have a current exercise regime it's safe to continue with that, or take up gentle exercise, such as swimming or walking, which are ideal before, during, and after pregnancy.

If you smoke, you should try to give up, as this is beneficial for your general health and, more specifically, reduces the risk of miscarriage, stillbirth, premature birth, low birth weight, and sudden infant death. Likewise, you should try cutting down on or stopping your alcohol intake. Current advice from the Department of Health recommends that you avoid alcohol completely while trying to get pregnant and once you are pregnant, as safe levels of alcohol intake are difficult to determine.

Checking your rubella status is a sensible measure as rubella can cause fetal abnormalities if you aren't immune and contract the infection in the first three months of pregnancy. If your immunity is diminished, you may be given a vaccine and should then wait three months before trying to get pregnant.

If you have a pre-existing medical condition or are taking medication, talk to your doctor or practice nurse about how these may affect a pregnancy.

Once you start trying to get pregnant, make a note each month of the first day of your period as this is one question your midwife or doctor will ask to determine your estimated due date.

Should I be taking folic acid before trying for a baby?

Folic acid has been shown to reduce the incidence of neural tube defects, such as spina bifida, in a fetus. If you are planning a pregnancy, you should take a daily folic acid supplement of 400 micrograms up to three months before conception and then continue with this until the 12th week of pregnancy. This supplementation is in addition to a well-balanced diet that includes green leafy vegetables and pulses, both of which are good natural sources of folic acid. Many breakfast cereals also contain folic acid, as do some fruits, such as oranges, papaya, and bananas.

Any woman with epilepsy who takes anti-epileptic drugs should take a higher dose (of 5mg) of folic acid supplementation.

I'm on the Pill but want a baby – what is the next step for me?

Whether you are taking the combined Pill, containing oestrogen and progesterone, or the mini Pill, which contains only progesterone, stop taking the Pill at the end of the packet. You will have a withdrawal bleed as usual and then your next bleed will be a natural period. Don't worry if your normal periods don't start immediately; for some women, it can take a few months for their menstrual cycle to return.

Some doctors recommend allowing a month or two for your natural cycle to return before trying to conceive. Others believe there's no point in waiting. However, it can help to wait for one natural period before trying to get pregnant, as this means the pregnancy can be dated more accurately and you can start pre-pregnancy care, such as taking folic acid and adopting a healthy lifestyle. Don't worry if you do get pregnant sooner, it will not harm the baby.

I'm a bit of a binge drinker. Is this OK as long as I stop once I'm pregnant?

It would be far better for your health and the health of a future baby to stop binge drinking before you conceive. The effects of alcohol on a developing baby or fetus are influenced not only by the amount

Honestly assessing your lifestyle can motivate you to make the changes necessary for a healthy pregnancy

of alcohol consumed, but by the pattern of drinking, with binge drinking in pregnancy considered particularly harmful. Binge drinking and alcohol addiction have been shown to affect the health of the developing baby, so if you know that you drink more than you should, consider how you can reduce your intake before conceiving. Government policies now advise total abstinence from alcohol, but do acknowledge that the occasional drink in pregnancy is unlikely to result in harm to the fetus.

Does smoking stop you becoming pregnant?

There is evidence that smoking compromises your menstrual and reproductive health. Women smokers who try for a baby can take up to two months longer to conceive than non-smokers. It is not clear how smoking damages women's fertility, but it may affect the release of an egg before fertilization or the quality of the eggs. It is thought to take around three months for fertility to improve after stopping smoking.

Giving up smoking is one of the single most important things you can do for yourself and for the health of a future pregnancy. If you currently smoke, then it is wise to consider giving up, or at least cutting down, even if you don't plan to have a baby straight away. The British Medical Association estimates that smoking and passive smoking are responsible for up to 5,000 miscarriages and 120,000 cases of impotence in men aged between 30 and 50 each year. Women who smoke are also more likely to have an ectopic pregnancy or miscarriage. Medical research has also shown beyond doubt that smoking affects the development of babies in the womb as they are starved of oxygen while they are growing.

Smoking remains one of the few potentially preventable factors associated with low birth weight, premature birth, stillbirth, and cot death.

My partner says soft drugs are OK – but should we stop now we're planning a baby?

By soft drugs, you may be referring to nicotine or cannabis. Tobacco smoke and cannabis smoke are highly likely to be harmful to fetal development and should be avoided by pregnant women and any woman who might become pregnant, or is planning to become pregnant, in the near future. A chemical present in cannabis known as THC is thought to reduce luteinizing hormone (LH) in the genitals. This hormone triggers ovulation in women and is involved in sperm production in men. So, as well as being potentially harmful to a fetus, smoking cannabis can result in a short-term decrease in reproductive ability.

Is it safe to take prescribed or over-the-counter medicines?

If you are trying to conceive, it's best to avoid taking any drugs, prescribed or otherwise. Some medicines can decrease fertility, so tell your doctor you are trying for a baby if you need a prescribed medicine. This is just as important for men as for women, as some prescriptions can affect sperm production or development. Talk to your doctor too if you are on long-term medication, as he or she may be able to prescribe an alternative if the original drug is known to have an effect on fertility. If you do require short-term pain relief, then a low dose of paracetamol is considered safe, but talk to your doctor or pharmacist if in doubt.

My partner had a vasectomy – can it be reversed?

Although the decision to have a vasectomy is usually considered an irreversible one, in some cases the procedure can be reversed. If a reversal is required, an operation called a vaso-vasostomy is performed by an urologist using microsurgery. The success of

Signs of ovulation

Ovulation occurs when an egg, or ovum, is released from the ovary. To become pregnant, sperm must meet and fertilize an egg and the resulting embryo must implant in the uterine wall. There are signs to look for that indicate ovulation:
* A change in cervical mucus from being sparse or thick and opaque to being clear, jelly-like, and stringy.
* A rise in your temperature (see right).
* Mid-cycle or ovulatory bleeding thought to result from the sudden drop in oestrogen that occurs at ovulation.
* Localized pain.
* Swelling of the vulva before ovulation, especially on the side that you ovulate.

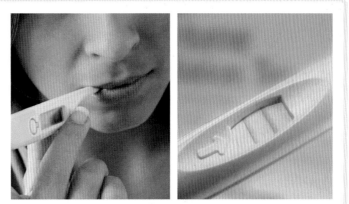

TOP LEFT: A change in your basal body temperature can indicate ovulation. Just after ovulation, your temperature rises between 0.3 and 0.9°C (0.5 and 1.6°F). **TOP RIGHT:** Ovulation kits can be purchased over the counter from chemists and supermarkets. These simple urine tests detect a surge in the level of luteinizing hormone (LH), which occurs just prior to ovulation.

the operation depends on many factors, but chiefly on the length of time since the vasectomy was performed, as the likelihood of the tubes becoming blocked increases with each year that goes by. However, the operation is successful in more than 80 per cent of men who have the reversal within 10 years after a vasectomy. Even if the vasectomy was done over 10 years ago, there is still a reasonable chance of success.

I don't seem to be falling pregnant – is it because I'm overweight?

Being overweight can affect your fertility. Estimating your body mass index (BMI) – a measure of your body fat based on your weight and height – helps you gauge whether you have a healthy weight for your height. A normal body mass index is 19–24; a BMI of 25–29 is considered overweight; 30–39 obese; and over 39 extremely obese.

Fertility rates appear to be lower and miscarriage rates higher in women who are overweight, so women planning a pregnancy are encouraged to maintain a BMI in the range of 20–25 to improve their reproductive health. The reasons for links between BMI and fertility aren't entirely clear, but the suggestion is that your hormonal balance becomes disrupted when your body has more fat-related weight than is optimal. If you are overweight, you also have a higher risk of complications during pregnancy, such as high blood pressure and diabetes, and the extra weight of pregnancy will put more strain on your joints.

Even a small weight loss can increase your ability to conceive and have a healthy pregnancy. If you're concerned about weight, you may find it useful to talk to your doctor or practice nurse for advice.

I like to be really skinny – will that stop me having a baby?

Being underweight, with a BMI of less than 19, can cause hormonal disturbances that disrupt ovulation and in turn affect fertility; this relationship between weight loss and lack of ovulation has been well

MIDWIFE WISDOM

Stopping contraception
ready for conception

When to stop contraception before conceiving is fairly straightforward, although for some methods a degree of planning is required.

* Barrier methods, such as the diaphragm and sheath, can be stopped immediately once you decide to start trying.
* If you have an IUD, you will need to make an appointment to have your coil removed; you can start trying straight away after this.
* If you are on the Pill, finish the packet before stopping (see p.16). Your cycle may take time to settle, although some women conceive as soon as they stop the Pill.

documented and observed in young athletes, ballet dancers, and gymnasts. Surprisingly, underweight women often find it difficult to believe that their weight is standing in the way of conception, since they are more likely to be rewarded by society for being thin. Suggestions that she should gain weight may be a thin woman's first encounter with being told that her health is not optimal. A recommended BMI of 20–25 is advised to avoid problems with ovulation, and you may need to take steps to try to gain weight in a sensible way. If tests show that you are not ovulating regularly, you may also be offered medication to deal with the problem.

I've had STIs in the past, but everything is fine now – will that stop me conceiving?

A previous sexually transmitted infection (STI) should not cause problems if it was found early and treated successfully. However, chlamydia and gonorrhoea can have long-term consequences if left untreated, especially in women. Untreated STIs also can be passed on to your baby.

Chlamydia is the most common sexually transmitted infection in the UK. Although it is curable, many people are not aware of the health risks it presents. Up to 70 per cent of chlamydia infections in women have no obvious symptoms, so a large number of cases are never diagnosed. The risk is that untreated chlamydia can cause pelvic inflammatory disease, which is the most common cause of female infertility. In a large number of investigations, there is a clear link between chlamydia infection and tubal infertility, whereby the infection causes adhesions and scar tissue to form on the Fallopian tubes, causing blockages in the tubes and increasing the risk of complications such as ectopic pregnancy.

In a Finnish research study, chlamydia antibodies were found in the semen of 51 per cent of infertile men compared to 23 per cent of fertile men, and the study therefore concluded that chlamydia may affect male fertility as well as female fertility.

The classical STIs, such as syphilis and gonorrhoea, are usually easier to recognize and subsequently diagnose and treat.

I'm 37 and would like to start trying for a baby – have I left it too late?

Increasing numbers of women are delaying their first pregnancy until they are in their late 30s and early 40s and, as with any life choice, this has advantages and disadvantages. The main concern for women is that their fertility does decrease with advancing age, and so for some women it may take a little longer to get pregnant, or they may find that they need to look at ways of assisting conception (see p.27). Also, the risk of conceiving a baby with a chromosomal abnormality such as Down's syndrome increases as you get older, rising from a 1 in 356 chance at 35 to a 1 in 240 chance at 37.

Fertility guidelines indicate that if you are over 35 and haven't got pregnant after six months of trying, then you should seek medical advice. If you do conceive, it is likely that you will be more closely monitored during pregnancy than younger women because of the increased risk of the baby being smaller than expected or other complications occurring in pregnancy and labour.

On the other hand, many older women have no problems conceiving, and there are positives to being an older mum. Older mums are more likely to breastfeed than younger mums and often feel more assured and confident in their own capabilities because of life experience.

Is my endometriosis preventing me from getting pregnant? We've been trying for two years.

Endometriosis occurs when cells from the lining of the uterus, known as the endometrium, spread to other areas, such as the Fallopian tubes, ovaries, and pelvis, which can cause scarring and blockages that can affect fertility. Although you have endometriosis, it won't be assumed that this is the only cause of your problem. The general advice for any couple who have been trying to get pregnant for over 18 months is to seek medical advice, and it is likely that you will both be offered investigations to determine if there is any specific reason why a pregnancy isn't happening.

There is some evidence to suggest that diet plays a part in the symptoms of endometriosis; it is thought that increasing the intake of vitamins C and E plus B_1, B_6, and B_{12}, together with increasing the intake of essential fatty acids, such as omega-3 and omega-6, and reducing the intake of red meat and trans fats found in processed foods, could help to reduce the symptoms of endometriosis and in turn improve the fertility of women with the condition.

Prepare mentally by having faith in your ability to conceive and each day visualizing your forthcoming pregnancy

ESSENTIAL INFORMATION: TRYING FOR A BABY

All about conception
The beginning of life

Conception occurs once an egg is successfully penetrated by one sperm. The journey of the egg and the sperm, although apparently simple, requires a whole complex chain of events to occur for fertilization and implantation to take place.

How is the egg released and fertilized? After menstruation, the body secretes follicle-stimulating hormone (FSH), which acts on the ovaries to mature a follicle containing an egg. At the time of ovulation, a rise in the level of luteinizing hormone (LH) triggers the release from the ovary of an egg, which travels into the Fallopian tube to await fertilization by a sperm. Up to 300 million sperm are released in each ejaculate, and of these only around 200 make it into the Fallopian tube. These remaining sperm swarm all over the egg and many sperm may bind to the egg's surface. At this stage, the

sperm then shed their bodies and tails and release enzymes to help them burrow down into the egg. However, only one sperm can penetrate the innermost part of the egg, which is known as the oocyte. Once the egg and sperm have successfully fused together, fertilization has taken place.

How are genes inherited? The sperm and egg each contain 23 chromosomes that carry the genetic material of the parents. As human cells contain 46 chromosomes, once the egg and sperm fuse, their chromosomes join to provide the fertilized cell with a full complement of chromosomes. Each egg and sperm carries its own unique set of genes in the chromosomes, which means that the resulting baby has its own individual genetic makeup. The exception is identical twins; they result from one egg and sperm and inherit the same genetic code.

How fertilization occurs

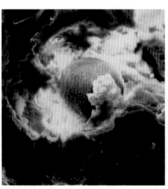

THE MOMENT OF OVULATION: At about day 14 of the menstrual cycle, a mature egg bursts from a follicle in the ovary and travels into the Fallopian tube.

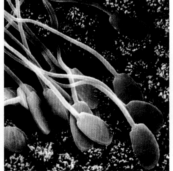

THE JOURNEY OF THE SPERM: At the point of ejaculation, sperm stream through the cervix and into the uterus to begin their journey to the egg.

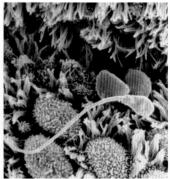

SPERM TRAVEL THROUGH THE FALLOPIAN TUBE: The Fallopian tubes have a frond-filled lining that helps to fan the sperm towards the egg.

From conception to implantation

The fertilized cell that results from the fusion of the egg and sperm is called a zygote, which divides into two identical cells and continues to divide as it begins its journey down the Fallopian tube until it forms a bundle of cells known as a morula. By the time it reaches the uterus, it forms a bundle of around 100 cells, called a blastocyst. About a week after fertilization, the blastocyst embeds itself in the lining of the uterus, the endometrium. At this point the pregnancy is established; the blastocyst develops into an embryo and the placenta develops. The hormone human chorionic gonadotrophin (hCG) is released; this stimulates the production of progesterone, which maintains the lining of the uterus.

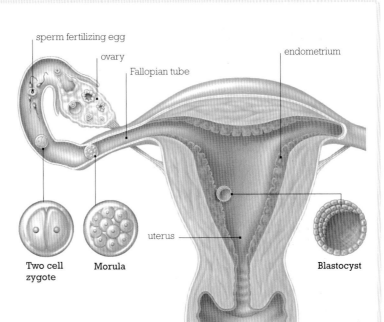

sperm fertilizing egg

ovary

Fallopian tube

endometrium

uterus

Two cell zygote

Morula

Blastocyst

THE JOURNEY TO THE UTERUS: From the moment the egg is fertilized in the tube to the implantation of the blastocyst in the lining of the uterus takes up to around seven days.

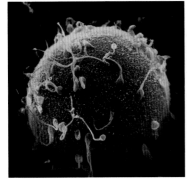

FERTILIZATION OF THE EGG: The surviving sperm swarm all over the egg, releasing enzymes to break down the egg's outer layer. One sperm penetrates the egg.

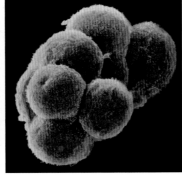

THE DIVISION OF CELLS: At about four days after conception, the fertilized egg has divided repeatedly to form a bundle of cells called a morula.

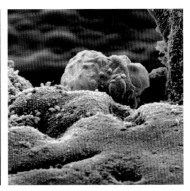

IMPLANTATION IN THE UTERUS: Now known as a blastocyst, made up of around 100 cells, the bundle burrows into the lining of the womb and an embryo begins to form.

I've had a miscarriage
why did it happen to me?

What is a miscarriage?

A miscarriage is the spontaneous loss of a baby at any time up until the 24th week of pregnancy. After 24 weeks the loss is referred to as a stillbirth. The signs of a miscarriage are vaginal bleeding and period-like cramps. As not all miscarriages follow the same pattern, there are various terms to describe what occurs:

* **A threatened miscarriage** occurs when there is bleeding and possibly pain, but the fetus survives.
* **An inevitable miscarriage** occurs when there is bleeding and pain due to contractions in the uterus, the cervix opens, and the fetus is expelled.
* **A missed miscarriage** occurs when the fetus dies but remains in the womb and either is expelled naturally later or removed in an operation.

The risk of miscarriage
What can increase the likelihood of a miscarriage?

There are several factors that can increase your risk of miscarriage.

Older women have an increased risk of having a miscarriage. It is thought that this is largely due to the fact that older women are more likely to have babies with chromosomal abnormalities, which may have problems developing and miscarry. Some underlying medical conditions can also increase your chances of miscarriage, such as polycystic ovary syndrome or fibroids. Other factors that can increase your risk are if you are particularly underweight or overweight, smoke, drink heavily, or take recreational drugs. Miscarriages are also more likely the more pregnancies you have had.

I've recently miscarried – why did this happen?

Miscarriage occurs in 10–20 per cent of pregnancies. In the vast majority of these the cause is never identified, but it's unlikely to be related to anything you did or didn't do. There are thought to be several reasons why miscarriages occur (see p.25). There may be a genetic problem, in which the baby or placenta doesn't develop normally; levels of the pregnancy hormone progesterone may be low; there may be an immune disorder in which the mother's immune system reacts against the pregnancy; an infection may be present; or there may be problems with the uterus or cervix. Miscarriages tend to be more common in older women.

The Miscarriage Association (see p.310) offers support and up-to-date advice and information about miscarriage. You may feel comforted to know that, statistically, any future pregnancy you have is likely to progress normally.

My period was late and now I'm bleeding really heavily – could I be having a miscarriage?

In the absence of a positive pregnancy test or a pregnancy confirmed by an ultrasound scan, it is difficult to know whether or not you were pregnant. If you have had unprotected intercourse in the time since your last period, it is possible that you could have been pregnant and this is a miscarriage. The lateness of your period may give a clue, but won't confirm one way or another. If you have any other symptoms of pregnancy it might be worth doing a pregnancy test as sometimes, even when there has been bleeding, a viable pregnancy is discovered.

However, it could also be a late period for no other reason than that this happens on occasion to everyone. A delayed period can be caused by weight loss or gain, stress, or if you have been taking the oral contraceptive Pill but missed a dose.

Talk to your doctor if the bleeding continues; you feel faint or experience palpitations; your period lasts for longer than seven days; you have more than six well-soaked pads a day; or if you have any severe abdominal pain. Your doctor can carry out a blood test to check your iron levels and possibly determine if you have been pregnant, in which case an incomplete miscarriage or ectopic pregnancy will need to be ruled out (see p.25).

One in four women miscarry in their first pregnancy. In most cases, women go on to have successful pregnancies

Q I'm 10 weeks pregnant and getting cramping pains. Do I need to rest to avoid a miscarriage?

Cramping pains on their own without vaginal bleeding or spotting can occur at this stage of pregnancy. Sometimes pain can be felt as the ligaments stretch when the baby and your uterus grows. There are also other possible causes for the pain aside from miscarriage, such as constipation or a urinary tract infection.

Many doctors advise rest to avoid a "threatened" miscarriage, but there is no strong evidence that this makes any difference to the outcome of a pregnancy. If you feel like resting because you are in discomfort from the cramping pains then do rest, but if you feel happy continuing as normal then that may be the best option for you. Soaking in a warm bath and practising relaxation techniques may ease the intensity of the pain. If the pain increases or you get any bleeding or spotting, contact your doctor.

Q Does bleeding in pregnancy mean that miscarriage is inevitable?

No, many women experience bleeding in early pregnancy and then proceed to have a healthy pregnancy and baby. Indeed, some women have intermittent bleeding throughout pregnancy. Despite this, any bleeding should be investigated. This is usually done with a scan to determine if the pregnancy is viable (going to continue) and to identify if there is any indication of where the

bleeding is coming from. In very early pregnancy, it can be hard to see the pregnancy on a scan and a blood test to measure levels of the pregnancy hormone human chorionic gonadotrophin (hCG) may be done, mainly to rule out the possibility of an ectopic pregnancy (see p.25). Unfortunately for you this is a time of waiting; the timing of any further scans is usually determined by the findings of the initial scan and blood tests and the symptoms you are experiencing.

Q I've had three miscarriages before and I'm scared of trying again – is there anything I can do?

It is understandable given your experiences that trying to get pregnant again is a scary proposition. Following a third miscarriage, it is usual for your doctor to offer you a number of investigative tests to see if a reason for the miscarriages can be found. In some cases, a cause is identified and treatment can be offered to help improve the outcome for subsequent pregnancies.

You are likely to be given a number of blood tests. These are to look for antibodies (proteins in the blood that fight any substance they recognize as foreign to your body), chromosomal abnormalities, and infection. You may also have a vaginal examination and swab and an ultrasound scan to check your womb and tubes. If a chromosomal abnormality is found, genetic counselling should be offered to discuss the implications for future pregnancies. The levels of the hormones progesterone and prolactin may also be checked as these can play a role in miscarriage. Sometimes, the cervix is found to be weakened and likely to open early. If this is the case, you may be offered a cervical stitch that acts like a drawstring on the cervix and hopefully prevents future miscarriage or premature delivery.

If you haven't already been offered these tests, talk to your doctor about them before trying to get pregnant again so that you can begin any recommended treatment as soon as possible.

Q My mum had two miscarriages – does that mean I am more likely to miscarry?

Ask your mum if she was given any particular reason for her miscarriages. If, for example, she knows that they were due to a chromosomal abnormality, such as sickle-cell disease, or if she had a medical condition, such as heart disease, then there is a possibility that the condition is hereditary and the risk of miscarriage may be the same for you too.

However, it's most likely that your mother's miscarriages were unfortunate chance occurrences for which no reason was found. If this is the case, then you are at no more risk of experiencing a miscarriage than any other woman your age. However, if you do become pregnant, it would be worth mentioning your mother's pregnancy history at your initial antenatal appointment, as your family medical history is an important part of your medical notes during pregnancy.

Talking about your experience of miscarriage rather than keeping it to yourself can help the healing process

Q I've had several miscarriages and my doctor has referred me to a genetic counsellor – why?

A genetic counsellor is a highly trained professional who supports families before and after conception. Quite often a miscarriage is caused by a genetic abnormality in the fertilized egg or embryo. This is usually a one-off and can affect any woman. However, if a woman has recurrent miscarriages, it may be that she is carrying a genetic condition.

Women and their partners are referred to a genetic counsellor if either partner has a condition that can affect future children or the chances of becoming pregnant or continuing with a pregnancy (as they may be more likely to miscarry or be offered a termination). For example, if there is a history of sickle-cell disease, a blood disorder that causes chronic anaemia and increases the risk of a preterm birth and health problems in the baby, it may be that either or both couples are carrying a gene that can affect a baby.

A genetic counsellor helps you understand how your genes could affect conception and pregnancy and about the tests available to determine if a fetus is affected. The counsellor will discuss a range of issues, including the moral and ethical issues related to genetic testing, as it is common for couples to feel stress, guilt, and confusion in this type of situation.

Q I lost my baby, but I want to get on and try again – is this OK?

Although there are no hard rules about when to try for another baby, it is important that you allow yourself time to grieve and your body to recover before trying to conceive again. Some women feel able to try again within a month, while others may not feel ready for at least a year. Whatever you feel, it's wise to let your hormones and body settle down after a miscarriage before considering another pregnancy. The usual advice is to wait for at least three months before trying to conceive again so that you feel both emotionally and physically prepared for another pregnancy. Your partner also needs to feel that the time is right for you both to try again.

ESSENTIAL INFORMATION: TRYING FOR A BABY

Possible causes of miscarriage
Losing a baby in pregnancy

About 1 in 4 first pregnancies ends in miscarriage, generally within the first 12 weeks. Often no cause is identified and it may not be investigated unless a woman has had three or more miscarriages in a row, known as "recurrent miscarriages".

Why has it happened? Some miscarriages occur because of a one-off genetic problem (caused by a faulty chromosome) when the baby does not develop properly. Genetic problems account for 60 per cent of early miscarriages. If you think this may have been the cause, you can request tissue tests from the baby. Based on these results, you may be able to receive specialist counselling to discuss the risk of it happening again (see p.24). After 12 weeks, the chances of you losing your baby because of a chromosomal disorder reduce to about 10 per cent; however, if

you are over 35, this risk is higher. Other less common causes of miscarriage include fibroids (non-cancerous growths), infection, problems with the uterus, hormonal imbalances, and immune system disorders. An ectopic pregnancy, below, occurs when the embryo implants in a Fallopian tube and needs to be removed.

What can cause late pregnancy loss? A late pregnancy loss (referred to as a stillbirth after 24 weeks) can be due to the cervix being weak (or "incompetent"), causing the cervix to dilate too early. This accounts for 15 per cent of repeated miscarriages. In future pregnancies, a stitch around the cervix can strengthen this muscle and prevent it opening early. Another cause of a late miscarriage can be if the placenta does not function properly and affects the baby's growth.

Ectopic pregnancy

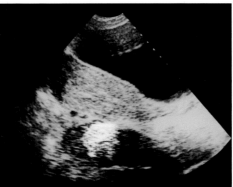

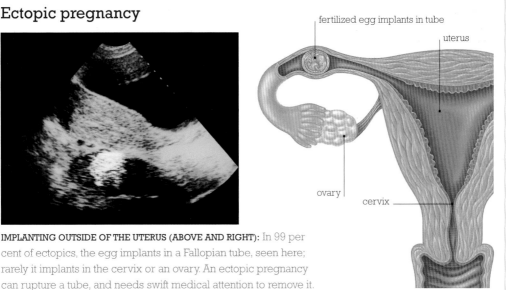

fertilized egg implants in tube

uterus

ovary

cervix

IMPLANTING OUTSIDE OF THE UTERUS (ABOVE AND RIGHT): In 99 per cent of ectopics, the egg implants in a Fallopian tube, seen here; rarely it implants in the cervix or an ovary. An ectopic pregnancy can rupture a tube, and needs swift medical attention to remove it.

We had a miscarriage at 20 weeks. Will the doctors find the cause so that we can move on?

Coping with the loss of a baby well into pregnancy is difficult and upsetting. Many women ask themselves why a miscarriage happened and feel unable to move on until that important question is answered. Unfortunately, unless this was a recurrent miscarriage of three or more, there may not be an investigation, although it may be suggested that you have a cervical stitch in future pregnancies to stop the cervix dilating too early (see p.24).

It may be worth talking to a counsellor who is trained to support women and families through such difficult times; your doctor or midwife may be able to refer you. You may find that discussing your miscarriage directly with a health professional helps to answer any concerns you or your partner have, and by communicating in this way you will have started to move forward and may begin to feel able to consider planning another pregnancy.

My partner had a miscarriage. I'm being supportive, but I'm devastated too. What should I do?

Dealing with a miscarriage is very difficult for both women and men, but often far more attention is given to a woman, and a man's feelings are simply ignored. However, it's important that you don't internalize your loss and do acknowledge your feelings, which may range from feeling scared, disappointed, and out of control, to blaming yourself for not being supportive enough and mourning the loss of your identity as a father. Although you want to support your partner, you also need to recognize your own need to grieve, as working through your emotions can help you to come to terms with your loss more quickly.

A good support network is important for both of you and it can help to find a sympathetic listener outside of your relationship. Initially, you may find discussing your feelings with another male easier than talking to your partner. You could also talk to your doctor, the midwife, or a counsellor, or contact the Miscarriage Association helpline.

MIDWIFE WISDOM

Talking to others
coming to terms with your loss

Losing a baby during pregnancy can be devastating, leading to feelings of grief such as anger, depression, guilt, and anxiety. Talking to others can help you to work through your feelings.

❋ Ask your midwife or doctor to put you in touch with a counsellor who specializes in pregnancy loss.

❋ Let close friends and family members know how you are feeling.

❋ The Miscarriage Association is a great source of support and advice (see p.310).

❋ Talk to your doctor or midwife about why the miscarriage may have happened.

What is a "D and C"?

D and C stands for dilation and curettage, a surgical procedure in which the opening to the uterus, called the cervix, is stretched (dilatation) and the tissue that lines the uterus is scraped away or removed (curettage). This procedure is sometimes carried out after a miscarriage to ensure that any of the remaining products of the conception and pregnancy have been removed.

There are advantages and disadvantages to consider before having a D and C. The procedure is usually completed within two hours and most women resume their usual activities within a week. However, the need for routine surgical evacuation, or a D and C, following a miscarriage has been questioned because of potential complications, such as bleeding and infection. Ask your doctor for advice. There are less invasive options than a D and C for dealing with a miscarriage. One method is simply to watch and wait to see if the uterus will spontaneously expel any remaining products of conception. Another option is a drug treatment that works by stimulating the uterus to contract and naturally expel pregnancy tissues.

We're not getting pregnant
what do we do now?

Q We've been trying to conceive for 12 months – can the doctor identify the problem?

There are many factors that can increase or decrease your chances of becoming pregnant, but if you have been trying for a year, it would be sensible to contact your doctor. After an initial assessment of your general health and lifestyle, your doctor will offer your partner a sperm test (see below) and you will be offered tests to see if you are producing eggs and check whether or not your Fallopian tubes are blocked. Blood tests will be carried out to check your iron levels, your red and white blood cell count, and to check how organs such as your liver and kidneys are functioning. In addition, couples are asked to agree to a sexual health screening to check for previous or current STIs, such as HIV and syphilis.

Q My wife has been tested and has the all clear – how can I tell if I'm causing our fertility problem?

You will be offered a semen analysis to determine your sperm quantity and quality – how sperm move (motility) and whether they are a normal form. A healthy sperm count should have a concentration of 20 million spermatozoa per millilitre of semen, with

75 per cent of these alive and 50 per cent of these "motile", or moving as well as possible. Differences can occur over time in both the quality and quantity of sperm, so if your first sample is poor, you will probably be tested again a couple of months later.

You are also likely to be advised to give up smoking, reduce alcohol intake to 1–2 units once or twice a week, and to wear loose-fitting underwear to avoid overheating the testes. If a problem is found, you will be referred to a specialist for a consultation. Try to avoid becoming stressed as this can also affect fertility. Learning relaxation techniques with your partner and practising these regularly will help.

Q We can't conceive naturally – what do we do now?

Assisted conception, or assisted reproduction, is the term used when women are helped to conceive without having intercourse. There are five main procedures available, listed below. Your consultant will go through each one with you, and together you can make a decision about which is most suitable depending on your problem. You can also contact the National Institute for Health and Clinical Excellence (NICE) for more information (see p.310).

✱ **Ovarian Stimulation (OS), or Super Ovulation (SO)**, involves injections of fertility hormones to boost egg production. This is followed by intra-uterine insemination (IUI) of sperm, whereby sperm are collected and sorted so that only the strongest remain and these are then artifically placed inside the uterus via a catheter. This is ideal for couples when the man's sperm is "slow" or the woman has problems ovulating, or there is a combination of both.

✱ **Gamete Intra-Fallopian Transfer (GIFT).** This is suitable for couples for whom no cause for infertility has been found. It involves stimulating the ovaries to produce eggs, which are removed, mixed with

> If you have been trying for a baby for over a year, it may be time to chat to your doctor – there may be a simple solution

ESSENTIAL INFORMATION: TRYING FOR A BABY

Conception problems
Conditions preventing conception

There are a range of reasons why a couple may have difficulty in conceiving. Investigations and tests may uncover specific conditions, which may be treatable, or you may be offered help to conceive.

What can affect a man's fertility? A semen analysis may reveal various reasons why sperm have difficulty in fertilizing an egg. The sperm count may be low (less than 20 million sperm per ml); the motility of the sperm (how they move) may be poor; and there may be a high percentage of abnormally formed sperm. Some men experience a failure to ejaculate at orgasm. There may also be damage to the tubes that connect the testicles to the seminal vesicles where sperm are produced, and this may have been present from birth or caused by a later infection.

What can affect a woman's fertility?
Conditions such as polycystic ovary syndrome (a hormonal imbalance that causes ovarian cysts) and endometriosis (see p.19) can disrupt fertility. Other hormonal imbalances, such as low levels of FSH and LH, can affect ovulation; or levels of progesterone may be too low to sustain a fertilized egg. Damaged Fallopian tubes, caused by an ectopic pregnancy (see p.25), surgery, endometriosis, or pelvic inflammatory disease, which may be caused by an infection such as chlamydia, can prevent conception. Damage to the ovaries can occur from scarring as a result of surgery or infection, or the supply of eggs may be low. Some women have an abnormally shaped uterus, or have uterine scarring, that can prevent the successful implantation of an egg.

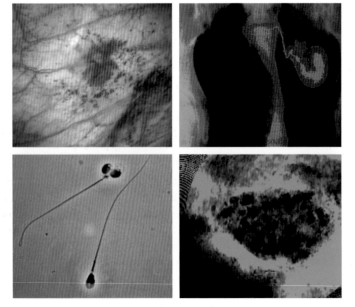

TOP LEFT: Endometriosis causes cells from the lining of the uterus to travel to other areas such as the ovaries and tubes, which can affect fertility.
TOP RIGHT: Here, a special dye injected through the cervix reveals a blockage in the left Fallopian tube as the dye has been unable to enter the tube.
BOTTOM LEFT: If the head, or cap, of the sperm is abnormally shaped it will be unable to fertilize an egg.
BOTTOM RIGHT: In polycystic ovary syndrome, cysts in the ovaries mean that the follicles are unable to mature and produce ripened eggs.

sperm and replaced directly into the Fallopian tubes, allowing conception to occur inside the body.

✱ In Vitro Fertilization (IVF). This is the most widely used treatment and involves a seven-step process (see below and p.30). This is ideal for most problems, including blocked tubes.

✱ Intra-Cytoplasmic Sperm Injection (ICSI). This is used if the man's sperm count is low, the motility of the sperm is very poor, or the woman is allergic to her partner's sperm. The treatment involves injecting just one viable sperm into an egg (see box, right).

✱ Artificial Insemination by Donor (AID). This is simply the injection of donated sperm into the cervix. This is used when a man is unable to maintain an erection or is sterile. Similarly, women may require an egg donation if they are unable to produce their own eggs, although this is more complicated.

Whatever treatment is provided, it is important that you and your partner are treated as a couple rather than separate patients. It is also essential that you are kept informed throughout the process and given information on any risks and benefits.

What does IVF involve?

IVF, or In Vitro Fertilization, involves the surgical removal of an egg, which is then mixed with sperm in a laboratory dish to fertilize and produce an embryo outside of the womb (see p.30).

IVF treatment occurs in cycles, as there are various stages that must be completed for it to be successful. Initially, a drug is used in the form of a nasal spray or injection to switch off the woman's natural cycle of egg production in the ovaries, known as "down-regulation". Fertility drugs are then given to stimulate the ovaries to produce more than one egg (ovulation induction). Mature eggs are collected from the ovaries using a fine needle guided by ultrasound. The procedure is usually uncomfortable rather than painful. On the same day, the partner's sperm is collected and then the eggs and sperm are mixed in a dish. Within a few days, one or sometimes two embryos are transferred into the womb. If an embryo successfully attaches to the inside of the womb and continues to grow, a pregnancy results.

ICSI
(Intra-Cytoplasmic Sperm Injection)

This procedure may be used when it is thought that the quality of the partner's sperm may be responsible for fertility problems.
If the sperm count is low or movement is poor, sperm may be "assisted" in fertilizing the egg. An individual sperm is injected directly into the egg and, if fertilization takes place, the resulting embryo is placed in the uterus.

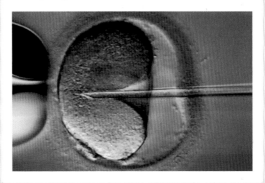

What are the success rates of fertility treatments?

Success rates for treatments vary, depending on the treatments used and the health of the couple. If you want to know the success rates of individual clinics, you can ask for their ratio of "live-births-per-cycle-started". This information is available from each clinic, but there are currently no nationally held data.

Overall, couples have a better success rate if the woman is aged 23–39 years, has been pregnant or has had a baby, and has a normal body weight (a body mass index between 19 and 24). The older a woman is, the less likely she is to get pregnant.

Figures show that for every 100 women who are 23 to 35 years, more than 20 will get pregnant after one IVF cycle; from 36 to 38 years, around 15 will get pregnant; at 39, around 10 will get pregnant; and in women over 40, around 6 will get pregnant.

ESSENTIAL INFORMATION: TRYING FOR A BABY

IVF treatment
The process of IVF

In vitro fertilization, or IVF, is a complex procedure with several stages, from the stimulation and harvesting of your eggs to the successful fertilization of the eggs, development of embryos, and transfer of the embryos into the womb for implantation. Undergoing IVF can be a stressful and time-consuming undertaking, but knowing in advance how the procedure works and what you can expect at each stage can reduce anxiety and help you and your partner to cope.

What happens first? To optimize the chances of success with IVF, more than one egg at a time is removed for fertilization. Normally, your body produces one egg each month. In IVF, you will inject yourself with drugs, such as clomiphene and hMG (human menopausal gonadotrophin) to stimulate your ovaries to produce several eggs. While you are undergoing this treatment, you will need to visit your clinic every one to two days over one or two weeks to monitor the development of the eggs. Once it is thought that the eggs are mature, you will be given a blood test to measure your levels of oestrogen, which is released around ovulation.

What happens next? Once your follicles are ripe and ready for ovulation, your eggs will be collected at the clinic using ultrasound or laparoscopy to guide a probe. Once the eggs have been collected, they will be mixed with your partner's sperm in a Petri dish in a laboratory ready for fertilization. Your partner needs to produce the sperm on the same day as the egg collection. He can either do this at home, or come into the clinic with you and produce the sperm while you are undergoing the egg collection procedure.

How eggs are fertilized

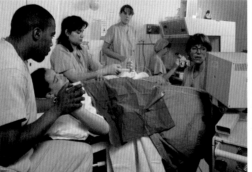

EGG REMOVAL: Your ripe eggs are removed in the clinic in a room similar to an operating theatre. You will usually be given a light anaesthetic and the doctor will use ultrasound guidance to collect your eggs with a probe.

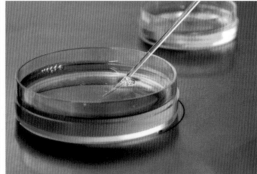

MIXING THE EGGS AND SPERM: Once your mature eggs have been removed successfully, they will be mixed with your partner's recently produced sperm in a special liquid in a Petri dish ready for fertilization. Any fertilized eggs will be monitored closely.

What happens in the laboratory? Once the egg and the sperm have been mixed, they are placed in the laboratory and monitored closely for the next few days. They will first be inspected around 18 hours later to see how many of the eggs have been fertilized and the clinic will usually pass this information on to you the day after the procedure. It's quite common for not all of the eggs to be fertilized and for only two or three to develop into embryos. The fertilized eggs are incubated in the laboratory over the next couple of days and their progress measured. The laboratory technician watches cell division under a microscope, waiting for the eggs to divide into two or more cells on their journey to becoming a blastocyst (see p.21).

If one or more fertilized eggs develop in the laboratory, you will be called back in for the embryo transfer. This is done by injecting eggs through a catheter into the uterus. No more than two eggs will be transferred and you will have the option to freeze any remaining embryos.

IVF procedures

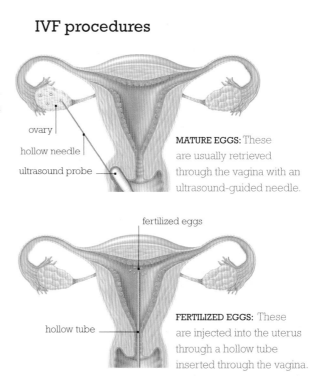

ovary
hollow needle
ultrasound probe

MATURE EGGS: These are usually retrieved through the vagina with an ultrasound-guided needle.

fertilized eggs

hollow tube

FERTILIZED EGGS: These are injected into the uterus through a hollow tube inserted through the vagina.

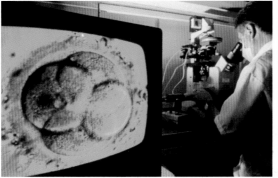

MONITORING THE EGGS: Over the next two to three days, the laboratory technician will keep a close eye on the development of the eggs. If one or more eggs starts cell division, you will be called back to have the developing eggs transferred into your uterus.

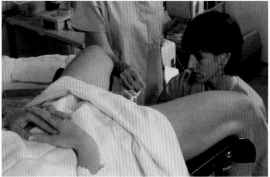

EMBRYO TRANSFER TO THE WOMB: In a procedure rather like a cervical smear test that does not require sedation, the fertilized eggs will be carefully transferred into the uterus through a catheter using ultrasound for guidance.

Surrogacy

A surrogate mother is a woman who reaches an agreement to carry a baby on behalf of another woman. She can either conceive the baby with the partner's sperm, in which case she is the maternal mother, or the infertile couple may fertilize their own egg through fertility treatment, which is then transferred into the uterus of the surrogate mother for her to carry the baby through pregnancy and deliver at birth. This process can be beset with problems: such as the conflicting emotions of both the surrogate mother and the receiving couple, or legal issues if, for example, the surrogate mother has a change of heart after the birth and wishes to keep the baby. For this reason, it is important that all parties entering into the agreement have carefully considered the implications and are confident and happy in their roles.

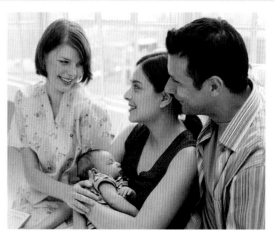

A GROWING BOND: Some couples develop a strong relationship with their surrogate mother, supporting her during the pregnancy and birth, and maintaining a close link with her after the baby is born.

IVF is so expensive – can we get help with funding?

Since April 2005, women between the ages of 23 and 39 are entitled to one free IVF cycle on the NHS. However, you must meet the eligibility criteria set by your local Primary Care Trust (PCT), which varies across the country and depends on factors such as your marital status, weight, and whether you or your partner smoke. Couples who can afford to, or who may have had one unsuccessful cycle already, often opt for a private clinic. Although these are regulated by the Human Fertilisation and Embryology Authority (HFEA), this cannot set costs, and a private course of IVF can cost from £4,000 to £10,000.

My partner is worried about producing his sperm sample. How can I reassure him?

As fertility problems affect 1 in 7 couples in the UK, reassuring your partner that this is not an unusual situation is always a good start. You could try leaving out a leaflet on fertility problems for him to read for more information. Try to empathize with

him as much as possible by sharing your experiences and the tests you have undergone.

Your partner may be worried about ejaculating at the required time, when he is already feeling anxious and is in a clinical environment. Some men require a sex toy, magazines, or video clips to help. For others, restraining from sexual intercourse for a few days can make ejaculation easier. If you live fairly close to the clinic, your partner may be able to produce the sample at home and deliver it.

Sometimes a medical condition such as diabetes prevents a man ejaculating. If this is the case, sperm can be obtained through "sperm recovery", whereby a small needle is passed through the skin of the scrotum into the testes and sperm is withdrawn.

The drugs I'm taking for IVF are giving me terrible mood swings. Is this normal?

The drugs used in IVF treatment are female hormones (see p.30) to stimulate your ovaries to mature more than one egg at a time, and progesterone, which helps to sustain a pregnancy.

Different levels of hormones can result in mood swings, as any woman who suffers with pre-menstrual tension (PMT) can testify, and this is also a common side effect of IVF treatment. It's worth considering too that couples undergoing IVF are under incredible stress, which has been linked to an increased risk of developing depression, so it's important to decide whether you are feeling "hormonal" or are in fact depressed. Your doctor can advise you and refer you if necessary.

My partner has a low sperm count – can you tell us what help is available for us?

Usually, two or three semen samples are taken to work out the average sperm count and to see if there are abnormal sperm present. A healthy semen sample of 2–5ml contains more than 20 million sperm per ml; a count below this is considered low. If your partner has abnormal sperm, further testing may be necessary. Lifestyle changes can boost sperm (see below). There are also hormonal treatments to improve sperm count and surgery to remove blockages. You may be reassured to know that even poor-quality semen can be used to fertilize an egg with IVF or with ICSI (see p.29).

Can lifestyle changes really improve sperm?

Poor-quality sperm has been linked to excessive drinking (more than three or four units of alcohol per day), smoking, and to wearing tight-fitting underwear,

The best way to improve your sperm count is to consider your lifestyle: eat healthily, drink less, and avoid tight pants!

which overheats the testicles and can affect their efficiency. Excessive stress and a poor diet are also thought to affect sperm. So yes, it is worth reviewing your lifestyle to see if improvements can be made. Jobs that may expose you to harmful agents, such as pesticides, may also affect sperm, so if you think your partner's job may pose a risk, it's worth investigating.

I'm pregnant using a donor – what happens if my child wants to trace her biological dad?

From April 2005, children who were conceived using donor sperm have had a right when they reach 18 years of age to find out their parent's identity. This also applies to children conceived using donor eggs and embryos. This right applies only to children conceived after this date and not retrospectively. Prior to this date, children had the right to know at 18 years of age if they were conceived using donor sperm, eggs, or embryos and to find out if they were related to someone they wanted to marry. The reason for this change in the law is that children conceived in this way are being given the same rights as adopted children regarding information on their genetic parents. However, some fertility experts fear that this will deter potential donors.

Is surrogacy allowed in the UK?

Currently, surrogacy is legal in the UK, although it is illegal to advertise it as a service. However, the law does not recognize surrogacy as a fixed agreement, which means that a surrogate can change her mind about the arrangement during the pregnancy and up to six weeks after the birth. It is usual for a surrogate to receive "reasonable expenses", although there is no definition of what is deemed as reasonable. Usually, this includes costs incurred by the surrogate relating to her pregnancy. If the father of the child is named on the birth certificate, this gives him equal rights to the child. If this is not the case, then six weeks after the birth the new parents can apply for a parental order that gives them full parental status. At this point, the surrogate gives up any parental rights to the child.

How will I know I'm pregnant?
confirming your pregnancy

Q I think I might be pregnant – what is the best way for me to confirm this?

By far the most accurate way to confirm a pregnancy is to perform a home pregnancy test. If used correctly, these are extremely accurate. Your doctor can offer a pregnancy testing service if confirmation is required. This may be the case if, for example, you test too early and get a false negative result (see below) and then lose faith in the home test. Apart from a home pregnancy test, pregnancy can also be confirmed with a blood test, although this is usually only done if there are possible problems such as irregular bleeding. Occasionally, ultrasound scans are used to confirm a pregnancy, particularly if there is a question mark about the dates, although an embryo cannot be seen on a scan until at least four weeks after conception.

Q I feel pregnant – how early can I do a test?

Pregnancy tests determine if you are pregnant by detecting a hormone called human chorionic gonadotrophin (hCG) in your urine. This pregnancy hormone is released when the fertilized egg is implanted in the lining of the womb and it rises significantly in the early stages of pregnancy. Most pregnancy tests can now detect hCG as early as the day you are due to have your period. If you have irregular cycles, use your longest recent cycle to determine when you should test.

Q My period is late but the pregnancy test was negative. Could I be pregnant?

If your test was negative and you still think you may be pregnant, wait for three days and perform another test; there may not have been enough hCG in your urine when the first test was carried out. If you have had two or three negative tests and still feel you may be pregnant, or your period has not arrived, ask your doctor for advice as there may be a number of medical reasons apart from pregnancy why your period has not arrived.

Q Are home pregnancy tests reliable?

If you follow the instructions carefully, home pregnancy tests are around 97–99 per cent accurate. When you are carrying out a home pregnancy test, it is advisable to use the first urine sample of the day and to not drink too much fluid the night before. This is to prevent the sample becoming too diluted, which could make it difficult to measure the levels of hCG.

Certain fertility medications can interfere with the results of a pregnancy test, so if you have been undergoing any fertility treatment and think this may apply to you, you should ask your doctor or fertility clinic for more information and advice.

Doing a pregnancy test too early in pregnancy can produce a false negative result, which means that the test reads negative but you are really pregnant. If you think this may be the case, repeat the test in three days' time.

> You may have missed a period or even feel different, but the best way to confirm you are pregnant is to do a test

First signs of pregnancy

The most obvious initial sign that you are pregnant is a missed period. Other common early pregnancy symptoms include feeling extremely tired and bloated, having increasingly tender breasts, experiencing an increased need to pass urine, and finding that you have a greater or lesser sex drive, although all of these symptoms can occur premenstrually. Some women also experience a small bleed around the time their period was due, which may be confused with a lighter period, that occurs when a fertilized egg implants in the wall of the uterus. There may also be a metallic taste in the mouth, nausea, or vomiting – described as morning sickness, although this can occur at any time of day. Some women don't experience any symptoms.

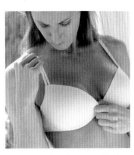

LEFT: Breast tenderness is a common symptom in early pregnancy.
BELOW: You may feel very tired in the early stages of pregnancy due to the effects of your hormones and changes to your metabolism.

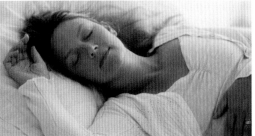

Q I'm on the Pill but my doctor has confirmed I'm pregnant. How can this have happened?

The oral contraceptive Pill is around 92–99.7 per cent effective, depending on the brand and how reliably it is taken. Although figures indicate that approximately 8 out of 100 women do become pregnant during the first year of using the Pill, other studies indicate that when the Pill is taken properly as instructed this figure falls to less than 1 out of 100.

Ideally, the Pill should be taken at the same time each day, although some types can be taken up to 12 hours late. If you forget to take even one Pill, you increase your chances of getting pregnant. If two or more Pills from the same packet are missed, this can dramatically increase the risk of pregnancy if no other contraception is being used.

Certain drugs, such as antibiotics, some herbal remedies, and other medicines, can interfere with the reliability of the Pill. Also, sickness and diarrhoea can reduce the Pill's effectiveness. Talk to your doctor, who will be able to help and advise you about what your options are next.

Q My girlfriend has told me she's pregnant – how can I be sure it's mine?

Unfortunately, the only way to be sure that you are the father of her baby is to take a DNA test, which can be carried out several weeks after the baby is born. To do this, you will need the consent of the mother, as samples of DNA will need to be obtained from the child (and possibly from the mother too). DNA (deoxyribonucleic acid) is found in our body cells and is responsible for our genetic makeup and hence our characteristics. DNA is identified in a blood sample or from a scraping of cells inside the cheek. Samples from the child and partner need to be obtained in the same way.

Q I drank and smoked quite a lot before I realized I was pregnant. Will this affect the baby?

As you are probably aware, it is not advisable to drink and smoke during pregnancy. There are, however, many women in your position who did not realize they were pregnant and continued to smoke

MYTHS AND MISCONCEPTIONS

Is it true that...

 Doing a headstand after sex helps you conceive?
There may be some truth in this! You don't have to do headstands after sex, but there are ways you can help your partner's sperm on its way up to the egg. Don't rush off to the gym straight after sex – stay in bed and let gravity do some of the work.

 Eating yams makes you more likely to have twins?
This is debatable. It seems that certain cultures have more twins than others, and also eat a lot of yams. Although there is no scientific proof, some yams contain a substance similar to oestrogen which may help some women in this culture have more twins.

 Acupuncture boosts your chance of IVF success?
This is still under debate. In a recent study, researchers said acupuncture increased success rates by almost 50 per cent in women having IVF treatment. The theory is that acupuncture can affect the autonomic nervous system, making the lining of the uterus more receptive to receiving an embryo. But the scientists admit they don't know for certain why the complementary therapy helped, and more studies are planned.

and drink. The important thing is to stop drinking and smoking now and take the best possible care of yourself and your baby. As many young women "binge drink", it is important for women of child-bearing age to be aware that alcohol does cross the placenta and is a toxic substance to the baby. Most women, once they realize they are pregnant, stop drinking immediately and this is the best course of action for you to take.

If a mother continues to drink heavily, the alcohol can adversely affect the developing fetus, especially between weeks 4 and 10 of pregnancy, and serious complications, such as fetal alcohol syndrome and fetal alcohol spectrum disorder, can develop. If one of these conditions develops, it can result in physical, behavioural, and learning disabilities that can have lifelong implications for the baby. Drinking in pregnancy also increases the risk of miscarriage and premature labour.

The harmful chemicals in smoke can restrict the baby's growth and cause dependency on nicotine even within the womb (see p.42) so give up now.

I haven't got any pregnancy symptoms yet – when are they likely to start?

Not everybody feels the full range of pregnancy symptoms as soon as they become pregnant, and it is not uncommon for some women to experience none at all. There are many factors that influence the range and intensity of pregnancy symptoms, such as your age, working environment, your state of health, diet, previous pregnancies, smoking, and how your body reacts to pregnancy hormones.

Nausea and vomiting are among the most common symptoms that women report, usually in the first three months and starting at around six weeks. These tend to improve by 12 weeks, but for some women can continue throughout the pregnancy.

Another early pregnancy symptom is breast tenderness, which is caused by changes in the levels of hormones that help to get your breasts ready for breastfeeding. The breasts may enlarge and become tender and heavier.

MIDWIFE WISDOM

A surprise pregnancy
dealing with an unexpected event

If your pregnancy was unplanned, you may have to work through feelings of shock and anxiety before coming to terms with this life-changing event.

✽ Be open with your partner about your feelings and reassure him that this is as much of a shock for you.

✽ Rather than feel anxious about your lifestyle, make positive changes straight away: adopt a healthy diet, stop smoking and drinking, and take folic acid (see p.15).

✽ You may feel overwhelmed, but rather than despair, just allow yourself time to adjust physically, mentally, and emotionally.

These early symptoms may settle around the middle of the pregnancy. A lack of symptoms is not indicative of how healthy your pregnancy is – you may just be one of the lucky few who sail through with no annoying side effects!

My partner doesn't seem as enthusiastic as me about the pregnancy – should I be worried?

Men and women can react to the news of a pregnancy in different ways and for many men, coming to terms with a pregnancy can take far longer. It's worth bearing in mind that during the early stages of pregnancy, men can find it hard to relate to the pregnancy as they have yet to see their baby on a scan or the changes in your body. On the other hand, you may be very aware that your body is undergoing many physical and emotional changes.

It's likely that your partner simply needs more time to adjust to the news. He may be concerned about the changes to your lifestyle and the financial implications of having a baby. Talking openly to each other can help to ease anxieties for you both.

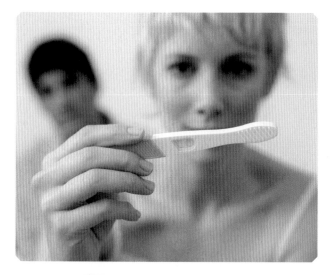
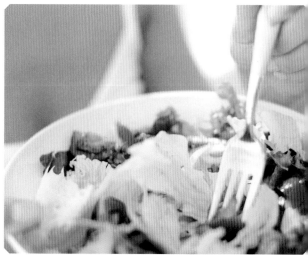
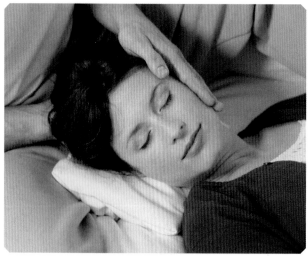
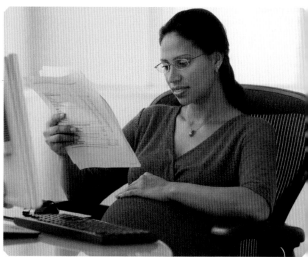
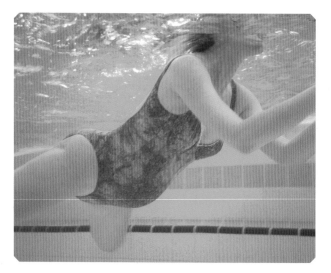
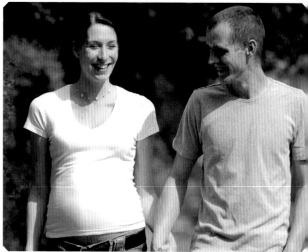

Now you're pregnant

* **My test is positive**
  what happens next?

* **Why is pregnancy so scary?**
  a safe pregnancy

* **What to eat... What not to eat**
  your diet in pregnancy

* **Should I go swimming?**
  keeping active in pregnancy

* **What do I tell my boss?**
  your rights and benefits

* **Will life ever be the same?**
  special situations

My test is positive
what happens next?

Q We've confirmed the pregnancy – when should we tell everyone?

This is down to personal preference. Many women wait until after their first scan at around 12 weeks before announcing their pregnancy. This is mainly because the chances of miscarriage are at their highest during the first trimester. This avoids having to break the news if you do miscarry. On the other hand, you may value others' support. Circumstances may dictate that you tell people earlier, for example, if pregnancy symptoms are pronounced. Some couples find that waiting to share the news allows them to adapt to the idea of parenthood without constant "advice" from others.

Q It's what we wanted, but now I feel unsure – am I just scared?

Finding out you are pregnant, even if it was planned, can feel overwhelming and what you are feeling is perfectly normal. The hormonal changes you are experiencing can also give you highs and lows, which you have to handle along with the physical changes of pregnancy. Talking to your partner, a trusted family member or a friend, or confidentially to your midwife, about how you are feeling may help relieve your anxiety. It's important to acknowledge that pregnancy is a period of enormous change – physically, emotionally, socially, and financially – and it takes time to adjust to these changes.

Q I want the baby but my partner doesn't – can he force me to have an abortion?

No, whether or not you proceed with the pregnancy is your decision. Your partner may simply need more time to adjust, but if he remains adamant that he doesn't want the baby, you need to decide about the future of your relationship.

Q My mum has strong opinions about pregnancy – how can I tell her I want to do it my way?

You could take your mother to an antenatal appointment so she can see how things have changed and your midwife can explain the reasoning behind your care. If she still interferes, have a frank talk. Tell her that although you love her and know she wants to help, you want to make your own decisions. Hopefully she will come round to your point of view.

Q We don't feel ready financially – how will we cope?

There are ways to cut costs when preparing for your baby. Although some items should be new, such as mattresses and car seats, many things can be bought second-hand or passed on from friends and relatives, who may also wish to buy an "item". There is a range of monetary and health benefits that you may be entitled to (see pp.62–3). Also, some families are eligible for a Sure Start Maternity Grant, a one-off payment that doesn't have to be paid back, and child benefit is paid to all people bringing up children. A child trust of £250 is also available for each baby born in the UK (see p.61). Your midwife can give you contact details for any benefits you are entitled to.

Q I'm pregnant by IVF – is there anything different I should do?

Some experts believe that once pregnant, providing there are no other risk factors, you should be treated the same as unassisted low-risk pregnancies. Others believe that you are already a higher risk because you needed help to conceive. Recent research suggests a link between IVF and growth problems, so regular scans may be sensible. Your hospital may have a policy for IVF pregnancies and you could speak to your midwife about consultant care.

How do I work out when my baby is due?

If you have a regular cycle, your due date is calculated at 40 weeks after the first day of your last menstrual period. Look on the chart for the month and then the first day of your last menstrual period (printed in bold type). Directly below it is the date that your baby is due – your estimated delivery date (EDD).

January	1	2	3	4	5	6	7	8	9	10	11	12	13	14	15	16	17	18	19	20	21	22	23	24	25	26	27	28	29	30	31
Oct/Nov	8	9	10	11	12	13	14	15	16	17	18	19	20	21	22	23	24	25	26	27	28	29	30	31	1	2	3	4	5	6	7
February	1	2	3	4	5	6	7	8	9	10	11	12	13	14	15	16	17	18	19	20	21	22	23	24	25	26	27	28			
Nov/Dec	8	9	10	11	12	13	14	15	16	17	18	19	20	21	22	23	24	25	26	27	28	29	30	1	2	3	4	5			
March	1	2	3	4	5	6	7	8	9	10	11	12	13	14	15	16	17	18	19	20	21	22	23	24	25	26	27	28	29	30	31
Dec/Jan	6	7	8	9	10	11	12	13	14	15	16	17	18	19	20	21	22	23	24	25	26	27	28	29	30	31	1	2	3	4	5
April	1	2	3	4	5	6	7	8	9	10	11	12	13	14	15	16	17	18	19	20	21	22	23	24	25	26	27	28	29	30	
Jan/Feb	6	7	8	9	10	11	12	13	14	15	16	17	18	19	20	21	22	23	24	25	26	27	28	29	30	31	1	2	3	4	
May	1	2	3	4	5	6	7	8	9	10	11	12	13	14	15	16	17	18	19	20	21	22	23	24	25	26	27	28	29	30	31
Feb/Mar	5	6	7	8	9	10	11	12	13	14	15	16	17	18	19	20	21	22	23	24	25	26	27	28	1	2	3	4	5	6	7
June	1	2	3	4	5	6	7	8	9	10	11	12	13	14	15	16	17	18	19	20	21	22	23	24	25	26	27	28	29	30	
Mar/Apr	8	9	10	11	12	13	14	15	16	17	18	19	20	21	22	23	24	25	26	27	28	29	30	31	1	2	3	4	5	6	
July	1	2	3	4	5	6	7	8	9	10	11	12	13	14	15	16	17	18	19	20	21	22	23	24	25	26	27	28	29	30	31
Apr/May	7	8	9	10	11	12	13	14	15	16	17	18	19	20	21	22	23	24	25	26	27	28	29	30	1	2	3	4	5	6	7
August	1	2	3	4	5	6	7	8	9	10	11	12	13	14	15	16	17	18	19	20	21	22	23	24	25	26	27	28	29	30	31
May/June	8	9	10	11	12	13	14	15	16	17	18	19	20	21	22	23	24	25	26	27	28	29	30	31	1	2	3	4	5	6	7
September	1	2	3	4	5	6	7	8	9	10	11	12	13	14	15	16	17	18	19	20	21	22	23	24	25	26	27	28	29	30	
June/July	8	9	10	11	12	13	14	15	16	17	18	19	20	21	22	23	24	25	26	27	28	29	30	1	2	3	4	5	6	7	
October	1	2	3	4	5	6	7	8	9	10	11	12	13	14	15	16	17	18	19	20	21	22	23	24	25	26	27	28	29	30	31
July/Aug	8	9	10	11	12	13	14	15	16	17	18	19	20	21	22	23	24	25	26	27	28	29	30	31	1	2	3	4	5	6	7
November	1	2	3	4	5	6	7	8	9	10	11	12	13	14	15	16	17	18	19	20	21	22	23	24	25	26	27	28	29	30	
Aug/Sept	8	9	10	11	12	13	14	15	16	17	18	19	20	21	22	23	24	25	26	27	28	29	30	31	1	2	3	4	5	6	
December	1	2	3	4	5	6	7	8	9	10	11	12	13	14	15	16	17	18	19	20	21	22	23	24	25	26	27	28	29	30	31
Sept/Oct	7	8	9	10	11	12	13	14	15	16	17	18	19	20	21	22	23	24	25	26	27	28	29	30	1	2	3	4	5	6	7

Q When will I have my first antenatal appointment and how many can I expect?

Your first appointment with the midwife, known as the "booking appointment", usually takes place between 8 and 12 weeks. This tends to be the longest one as its purpose is to obtain your medical history and carry out a series of checks (see p.74) so that your care during pregnancy and birth can be planned.

For a first pregnancy with no complications, 10 appointments are usual, and for subsequent pregnancies, 7 visits are adequate. You can contact your midwife between appointments if you have any concerns or questions.

Q I got pregnant straight away – are we super-fertile?

If you have intercourse around ovulation time and neither of you has fertility problems, you have a 25 per cent chance of conceiving. So I'm afraid this just indicates that intercourse was well timed!

Q My partner treats me as if I'm made of glass. How can I show him that this isn't necessary?

Discuss your feelings and allow him to voice his concerns. Ask him to come to an appointment, as the more he understands, the better equipped he will be to provide more appropriate support when needed.

Why is pregnancy so scary?
a safe pregnancy

Q Is it OK if I cut down on smoking, rather than give up?

Although you may be tempted just to cut down, many smokers inhale more deeply when smoking fewer cigarettes and so their intake of damaging toxins increases. The carbon monoxide, nicotine, and other substances that you inhale pass out of your lungs, into your bloodstream, and cross the placenta. Nicotine makes your baby's heart beat faster as he struggles to get oxygen, which can affect his growth rate. Smoking increases the risk of miscarriage, premature birth, and low birth weight, and exposure to tobacco chemicals makes your baby more likely to suffer from conditions such as asthma and chest infections after the birth, which may be bad enough to warrant a hospital stay. There is also a higher risk of cot death if you or your partner smokes.

Q Can passive smoking affect my unborn baby?

In a word, yes. If you live with a smoker, you will be inhaling thousands of toxic carcinogenic chemicals that are released into the air around you from the burning end of the cigarette and the exhaled smoke. Several studies have confirmed that passive smoking can result in health problems and increase the risk of miscarriage and premature birth. There has also been a link between passive smoking in pregnancy and an increased risk of central nervous system tumours in children and a reduced IQ.

Q I've been told that sunbeds and jacuzzis can harm my baby. Is this true?

Although there is no evidence that sunbed or jacuzzi use cause harm to the unborn baby, it has been reported that a rise in the mother's temperature, which can happen while on a tanning bed, or in a hot tub or sauna, may in turn increase the temperature of the fetus. A temperature above 39°C (102°F) has been associated with spinal malformations in developing babies, and if a rise in temperature is maintained for long enough, it has been suggested that it can cause brain damage. The temperature of the amniotic fluid around the baby can also increase and it is thought that an extreme rise in your body temperature can cause problems with the flow of blood to the baby, particularly in the first 12 weeks of pregnancy. Generally, the advice is to limit sunbed use and sunbathing because of the risk of skin damage leading to skin cancer. In pregnancy, it would be best to stop or limit sunbed and jacuzzi sessions, and take extra precautions when sunbathing.

Sunbeds may become a thing of the past as they pose health risks for everyone, not just pregnant women

Q Is it safe to use a microwave?

Microwaves use electromagnetic radiation, which causes water molecules in food to vibrate to produce heat. The radiation levels in modern microwave ovens are low and not thought to pose a risk to the health of either a woman or her unborn baby, although there hasn't been extensive research. It is best not to use a microwave if it is very old or is not working properly, as there is a slight risk of radiation leakage. Always follow the instructions.

Taking medicines in pregnancy
What is safe to take?

The advice to pregnant women is to avoid taking any medicines in pregnancy if at all possible. If you do need to take medication, check with your midwife or doctor first, or ask your pharmacist for information on over-the-counter drugs. The list below offers some guidance.

Antiemetics: For women with severe morning sickness, an antiemetic drug may be suggested. Your doctor will recommend one that is safe to take in pregnancy.

Antihistamines: Most of these should be avoided in pregnancy. If you have hay fever, try to avoid known triggers and allergens, or talk to your doctor about safe medications in pregnancy.

Painkillers: If natural remedies, such as a head massage to relieve a headache, or a warm bath to ease backache, don't work, then paracetamol is generally considered safe for short-term use in pregnancy, although it should be avoided if possible. Ibuprofen should be avoided altogether, as should aspirin (unless specifically prescribed by your doctor).

Antibiotics: There are antibiotics that are safe for use in pregnancy. Penicillin-based ones are usually prescribed, or if you are allergic to these there are other safe alternatives. The following ones should be avoided in pregnancy:
* **Tetracylines** can affect the development of a baby's bones and teeth and may cause discolouration of the teeth.
* **Streptomycin** can cause damage to the ears of the growing fetus and result in hearing loss and so should be avoided in pregnancy.

* **Sulphonamides:** These cause jaundice in the baby and should not be given in pregnancy.

Laxatives: If you are suffering with constipation, try natural dietary remedies first, such as eating lots of fibre and drinking plenty of fluids. If these don't work, then over-the-counter laxatives are safe to take in pregnancy. Ones that contain bulking agents are the best.

Antacids: Heartburn is a common problem in late pregnancy due to the pressure of the baby on the stomach. Antacids are generally safe to take, but avoid sodium bicarbonate as the sodium is absorbed into the bloodstream.

Diuretics: These should be avoided. If you experience sudden swelling in the face, hands, or feet, you should talk to your doctor or midwife, as this is one of the signs of pre-eclampsia (see p.89).

Cold and flu remedies: As these remedies often contain a variety of ingredients, which can include antihistamines and other decongestants that are best avoided in pregnancy, it's important to check the label carefully and talk to your doctor or pharmacist before taking any of these. Try natural remedies, such as steam inhalations, before resorting to medicines, or simply take paracetamol for a short time.

Steroids: Anabolic steroids should not be used in pregnancy. It's safe to use mild steroid creams short term for eczema, although avoid using these over a large surface area. Steroid asthma inhalers are safe, as are steroids prescribed for other conditions if your doctor knows you are pregnant.

Q My friend says it's dangerous to dye my hair while I'm pregnant. Is she right?

A concern is that chemicals in hair dye could be carried via your bloodstream to the baby. However, hair dyes are not thought to be highly toxic, and women who colour their hair are exposed only to low amounts of chemicals. Any risks, if there are any, are lowered after the first 12 weeks, when the main organs and systems of the baby's body have formed. If you are dyeing your own hair, wear gloves, don't leave the dye on for longer than needed, rinse your scalp thoroughly with fresh water afterwards, and use the dye in a ventilated room. You could try alternatives such as henna, or opt for highlights where the dye doesn't come into contact with skin.

Q Is it safe to take over-the-counter painkillers while I'm pregnant?

Many women are concerned about the safety of medications in pregnancy (see p.43). Any medicine taken by a pregnant woman can cross the placenta and enter the baby's bloodstream; the effects on the baby depend on what the medicine is and at what stage of pregnancy it is taken. As the first 12 weeks is a critical time for the fetus when its limbs, organs, and systems are forming, many women choose to avoid all but the most essential medication at this time. Most experts believe that paracetamol is safe on an occasional basis, but that aspirin and ibuprofen should be avoided. Codeine-based painkillers are thought to be safe in small amounts but should be approved by a doctor. Any persistent pain should be brought to the attention of your doctor or midwife.

Q Since I've been pregnant, I've had terrible headaches. Could computer work be the cause?

Tension headaches and migraines are common in pregnancy, probably due to fluctuating hormones. Also, it is not uncommon to have severe headaches with prolonged computer use. This could be due to eye strain and the fact that you are immobile, which can cause tension. Minimizing computer use and taking breaks may reduce the risk of headaches. If this doesn't help, talk to your manager about moving to a different area of work at least until later in pregnancy (headaches are often worse in the first trimester). This is your right as a pregnant woman.

Natural pain relief

Try exploring natural remedies to relieve pregnancy aches and pains before resorting to medication. A head massage, drinking plenty of clear liquids, or resting in a darkened room can help relieve a tension headache. Gentle stretching exercises, or a warm bath can relieve backache. Various complementary therapies can be used in pregnancy, for example, reflexology can relieve back pain and circulatory problems, and homeopathy can treat pregnancy symptoms such as nausea and indigestion. Before using any type of complementary therapy in pregnancy, consult your doctor and a registered practitioner.

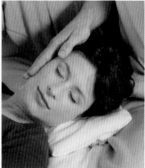

HEAD MASSAGE: A gentle head massage may be sufficient to ease a tension headache and avoid the need for medication.

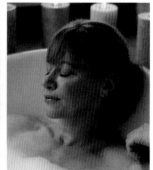

RELAXING BATHS: Taking time out to switch off and enjoy a long soak in a warm bath can help relieve problems such as backache.

Q I've been told I should wear gloves when gardening. Why?

The main concern for a pregnant gardener is toxoplasmosis. The parasite *Toxoplasma gondii* can be found in soil, usually from cat faeces, and can be passed from hands to mouth or eyes. Although toxoplasmosis doesn't affect healthy adults with good immune systems, if contracted in pregnancy it can have serious consequences. There is a 40 per cent chance that the infection will be passed to the baby, causing miscarriage or stillbirth, blindness, brain damage, or other health problems later. However, contracting toxoplasmosis in pregnancy is rare – only about 1 in 500 pregnant women in the UK contract it.

There are simple precautions to make gardening safe in pregnancy, such as wearing gloves when touching soil or plants, washing your hands with soap and water after gardening, even if you wore gloves, and not touching your face or eyes while gardening or until you have washed your hands. Wear gloves too if you have to change cat litter.

Q I work for a dry cleaner. Could the chemicals harm my baby?

Concerns about dry cleaning chemicals stem from research showing that women who operated dry cleaning machines had a higher risk of miscarriage. If touched or inhaled, some organic solvents used in dry cleaning machines can pass through the placenta and some are thought to increase the risk of miscarriage or birth defects. In pregnancy, try to limit your contact with organic solvents and industrial chemicals. Your employer should carry out a detailed risk assessment and it may be necessary to change your duties for the duration of your pregnancy.

Q Should I worry about pollution?

There have been studies on the effects of pollution on unborn babies. The WHO (World Health Organization) reviewed the evidence in 2004 and concluded that pollution can negatively affect lung growth in unborn babies, leading to respiratory problems. One study found a link between pregnant women being exposed to high levels of carbon

> Being aware of, and avoiding, environmental hazards is a sensible precaution to take during your pregnancy

monoxide and ozone in the second pregnancy month and an increased risk of heart defects in the baby. Another study found a link between nitrogen dioxide pollution and an increased risk of premature birth. All studies stated that further research is needed in order to provide conclusive evidence.

Simple measures can reduce your exposure to pollution during pregnancy, such as avoiding busy streets, avoiding exercising near traffic, standing back from the kerb when crossing a road, and avoiding having to stand for too long on central reservations. Try not to travel during "rush hour" and, if you live in a town, spend some time in the countryside. Keep your home ventilated, and use a doormat to trap outdoor pollutants.

Q I'm asthmatic. Can I use my inhalers during pregnancy?

It is essential that you keep asthma under control in pregnancy, which means continuing to use your inhalers, as the risks from uncontrolled asthma are greater than any risk from taking asthma medication. If asthma is uncontrolled, it can mean that not enough oxygen gets to the baby, leading to a low birth weight and increasing your risk of pre-eclampsia (see p.89). One of the best ways to control asthma, in addition to taking medication, is to avoid "triggers", such as pet fur and dust mites. Use air filters, vacuum and damp dust, and use duvet and pillow protectors. Sometimes, pregnancy reduces the severity of asthma. However, if you feel wheezier than usual, talk to your doctor about reviewing your medication.

Travelling abroad

Enjoy hassle-free travel in pregnancy by planning ahead and taking sensible precautions. If you need to fly, check the airline's guidelines; many require a doctor's note after about 28 weeks to say that you are fit and most won't take pregnant women from around 34 weeks.

✱ Check whether immunizations or other precautions, such as anti-malaria treatment, are needed.

✱ When flying, take frequent sips of bottled water, move your legs and ankles to lessen the risk of a blood clot, and wear support stockings.

✱ When abroad, drink only bottled water and wash your hands before eating.

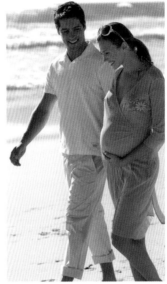

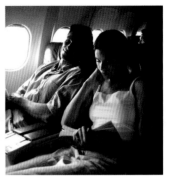

ABOVE: Make sure you have some room to move your legs during flights. **LEFT:** Taking sensible precautions against sun damage is particularly important in pregnancy when skin tends to darken quickly (see p.105).

Is it safe to sleep on my back?

This is more of a problem in late pregnancy when lying on your back can cause the baby to press on the large blood vessels that carry blood to and from the heart, making you dizzy. However, in a healthy pregnancy, you are unlikely to harm yourself or the baby by sleeping on your back for brief periods. If you stayed on your back for long, you would wake feeling uncomfortable and change position anyway.

Often, the best sleeping position is on your side, preferably on the left to make it easier for the heart to pump blood around. A pillow under your tummy and one between your knees can increase comfort (see p.111). If you want to sleep on your back, put a pillow under one side to tilt your body and take the pressure off the large veins and lower back.

We're renovating an old house. Could dust from old lead paint harm my baby?

You are right to be concerned about exposure to lead. Lead was a common ingredient in paint before the mid-1970s. It's unclear exactly what the risks are, partly because it's difficult to measure how much the body absorbs substances, and partly because of the lack of research on the effects of lead in pregnancy. However, lead has been linked with a higher risk of miscarriage, prematurity, low birth weight, and early infant death. You're exposed to lead if you scrape or sand lead paint, causing you to inhale lead dust. Get professionals to remove lead-based paint while you are out, and air rooms thoroughly afterwards.

My partner works with pesticides – is this a problem?

A pesticide is a substance or organism used to control or destroy a pest and is generally toxic to the human body. It is possible that exposure to harmful substances could affect a man's fertility, but there is no evidence that substances in the semen interfere with the normal development of a baby, or that substances on a father's clothes or shoes can affect the mother prior to or during pregnancy. If your partner's workplace is properly regulated, he should be wearing protective clothing and practising good hygiene to reduce his exposure to toxins.

What to eat...What not to eat
your diet in pregnancy

Q I love seafood and eat it regularly. Can I continue to eat it during pregnancy?

Eating raw or undercooked shellfish is risky and should be avoided as they can contain harmful viruses and bacteria. Raw oysters can carry a virus called Norovirus, which causes nausea, abdominal pain, and diarrhoea, and raw or partially cooked shellfish can contain hepatitis A, a virus that affects the liver. However, eating well-cooked prawns, lobster, oysters, clams, cockles, scallops, or crab is now considered safe, as cooking kills any bacteria or viruses. Nutritionally, too, cooked shellfish are beneficial as they are low in fat, high in proteins, and rich in minerals. A well-cooked prawn or lobster turns red and its flesh opaque, while a cooked scallop is opaque, white, and firm to touch. Clams, mussels, and oysters open their shells when they are well cooked – throw away any that don't open. Make sure you buy shellfish from a reputable source.

Q My midwife said I should avoid pâté. Why?

All pâtés, including those made from vegetables or fish, should be avoided during pregnancy unless they are tinned or have been heat-treated. This is due to the risk of listeriosis, a rare infection caused by the bacterium *Listeria monocytogenes* found in pâtés, blue-veined and some soft cheeses, unwashed salads, and ready-to-eat foods. Listeriosis resembles a mild "flu", with symptoms such as aching, sore throat, and a raised temperature. However, even a mild infection can cause miscarriage, stillbirth, or severe illness such as meningitis or septicaemia in the newborn. Another reason to avoid liver pâté (and also fish liver oils, liver sausage, and liver) is that it contains high levels of vitamin A, which has been linked to birth defects.

Q I like to eat rare steaks – are they allowed in pregnancy?

No. You should make sure that you eat only meat that has been well cooked, as raw meat contains bacteria that can cause food poisoning. This is especially important with poultry and products made from minced meat, such as sausages and burgers. Meat should be cooked until it is piping hot all the way through, there is no pink meat, and the juices run clear. Wash your hands after handling raw meat, and keep it separate from foods that are ready to eat. You should also avoid eating raw eggs and undercooked poultry because of the risk of salmonella.

Q I eat a lot of mozzarella, but is it counted as one of the "soft cheeses" to be avoided?

Cheese is one of the top worries for pregnant women, according to a health research charity. However, soft processed cheeses, such as mozzarella, cottage cheese, and cream cheese, are safe to eat throughout pregnancy. The advice is to avoid cheeses such as Camembert, Brie, or Chèvre (a type of soft goat's cheese), or others that have a similar rind, and blue-veined or mould-ripened cheeses, as these could contain listeria, a type of

Try not to feel daunted by the seeming barrage of information on offer; in reality, just a few dietary precautions are needed bacteria that could harm your baby (see above). According to the Food Standards Agency, cooking should kill any listeria, so it should be safe to eat food containing soft, mould-ripened, or blue-veined cheeses, provided it has been properly cooked and is piping hot all the way through.

Q I've started to crave chocolate all the time – is this likely to harm my baby?

It's not unusual for women to experience cravings in pregnancy. Most are "normal", while others, such as urges to eat earth, coal, chalk, or soap, are not, although they do sometimes happen!

Normal cravings can include a desire to eat anything from pickled onions and ice cream to chocolate. Do mention this craving to your midwife as she may want to check that you are not deficient in magnesium, B vitamins, or iron, all found in dark chocolate. A little indulgence is fine, but giving in to a pregnancy full of chocolate could cause nutritional deficiencies if it stops you eating a well-balanced diet, and lead to excessive weight gain.

However, eating chocolate in pregnancy has been linked to contented babies; this may be due to a high intake of phenylethylamine, a mood-enhancing chemical present in chocolate (also present in larger quantities in tomatoes and fruit), or it may be due to happy, relaxed mothers who have indulged!

Q I love spicy foods but have been told these may trigger an early labour – is this true?

Many people believe that eating a curry encourages the start of labour, but this is completely untrue. Although the reasoning behind this sounds logical, the theory does not work. One of the less talked about first signs of labour is a loose bowel motion or even diarrhoea. This occurs because the cervix (neck of the womb) and part of the bowel have a common nerve supply. As the cervix starts to soften in readiness for labour, so the bowel is stimulated. This may cause faster movement of food and more frequent, looser bowel motions. Labour may follow in the next few hours or it may not happen for a day or so. Some people think that if you eat an extra hot curry, for example, to bring on a bout of diarrhoea, this will stimulate the cervix and labour will start. Unfortunately, the process doesn't seem to work reliably in reverse. Labour following self-induced diarrhoea is probably coincidental, and the side effects of abdominal cramps, diarrhoea, and soreness are disagreeable.

However, if you regularly eat curries and spicy food, and have not been suffering from heartburn or indigestion, then there is no harm in treating yourself every now and then.

Q I'm fed up with people telling me what I should and shouldn't eat and drink – what do you say?

While no health promoter wants to be prescriptive, there is plenty of research highlighting the ill effects of poor nutrition, smoking, alcohol, and drug misuse on the fetus. Members of the health profession, and even friends and family, may have personal experience of babies born with low birth weights, birth defects, syndromes, withdrawal symptoms, or infants who go on to develop allergies in childhood, such as eczema and asthma. The reason people are offering advice is because they want what is best for you and your baby. In the first three months in particular, while your baby's organs are developing, lifestyle choices carry a risk. If you can, try to take on board this advice as long as you are sure it is correct, current, and evidence-based.

One of the most sensible approaches to eating in pregnancy is to allow yourself most things in moderation

Non-alcoholic drinks

It's important to stay well hydrated in pregnancy to combat fatigue and avoid constipation, which is a common side effect of pregnancy due to a sluggish digestion brought about by hormonal changes in your body. The advice is for you to aim to drink around two pints of fluid every day. This fluid should come mainly from water, but there are other good sources of fluids including herbal teas (avoid raspberry leaf tea until later in pregnancy, see p.144), fruit juices, and milk. However, try not to drink too much milk as it has a fairly high calorie content (stick to skimmed or semi-skimmed). Avoid, or limit your intake, of drinks containing caffeine, including tea, coffee, and carbonated drinks, as caffeine interferes with your absorption of vitamins, and high levels of caffeine have even been linked to an increased risk of miscarriage.

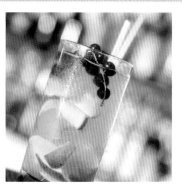

STAYING HYDRATED: A fruit cocktail is a delicious treat and a satisfying alternative to a glass of wine.

I'm really overweight – could this affect my pregnancy?

The medical concensus is that women with a high body mass index prior to pregnancy (see p.18) should try to limit the amount of weight they gain, as putting on too much weight increases the risk of developing high blood pressure, gestational diabetes, and having a big baby. The recommended weight gain in pregnancy is 10–12.5 kg (22–28 lb). If you gain weight within this range, you have a lower risk of complications during labour and birth.

However, pregnancy is not the time to go on a diet. Research shows that, for a pregnant woman who is overweight, a low-calorie diet does not reduce her chances of developing high blood pressure or pre-eclampsia and doesn't benefit the baby. Instead, you should seek advice from your midwife or doctor about how to eat a healthy, well-balanced diet that will ensure you don't pile on the pounds, but which keeps you and your baby healthy (see p.50).

I want to get back into my jeans right after the birth. How can I make sure I don't get too fat?

These days, it is almost impossible to pass a newspaper stand without seeing the latest celebrity who has not only fitted straight back into her clothes after having her baby, but who actually weighs less than she did before her pregnancy. However, this is concerning for health professionals, as a dramatic weight loss after the birth is not good for the mother or for her baby. The average weight gain during pregnancy is 10–12.5kg (22–28lb) (see p.107). Your baby (including the placenta and the waters surrounding the baby) makes up approximately 5kg (11lb) of this, with 6 kg (13lb) gained from increased fluids, fats, and an enlarged uterus. Much of this extra weight will be lost as soon as your baby is born. Also, after the birth, some of this extra weight provides nutrients for breastfeeding, which uses up to 500 calories a day.

The most sensible approach to controlling your weight during pregnancy is to eat a healthy diet and take gentle exercise to ensure that weight gain is not too dramatic. You should be eating around 2,100–2,500 calories a day, increasing this by 200 calories in the last trimester – the equivalent of a couple of slices of toast with low-fat spread and a glass of milk.

It is important to be realistic about postnatal weight loss. A sensible guide is "nine months on, nine months off" and most dieticians recommend losing no more than 0.9kg (2lb) a week. This may not seem much, but adds up to 6kg (14lb) in seven weeks – achievable with healthy eating and exercise.

Pregnancy diet
Eating for you and your baby

A healthy diet is important at any time, but is especially crucial during pregnancy to ensure that you and your baby have all the right nutrients needed; it will help your baby develop and grow, and help you to keep fit and well. Eat a wide variety of different foods each day to get the right balance of nutrients, and avoid certain foods that may be harmful to your growing baby (see p.47).

Fruit and vegetables Aim to eat at least five portions of fruit and vegetables each day, especially iron-rich leafy green vegetables. These provide essential vitamins and minerals and fibre, which helps digestion and prevents constipation. Ideally, eat them lightly cooked or raw. Frozen, tinned, and dried fruit and vegetables are good standbys.

The importance of iron Iron is essential for the production of haemoglobin, and you will need to up your intake in pregnancy to support the increase in your blood volume. If you are short of iron, you are likely to feel very tired and may suffer from anaemia (see p.81). Lean meat, green leafy vegetables, and dried fruit and nuts all contain iron.

Starchy foods Starchy foods, such as bread, potatoes, rice, pasta, yams, and breakfast cereals, should form the main part of any meal and are an important source of vitamins and fibre. Try eating wholegrains – bread, cereals, and pasta – as these contain more fibre and can prevent constipation.

Proteins You should have at least two servings of fish per week and eat a portion of eggs (well cooked), beans, lentils, lean meat, or thoroughly cooked chicken each day. Avoid liver (including liver pâté) as it contains high levels of vitamin A, which can increase the risk of birth defects.

Recommended daily servings

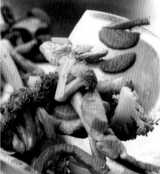

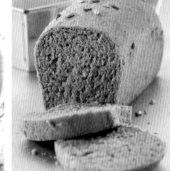

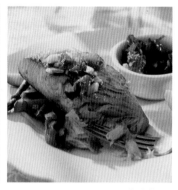

3–4 SERVINGS OF VEGETABLES: A helping of raw or lightly cooked vegetables provides vital vitamins and minerals.

4–6 SERVINGS OF CARBOHYDRATE: Wholemeal breads and other complex carbohydrates help sustain energy levels.

2–3 PORTIONS OF PROTEIN: A daily intake of protein, such as meat, fish, pulses, or cheese, ensures the healthy functioning of cells.

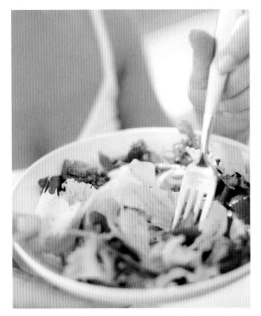

LIGHT MEALS: A freshly prepared salad is an ideal light meal during pregnancy. Unlike "bulky" foods, it is easy to digest and also boosts your intake of essential vitamins and minerals.

Dairy foods Foods that contain milk, such as cheese and yogurt, provide calcium, which is essential for healthy bones. It is important that your calcium intake is high before and during pregnancy. Avoid non-pasteurized soft cheeses (such as Camembert, Brie, and Chèvre) and blue cheeses, as these can contain the harmful bacteria listeria (see p.47).

Fluids During pregnancy your blood volume will increase, so it is important to keep up your fluid intake. Water is best, although fruit juices are also good (see p.49). Try to restrict your tea drinking to six cups per day, and coffee to three cups per day. Alcohol is not recommended (see p.53).

Foods to cut back on Limit your intake of sugar and sugary foods, such as sweets, cakes, biscuits, and fizzy drinks, as they contain calories but no nutrients. Also limit your consumption of high-calorie fats and fatty foods.

Vegetarian diet This needs to provide a sufficient intake of iron, calcium, vitamin B_{12}, and protein. Include dairy products, pulses and beans, fortified cereals, eggs, seeds and nuts, and green leafy vegetables in your diet, and talk to your doctor about taking a supplement if necessary.

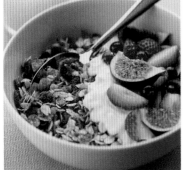

1–2 SERVINGS OF EGGS OR CEREALS: Including foods that are rich in iron is important in pregnancy to prevent anaemia (see p.81).

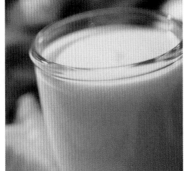

2–3 SERVINGS OF LOW-FAT DAIRY: Dairy products, such as low-fat milk, are an excellent source of calcium, fats, and protein.

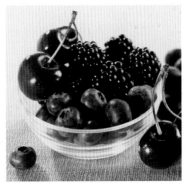

5 PORTIONS OF FRUIT: Include a range of different fruits. These are rich in antioxidants, which protect against damaging free radicals.

MYTHS AND MISCONCEPTIONS

Is it true that...

 ### You lose a tooth for every baby?

Pregnancy doesn't have to ruin your teeth. There was some basis for this myth back when nutritional deficiencies meant that women might have insufficient calcium to support an unborn baby's needs. Calcium is vital for all women, and your midwife or doctor may recommend you take a calcium supplement. Good food sources of calcium include: dairy products, leafy green vegetables, canned sardines with the bones, fortified tofu, and fresh fruit juice. Do arrange a checkup and tell the dentist that you're pregnant.

Sweet cravings mean it's a girl, sour cravings mean it's a boy?

Many people believe that cravings can predict the sex of your baby. So, if you can't get enough chocolate, you're having a girl, but if you crave straight lemon juice then you're having a boy. However, according to some scientists, cravings don't even exist! There is also the myth that if your partner puts on weight during your pregnancy, then you will be having a girl. If he doesn't put on a pound, then you're carrying a boy.

Heartburn means hair?

Heartburn is very common in pregnancy – chalk it up to pregnancy hormones loosening the muscles of your oesophagus. But no, it doesn't mean that your baby will be born with a full head of hair!

Q Is it alright for me to have the occasional glass of wine throughout my pregnancy?

This is really a personal choice you need to make in pregnancy. Although experts do not agree on the exact level of alcohol needed to cause harm to babies during pregnancy, the general consensus is that drinking has to be heavy and regular to cause a dangerous condition known as fetal alcohol syndrome (see p.37).

However, you should be aware that alcohol crosses the placenta to your baby very easily and quickly, and that drinking during pregnancy could potentially damage your baby and your own health. The government's official advice is not to drink alcohol when you are pregnant or trying to conceive. If you do decide to drink, make sure it is no more than one or two units, just once or twice a week. Many women give up alcohol during pregnancy and you may feel that you simply no longer enjoy the taste. It's also worth noting that although alcohol doesn't contain fat, it's high in calories, with a glass of dry white wine containing over 100 calories.

Q I have a really sweet tooth – is it OK to indulge this during pregnancy?

While occasional treats of sweets or crisps are fine, processed foods usually contain hidden fats and sugars and provide few nutrients, so it's best to try and curb the amount of sweet foods you eat. Read food labels and look for alternative foods containing less fat and added sugars. Just as you would consider carefully how you wean and feed your growing child, you should look after yourself in the same way.

One of the best ways to curb your sweet tooth is to eat regular meals throughout the day. This helps to steady your blood sugar level and reduce sweet-tooth cravings. Try not to go longer than three hours without eating and, if you are hungry, have a healthy snack between meals, such as malt loaf, a cottage cheese sandwich, chicken or lean ham, a low-fat yogurt, or fruit, including fresh, tinned, or dried, such as raisins or apricots. Also, try to ensure that you

drink about two litres of water a day, as perceived hunger is often really dehydration. If you can't give up sweet drinks, you could try artificial sweeteners, such as saccharin. There is no evidence that small amounts of these are harmful during pregnancy or while breastfeeding.

Q Should I be taking vitamin supplements during my pregnancy?

There is still uncertainty about whether women who have a well-balanced diet need dietary supplements during their pregnancy. If you do decide to take a supplement, it is important to choose one that is designed specifically for pregnant and breastfeeding women and which contains the appropriate mix of vitamins and minerals. A good pregnancy supplement contains more folic acid, calcium, and iron than a general multivitamin and no vitamin A.

If you do take a supplement, it's still important to eat a varied, well-balanced diet. If you are unsure at all about which medicines and supplements are safe during pregnancy, your local pharmacist will be able

---

MIDWIFE WISDOM

✳ Cravings
should you give in to a food craving?

No-one is really sure what causes food cravings in pregnancy, although it may be a mixture of hormonal, physical, and psychological factors.

✱ The most common cravings are for sweet or salty foods; these are OK to indulge now and then, but are lacking in nutrients so try to limit your intake.

✱ Cravings for foods such as fruit or fish may be a natural desire to eat as healthily as possible in pregnancy.

✱ Strange cravings, known as "pica", for items such as chalk, may indicate an iron deficiency – and should not be indulged!

to advise you. You can buy antenatal supplements at almost any chemist, or your doctor may prescribe them if he or she feels that your diet is providing insufficient nutrients.

Q I don't have a very balanced diet – does this matter?

Maintaining a balanced diet is important and especially so in pregnancy. Now is a time when you need to make sure that your diet is providing you with enough energy and nutrients for the baby to grow and develop, and for your body to deal with the changes taking place. So yes, your diet does matter.

Your daily intake should include foods in approximately the following proportions: a third fruit and vegetables (at least five portions a day); a third carbohydrate-based foods like bread, potatoes, cereals, and pasta; a sixth of protein foods like meat, poultry, pulses, cheese, and other dairy products; a small amount of sugar and fat; and at least eight glasses of water each day. It's a good idea to cut down on foods such as cakes and biscuits, which are high in fat and sugar, to avoid putting on too much weight. If you feel you need some advice, discuss your diet with your midwife or doctor, who may also recommend that you take vitamin supplements in addition to your food (see above).

Q Is it safe to eat peanuts or foods containing peanuts during my pregnancy?

Some experts feel that if a child is at a particular risk of developing a peanut allergy, the problem may have started to develop before birth, when a sensitivity to peanuts may have started due to exposure in the womb from the mother's diet. However, some recent studies have suggested that avoiding peanuts may actually be increasing the incidence of allergies, pointing to countries where peanuts are a staple food and allergies relatively rare.

Your baby may be at risk of a peanut allergy if you, or your partner, or your baby's siblings suffer from asthma, eczema, hay fever, or other allergies. Official government advice is that if you fit into any of

Ensuring the future health of your baby starts now, at the beginning of life. Eat healthily to do what is best for you and your baby

these groups, you should not eat peanuts, or peanut products, in pregnancy or while breastfeeding. There is no need to avoid peanuts if your baby is not at risk of peanut allergy. Other nuts, such as hazelnuts, Brazil nuts, and walnuts, are safe to eat during pregnancy.

Weaning information has also changed, with "at risk" families being advised to delay the introduction of peanuts until the age of three.

Q Does what I eat in pregnancy influence my baby's long-term health?

There are reasons to believe that what you eat during your pregnancy can influence your baby's health long term and possibly her tastes too. Some experts have suggested that problems that occur later in life, such as obesity, diabetes, and other health problems, may be caused not so much by what a person eats during their own lifetime, as by what their mother ate while she was pregnant.

Also, there have been studies that have looked at links between a pregnant mother's protein and carbohydrate intake and a baby's blood pressure.

Research undertaken at Tommy's Maternal and Fetal Research Unit (see p.310) suggests that a mother's diet in pregnancy and while breastfeeding does influence the health of her offspring throughout their lives. Studies reveal that pregnancy diets rich in fat have been associated with the later development of breast cancer in children and further research is being carried out. Talk to your midwife for advice on eating a varied, well-balanced diet (see p.50).

Should I go swimming?
keeping active in pregnancy

Q I regularly go to the gym. I've just found out I'm pregnant – can I still go?

Many forms of exercise are safe during pregnancy. Regular exercise keeps you fit and healthy, so if you currently exercise then it's fine to carry on as before. Although you can continue to take part in most activities during the first trimester of your pregnancy, you may need to stop more vigorous exercise as your pregnancy continues. Do tell your fitness instructor that you are pregnant, so they can tailor your programme accordingly – pregnancy is not the time to break records or go for personal best! Ideal exercise gets your heart pumping, keeps you supple, manages weight gain, and prepares your muscles for the hard work of labour and delivery without causing undue physical stress for you or your baby.

Being active during your pregnancy can also reduce the physical discomforts of backache, constipation, fatigue, and swelling, as well as improve your mood and even help you to sleep more soundly. The Royal College of Obstetricians and Gynaecologists (RCOG) states that weight-bearing exercise in pregnancy can reduce the length of labour and may decrease delivery complications. So continue if you can.

Other forms of exercise recommended in pregnancy include swimming, walking, aquanatal classes, yoga, and pilates, as these are not high impact so are less likely to injure your joints.

Q What's the best type of exercise during the third trimester?

Swimming is an excellent form of exercise and can be maintained safely throughout pregnancy. It improves circulation, increases muscle tone and strength, builds endurance, and is favoured in late pregnancy as it makes you feel almost weightless. Many women find aquanatal classes enjoyable – exercising while standing in water is gentle on the joints and helps reduce swelling in the legs, common in late pregnancy. Aquanatal classes may be run either by a local midwife or by an exercise teacher trained to teach pregnant women.

Walking is a good form of exercise for this later stage of pregnancy as it keeps you fit without jarring your knees and ankles. Take some water to drink to avoid dehydration. Yoga and pilates are good if you can find a registered practitioner experienced in dealing with pregnant women. Yoga teaches breathing and relaxation techniques that can help with the demands of labour and birth. Many pilates exercises are done in a "hands and knees" position, which is ideal for pregnancy as it takes stress off the back and pelvis and, towards the end of pregnancy, can help to position your baby ready for delivery.

MIDWIFE WISDOM

✱ Benefits of exercise
why you should aim to stay fit in pregnancy

There is no doubt that exercising during pregnancy offers numerous benefits to both mother and baby.

✱ Regular exercise increases flexibility and suppleness, which will benefit you in labour.
✱ Aerobic exercise, such as swimming, increases stamina, improving blood circulation and preparing you for labour.
✱ Exercise releases endorphins, the body's natural painkillers, helping you to relax and lifting your mood.
✱ Exercise keeps backache at bay.
✱ An exercise regime will help you to recover more quickly after the birth.

ESSENTIAL INFORMATION: NOW YOU'RE PREGNANT

Safe exercise
Taking care in pregancy

Although exercise is highly recommended during pregnancy, this is a time when you may have to moderate your usual programme, especially as you get bigger, and avoid types of exercise or situations that may put you or your baby at risk.

What safety precautions should I take? If you are taking up exercise during pregnancy, be sensible about which type of exercise you choose. Avoid any type of exercise that is too strenuous and opt for low-impact activities, such as walking and swimming. Always do warm-up stretches before exercising and build up your stamina and fitness gradually. This is especially important as hormones in pregnancy relax joints and ligaments in preparation for labour (see opposite), which means that you are more susceptible to injury. Avoid exercising in very hot conditions as this may be harmful to the baby; in hot months, exercise early in the morning or indoors. Also, avoid exercising near traffic as you are more likely to be affected by pollution while exercising. Your centre of gravity changes in pregnancy, so avoid high-impact, fast-moving sports, such as tennis.

Should I stop exercising at any time? You should stop exercising straight away if you feel dizzy or short of breath; if you feel that you are overheating; if you are experiencing pain in your back or pelvis; or if you feel exhausted.

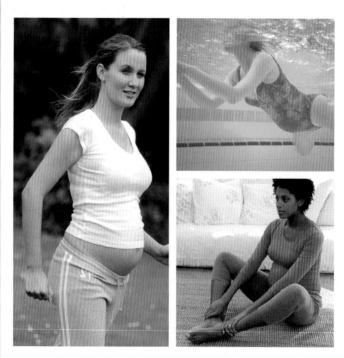

FAR LEFT: If you are used to jogging, it is safe to continue with this in pregnancy unless you have had problems in this pregnancy or previous ones.
TOP LEFT: Swimming is the ideal exercise during pregnancy, providing a moderate aerobic workout, toning muscles, and helping you to feel weightless.
BOTTOM LEFT: Yoga and relaxation classes are beneficial in pregnancy, helping you to focus on your breathing and increasing your suppleness.

I've had a previous miscarriage – should I avoid all kinds of exercise?

Many doctors feel that it is best to avoid all but the gentlest forms of exercise in the first 12–16 weeks of pregnancy if you have had two or more miscarriages, or have had vaginal bleeding during this pregnancy.

I'm not terribly fit, but would like to start an exercise regime – any advice?

If you are unused to exercise, then moderate activities, such as walking and swimming, would probably be best for you and beneficial for your baby, whereas starting a new competitive sport or vigorous exercise programme would not be ideal. Your body is already undergoing huge changes with your heart, lungs, kidneys, and virtually every other major body organ beginning to work much harder. Also, the pregnancy hormones progesterone and relaxin are softening the muscles and ligaments, so soft tissue injuries, back injuries, and abdominal strain become more likely, especially if you haven't exercised much before. Contact sports, vigorous team sports, and activities like diving and gymnastics carry the further risk of direct injury to your abdomen and uterus – especially as your uterus grows and rises out of your pelvis.

Is it safe to go jogging when you're pregnant?

Exercise is recommended in pregnancy to improve your circulation and energy levels, boost the immune system, and increase your stamina for labour. Although low-impact activities, such as walking, swimming, and gentle toning and stretching, are ideal, if you are used to jogging and your pregnancy is straightforward, it is fine to continue in pregnancy. However, it is not advisable to take up jogging for the first time now, particularly as there is a risk of falling and hurting your abdomen, and you should avoid jogging if you have a high-risk or multiple pregnancy. Other sports and exercises to avoid include gymnastics, horse riding, skiing, and squash.

Pelvic floor exercises
Strengthening the muscles that support pelvic organs

Learning how to exercise your pelvic floor muscles is vital in pregnancy to help you avoid stress incontinence (leaking urine).
This discreet exercise can be practised any time. Pelvic floor exercises involve squeezing your buttocks in and pulling in your tummy muscles, then holding for 5 seconds and releasing. Repeat this 5–6 times several times a day. You could imagine your pelvic floor going up like a lift, contracting your muscles a little more at each floor.

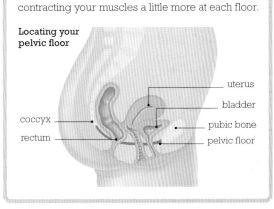

Locating your pelvic floor

coccyx

rectum

uterus

bladder

pubic bone

pelvic floor

When should I start doing pelvic floor exercises?

Pelvic floor exercises (see above) can be started at any stage of your pregnancy, but the earlier you start them the better. These exercises strengthen the pelvic floor, which is the network of muscles that support the bladder, womb, and bowel. Strengthening these muscles helps to reduce the risk of leaking urine while coughing or sneezing, known as stress incontinence. It is important that you know how to do these exercises and practise them regularly throughout your pregnancy.

As well as practising the exercises shown above, another way to exercise your pelvic floor muscles is by inserting a finger into your vagina and tightening the muscles around it.

Q **I'm very desk-bound in my job – is it dangerous to sit for long periods of time?**

During pregnancy, your circulation slows down and if you sit for long periods of time with the lower leg vertical, it can make it hard for blood to travel upwards. Although this may increase the risk of a blood clot, known as deep vein thrombosis (DVT), sitting for long periods in itself is unlikely to cause a clot. Your degree of risk also depends on your level of activity at other times. Exercise is the best way to minimize the risk of a blood clot and taking a brisk daily walk is ideal as it exercises your legs. There are also simple measures you can take while at work to reduce the risk of developing a clot. Try ankle movements every hour, get up and walk around every 3–4 hours, take the stairs rather than the lift, and walk over to see a colleague rather than email.

If you are especially concerned, talk to your midwife or doctor about wearing special stockings that are designed to improve circulation. However, it is important that you get the right size, as stockings that are too tight can add to the problem.

MIDWIFE WISDOM

Exercise in late pregnancy
adapting your routine to suit your changing needs

Towards the end of pregnancy, you will inevitably slow down, but you may not want to stop altogether! There are sensible ways to modify your exercise regime to ensure you stay safe and fit.

✱ In later pregnancy, avoid exercises that involve sudden movement, such as tennis, as your balance is less steady now.

✱ Swimming is perfect in late pregnancy and aids relaxation. You may need to modify your stroke and enjoy more floating.

✱ Reduce the intensity and length of your workout to avoid exhaustion.

Q **I've been getting lower back pain – could it be due to bad posture? I'm eight months pregnant.**

In a recent review of current research, more than two-thirds of pregnant women reported back pain. This pain increased with advancing pregnancy, interfering with work, daily activities, and sleep. Lower back pain is caused by the forward pull of the growing abdomen, so as your baby increases in size and gestation, the strain on your back is greater. So although bad posture may not be the sole cause, adopting a good posture is important to reduce the strain. Gentle exercise also helps to reduce the pain, and water aerobics is particularly beneficial.

Some women use a Transcutaneous Electrical Nerve Stimulation (TENS) machine in late pregnancy (see p.175), which helps to block the pain nerve impulses to the brain and stimulates the release of natural painkillers called endorphins. Other tips for lower back pain include a warm hand massage using a base oil, a warm deep bath, and using cushions to support you when relaxing and in bed.

Q **I'm seven months' pregnant now and quite big. Should I adapt my swimming style?**

You may find that as you get very large towards the end of pregnancy, you need to alternate your swimming style to find the one that is most comfortable for you. Apart from this, a low-impact activity like swimming is ideal as the water provides resistance, there is a low risk of injury, and the mass of water relieves pressure on the abdomen and helps to ease lower back pain.

Q **My midwife is running aquanatal classes at our local pool – are they safe?**

Yes, low-impact activities such as aquanatal classes are fine in pregnancy. You are fortunate to have this facility as not all areas are able to provide classes. The trainer or midwife conducting the sessions should be able to advise you about the range of movement recommended to minimize any risk.

Gentle, strengthening exercise, such as a brisk walk each day, can provide you with more stamina for labour and birth

As well as the benefits from exercise, these sessions help you to meet other pregnant women and build new friendships in pregnancy. Many trainers offer follow-on aquanatal classes after the birth, which can be helpful for postnatal pelvic floor toning.

What is pilates?

The pilates method of exercise was developed in Germany by a man called Pilates. This type of exercise is a core muscle workout that builds your strength without bulking muscles and teaches you to balance strength with flexibility. The idea is to achieve harmony between mind and muscle, and it is taught using eight basic principles: relaxation, concentration, coordination, centring, alignment, breathing, stamina, and flowing movements.

Pilates is a good exercise to do in pregnancy as it heightens your body awareness and is useful for control and confidence in labour and the postnatal period. It also incorporates pelvic floor exercises (see p.57), which are especially useful. It's best to avoid lying flat on your back in the second and third trimesters as this can reduce the blood supply to your baby. If you are going to take classes, speak to your instructor about using a wedge, pillow, or bolster to keep your head higher than your belly while performing the exercises.

Is there an exercise that helps you to avoid varicose veins?

Varicose veins are swollen, twisted, painful veins that are filled with an abnormal collection of blood that causes swelling (oedema) in the affected area, which is usually the lower leg and calf (see p.86). They are more common in women than men, with an increased incidence in pregnancy, and they also tend to be inherited. The most common symptoms of varicose veins and oedema are pain, night cramps, numbness, tingling, heaviness, and aching. You can lessen the risk of varicose veins by taking regular exercise, such as a brisk walk, and try building pockets of exercise into your daily routine, such as using the stairs instead of a lift, or parking further from your destination if you are a regular car driver.

I booked a skiing holiday before I found out that I'm pregnant. Should I cancel?

Skiing is really not recommended during pregnancy, particularly if it is downhill skiing (although if you are used to the sport, moderate cross-country skiing may be fine). This is because of the high risk of a fall and subsequent trauma to your abdomen and the baby. The same risk is associated with ice skating too. During the first trimester of pregnancy, your baby's vital organs are developing and so it is important that this process is not interrupted by any trauma to the abdomen, such as a fall.

In the second and third trimesters, your baby is growing and your womb is higher up and no longer has the protection of the pelvis, so an abdominal trauma could have serious effects on the baby and the placenta. Also in later pregnancy, falling on your abdomen can cause premature labour or separation of the placenta from the wall of the uterus, which is an emergency requiring prompt delivery of the baby.

Can I go horse riding while I'm pregnant?

Horse riding is one of the activities that is not recommended in pregnancy. Even if you are an experienced rider, it is best avoided, particularly as a horse can be unpredictable if startled in any way. There is the risk of injury if you fall off, and there is also the possibility that the jerky motion when riding could strain the ligaments supporting the uterus.

Antenatal yoga

Practising yoga in pregnancy is hugely beneficial. As well as strengthening and toning muscles, which will help you in labour and birth, yoga aims to bring about a greater awareness of your breathing rhythms, providing a perfect relaxation tool in pregnancy and preparing you to breathe through the contractions. Find an accredited teacher experienced in teaching pregnant women or attend an antenatal class.

RIGHT: Standing poses in yoga focus on achieving core stability and a firm foundation. This is beneficial during pregnancy when the additional weight you are carrying can affect your balance and cause unsteadiness.

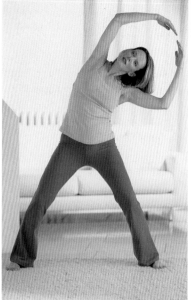

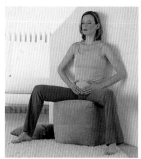

ABOVE: Calming sitting poses that concentrate on aligning your spine help you to focus on steadying your breathing and to centre yourself. Using a wall for guidance helps you to feel supported and brings your attention inwards to your breath.

We love going clubbing; will the loud music be OK for my baby?

There is evidence to suggest that babies can hear in the womb from about 16–20 weeks. However, your baby is protected by the amniotic fluid surrounding him, so most noises do not affect him. The ears of a fetus are often full of a protective greasy coating produced by the skin, known as vernix, so external loud noises would be muffled by the time they reach your baby. Your baby is most likely to respond to your reaction to loud music rather than the music itself.

There is a study that suggests that constant or regular exposure to noise can increase the risk of a small-for-dates baby, meaning your baby's growth is smaller than expected for his gestation. However, it is more likely that it is the environment and its effect on the mother that contributes to the baby's weight rather than the actual noise. Too much clubbing may mean you are getting too little rest and you may be drinking more alcohol than you should. You should probably consider whether you are getting enough quality rest and ensure that you are reducing or stopping your alcohol intake, as this is more harmful to your baby than loud music.

We like walking, but should I cut down on the number of miles now that I'm pregnant?

Walking is ideal in pregnancy as it is low-impact exercise and can be maintained throughout your pregnancy. If you plan to continue lengthy walks and like to walk briskly, try combining this with a slower, more leisurely pace. It's important to control your body temperature so that you don't overheat and feel uncomfortable. To do this, drink plenty of water to avoid dehydration and wear layers that you can take on and off as required. As your tummy grows, you may find hill climbing causes physical instability, as may trekking over uneven terrain, so stick to more level paths. If you find yourself getting breathless, take frequent breaks.

What do I tell my boss?
your rights and benefits

Q My manager said I can't have time off for my antenatal clinic, is this true?

All pregnant women are entitled to paid time off to attend antenatal appointments as required by a registered medical practitioner, midwife, or health visitor. The employee must show a certificate issued by one of the above professionals to confirm they are pregnant, together with proof of the appointment. You are not expected to do this for the first appointment as this will be when you ask for the documentation. Antenatal appointments include childbirth preparation or relaxation classes, as these are an important part of your care. If your employer is refusing to allow you time off, start by talking it through with him or her. If this doesn't help, seek advice from your human resources department or another senior member of staff. You can also contact trade union representatives, the Advisory, Conciliation, and Arbitration Service (ACAS), or the Citizens' Advice Bureau (see p.310).

Q When is the best time to tell my employer that I'm pregnant?

As soon as your employer knows that you are pregnant, the employment laws that protect you will apply, so it's a good idea to tell him or her straight away. It is recommended that you inform your employer in writing with details of your expected due date. Your employer should then conduct a risk assessment for you in your working environment. Any risks identified should be removed or, if this is not possible, alternative arrangements should be made for you. You can also discuss when your maternity leave will start, when you can take any outstanding holidays, and if there are any other entitlements. If your baby is born early or your maternity leave starts earlier than planned due to illness, the arrangements can be altered at short notice. Your employer should respect your right to confidentiality, so by telling them, this should not mean that everyone else at work will know. If you wish the issue to remain confidential until a certain date, you could add this to your letter.

Q Can you tell me about the new baby funding from the government?

The government introduced the Child Trust Fund for children born after the 1st September 2002. This is a voucher of £250 that is to be used to set up a tax-free savings account. The account will be for the child alone and can only be accessed by them when they reach the age of 18, although they can start to plan what to do with the money from the age of 16. Once the account has been set up, family and friends can add to the savings to a maximum of £1,200 each year. When your child is 7 years old, a second payment of £250 is made and children of low-income families will receive an additional £250 around the same time that will be paid directly into their bank account. There are three types of account that you can choose to set up for your baby: a savings account, an investment account, or a stakeholder account. Talk to a bank or building society about which account they would recommend.

Have the confidence to find out about your rights and talk to your employer about what you think will work best for you

Maternity benefits
Your rights in pregnancy

There is a range of benefits available to pregnant women and what you are entitled to depends upon your individual circumstances and your employment status. These benefits have improved considerably over the years. Check your company's policy, as individual companies may also offer their own, more generous, maternity package.

Ordinary maternity leave All pregnant employees are entitled to take 52 weeks of maternity leave, regardless of the amount of time they have worked for an employer and their salary. You can start your leave up to 11 weeks before the baby is due. You can choose to work up to your due date, although if you take any time off sick in the four weeks before your due date, your employer can start your leave from that date.

You are obliged to give your employer a minimum of four weeks' notice of when you intend to start your leave and a minimum of four weeks' notice of when you plan to return. You are also legally obliged to take a minimum of two weeks' leave after the birth of your baby. You may need to inform your employer in writing of your intention to take leave. Tell them the date when the baby is due and the date you want to start your maternity leave. If you meet certain criteria (see right), you may be entitled to statutory maternity pay for 39 weeks of your maternity leave, after which time you will be taking unpaid maternity leave.

What are my rights while I'm on leave?
You have the same employment rights and benefits (with the exception of your wages) while you are on maternity leave. However, while on additional maternity leave, some of your rights, such as contributions to a pension, may be temporarily

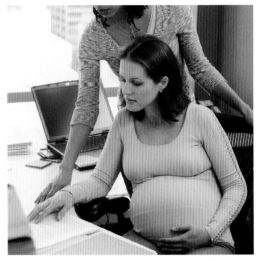

WORKING THROUGH: You can work until late in your pregnancy, but it's wise to allow yourself some time off before the birth to have a break and relax.

suspended. While on leave, you are also entitled to build up your minimum holiday entitlement, which you can add on to your leave either at the beginning or the end.

Statutory maternity pay If you have been in full-time employment, or work part-time or on a fixed contract for over six months, you are entitled to receive statutory maternity pay (SMP). You are eligible for this benefit if you have worked for the same company for 26 weeks, by the end of the 15th week before the expected week of the birth. This is paid at 90 per cent of your weekly earnings for the first six weeks and then at the lesser of £112.75 or 90 per cent of your weekly average for the next 33 weeks. This is not dependent on whether or not you plan to return to work, and you do not have to return the money if you change your mind about returning to work. Your employer will deduct your tax and National Insurance contributions, and then your employer reclaims around 90 per cent of your pay from the Inland Revenue.

Maternity allowance If you are self-employed, have changed your job, or have had periods of unemployment during pregnancy, you are entitled to maternity allowance, which is a tax-free benefit from the government that is also dependent on your National Insurance contributions.

Maternity allowance is paid for 39 weeks at a rate of £112.75, or 90 per cent of your average weekly earnings if your earnings are below this figure. To be eligible for maternity allowance, you will need to have been working for at least 26 weeks out of the 66 weeks before your baby's estimated due date, and have average weekly earnings of around £30. You can begin to claim your maternity allowance up to 11 weeks

before your baby is due, and the latest you can claim this allowance is the day after your baby is born.

Time off for antenatal care Your employer is legally obliged to allow you to take a reasonable amount of time off to attend any antenatal appointments, which can include time off to attend antenatal relaxation classes or hospital antenatal classes.

Additional benefits There is a range of other benefits that are not linked to employment, which pregnant women are entitled to claim. All pregnant women are entitled to free NHS dental care during pregnancy. They are also entitled to free eye treatment and free prescriptions. You continue to be entitled to free dental care and prescriptions for you and your baby for a year after the birth. You will need to obtain your exemption certificate from your health authority and your midwife or doctor will give you the application form when you have your booking in appointment.

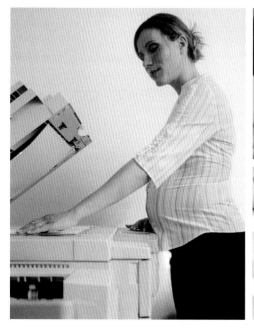

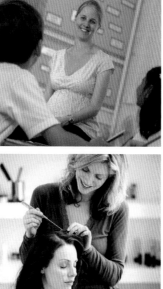

FAR LEFT: If you spend much of the day desk-bound, try to get up and move around regularly, even if it's just a walk to the photocopier, to avoid sluggish circulation. **TOP LEFT:** If your job involves standing for long periods of time, you may need to build in regular breaks towards the end of pregnancy or find ways to rest while working. **BOTTOM LEFT:** If you work with substances, make sure your employer has done a risk asssessment and that you are aware of anything you should avoid.

Q Since I told my boss I'm pregnant he has been really dismissive – what should I do?

The law protects you from being unfairly treated as a result of you being pregnant. This includes dismissal on the grounds of being pregnant or a reason that is connected to pregnancy. If you feel that your boss is treating you unfairly, try to resolve this with him first.

To protect yourself, it is advisable that you keep your manager informed of your maternity leave, return date, and antenatal appointments. Always confirm appointments in writing or provide official documents that show appointment times. You should also ask your manager about any additional benefits the company may have and when you will have your risk assessment. If your manager does not respond satisfactorily to these requests, seek advice from your human resources department, a senior member of staff, trade union representative, ACAS, or the Citizens' Advice Bureau.

Q Am I sure to get my job back after having my baby?

The law states that all employees on ordinary maternity leave (52 weeks) are entitled to return to their original job. This is regardless of how long they have worked there or what hours they work. Exactly the same terms and conditions should also apply. If a member of staff returns after parental leave (see right), then they should return to the same job where possible, if not a suitable alternative should be given. You have to notify your employer, usually in writing,

Some mothers have a change of heart about work when their baby arrives. Don't be afraid to change your mind

when your maternity leave is planned to start. When they receive this letter, they have 28 days to write and confirm your return date. You do not need to give notice if this is the date you plan to return, but if the planned date is different or changes, eight weeks' notice is required. You cannot work for the first two weeks (or four weeks if in a factory) following the birth of your baby.

Q How long can I stay at home after I've had my baby?

The law changed in April 2007. All pregnant women can now take up to 52 weeks as maternity leave, regardless of their length of continuous service at their place of work. Notification to your employer must be given before the 15th week before the baby is due (25 weeks' pregnant).

Statutory maternity pay is paid for 39 weeks to pregnant women earning at least £87 per week with 26 weeks continuous service into the 15th week before the baby is due. You need to give written notice to your employer 28 days before the start of statutory maternity pay. If you do not qualify for this benefit, you may receive maternity allowance for 39 weeks (see p.62).

Q Am I allowed to take additional time off unpaid after my paid maternity leave ends?

You can take parental leave after maternity leave and will be entitled to the same terms and conditions as if you were taking "additional" maternity leave of 52 weeks (see above). This means you can return to the same job, where possible, or a suitable alternative should be found. Parental leave is a separate entitlement for employees who have worked for the company for one year and must be used to care for the child or to find suitable childcare arrangements. Each parent can take 13 weeks for each child and it is unpaid. If you have twins, this means you will get 13 weeks for each twin. If you do not qualify for parental leave, you could take paid holiday or ask your employer for unpaid leave. It may be worth discussing flexible working options with them, too.

Paternity leave
Rights for fathers

Paternity leave can be granted for an employee who is the biological father or the partner or person who will be responsible for the child's upbringing.

To qualify for paternity leave, an employee must have had 26 weeks' continuous service at the end of the 15th week before the baby is due and the employer should be notified, in writing, by the end of the 15th week before the baby is due. The amount of leave granted is usually around one or two weeks, which can be taken together, but not as separate days. This time off must be taken within 56 days after the birth. Statutory paternity pay will be paid if an employee earns at least £87 per week. It will be worked out as the lesser of £112.75 a week or 90 per cent of the average weekly earnings. This is the standard paternity leave package, but individual companies may offer more generous terms and conditions.

Can I refuse to do tasks during pregnancy if they might put my health or the baby's health at risk?

An employer has a duty to comply with health and safety laws, and when you are pregnant your employer must carry out a risk assessment for you within the workplace. The sooner you tell your employer in writing that you are pregnant, the sooner this check will be conducted. Your employer has an obligation by law to tell you of any risks known to the company that may affect your pregnancy. Common risks to you or your unborn child are: exposure to toxic or harmful substances; lifting heavy loads; standing, sitting, or twisting for long periods of time; long working hours; or certain shift patterns. Your employer has a duty to either remove the risk or, if this is not possible, remove you from exposure to the risk. This may involve a suitable alternative job or suspension on full pay.

The company is talking about redundancy – can they get rid of me when I'm on maternity leave?

Your employer is breaking the law if they make you redundant because you are pregnant or taking maternity leave. This is an example of sexual discrimination, as they could not treat a man in the same way. However, if the reason is a legitimate one unconnected with your pregnancy, and they have not treated you any less favourably because you are pregnant, then this is allowed.

Apart from unfair redundancy, how else can I be discriminated against during pregnancy?

Other discriminatory issues during pregnancy include giving you unsuitable work (you should have had a risk assessment carried out, see above), changing your hours of work without your agreement, using pregnancy-related illness as a disciplinary issue, and giving you poor staff reports because you are pregnant.

My friend came back to work and was demoted – are they allowed to do that?

Under the Sex Discrimination Act (1975), it is against the law for an employer to discriminate against an employee on the grounds of gender, marriage, pregnancy, or maternity leave. This can be classified as direct or indirect discrimination. An example of indirect sex discrimination may be less favourable treatment of part-time workers, which may affect women in particular as more women tend to work part time than men. All employees on ordinary maternity leave (52 weeks) are entitled to return to their original job, however long they have worked at the company. If an employee returns after additional parental leave, they should return to the same job where possible, or if not to a suitable alternative. If it is felt that an employee has been demoted due to maternity leave, advice should be sought by the human resources department, a trade union representative, ACAS, or the Citizens' Advice Bureau.

Q I want to work part time after my baby is born – do I have that right?

Currently the law states that parents of children under the age of 6, or disabled children under the age of 18, have the right to apply for flexible working, which can include different shift patterns, when you work, how long you work, and where. You must make your request in writing. Your employer is duty bound to consider your request and must be able to demonstrate why this is not possible if it is refused. You are entitled to take a colleague with you to any meetings regarding this issue, which may be your trade union representative if you have one.

If at any point you feel that your employer has not reasonably demonstrated why the company cannot accommodate your request, you can seek the advice of a trade union representative, the human resources department, or another senior member of staff. Also, as previously mentioned, organizations such as ACAS and the Citizens' Advice Bureau may be able to offer advice and information.

Q What is maternity allowance and will I be eligible for it?

Maternity allowance is a benefit for women who have changed jobs during pregnancy, are self-employed, or who have had low earnings or unemployment during their pregnancy (see p.63). Your midwife should be able to advise you on what you are entitled to and can give you a certificate to confirm your pregnancy, which is known as a maternity certificate or Mat B1, which you will need to claim your maternity allowance.

Q What happens if I decide to be a stay-at-home mum – do I have to give my maternity pay back?

If you decide that you don't want to go back to work after the birth, you must give your employer at least the amount of notice your contract requires for leaving your job, and more notice if possible. You are still entitled to receive your maternity pay for up to 39 weeks even if your employment ends, and as long

Deciding exactly when to return to work is hard. Try not to feel pressured and do what feels right for you and your family

as you do not begin another job, and you do not have to pay any of this back. However, if you had additional maternity pay or benefits, you may be required to pay some or all of these back.

Q I want to work right up to the birth – is that allowed?

Yes, you can do this, but you may need a doctor's medical certificate to confirm that you are fit to do so, and you should tell your employer at least 15 weeks before your baby is due when you want to start your maternity leave. Think carefully before making this decision. Late pregnancy is extremely tiring and, if your job is mentally and/or physically taxing, it may be better to begin your leave a few weeks before your due date. You will also need time to prepare for the arrival of your baby.

Q I want to go back to work very quickly – how soon can I start?

Legally, you can return to work anytime from two weeks after the birth, or four weeks if you work in a factory. However, on a practical and emotional level, returning so soon may not be a good solution. Most women find that it takes around six weeks to recover after the birth. Breastfeeding takes around six weeks to become established too. Even if you bottlefeed, it is probable that your hormones, together with the natural exhaustion that follows having a baby, prevent you from concentrating. You may find that it is hard to be apart from your baby for long periods and you need to think about your baby's needs too.

Will life ever be the same?
special situations

Q I don't have a partner, but I want this baby – will I be OK if I go it alone?

This may be a worrying time for you, but you might find it reassuring to know that many women do have babies on their own. Although it would be wrong to pretend that this is as easy as it is with two parents, with additional support it is possible. You may also have very strong reasons why you want a baby, for example, increasing age, and this determination will give you strength and focus.

It will be a great help too if you can find someone to talk to and confide in. This could be your mother, a close friend or relative, or perhaps a tutor. As you are making far-reaching decisions about your future, it's important that you have support, accurate information, and time to think things through without

fear, panic, or pressure from others. Finding somebody you really trust and who you know can give you support when you need it, especially in labour, may help to relieve a lot of the pressure you are under and enable you to think more calmly and clearly about your situation and make plans as to how to proceed. A confidential service known as Care Confidential (see p.310) offers support, advice, and information for women during pregnancy.

It's worth bearing in mind too that your birthing partner doesn't have to be the baby's father; they can be anyone you choose.

Q I'm pregnant and still at school, will I have to leave school?

No, you will not have to leave school, and in fact you are expected to complete your schooling to the normal school-leaving age at the end of year 11. You should tell a senior teacher about your situation as soon as possible so that you can plan your education during your pregnancy. It may be possible to alter your timetable as you get further into your pregnancy, and you will probably get some home tuition for the few weeks just before and after the baby is born. You are allowed to take time off school for antenatal appointments, but if you are not well enough to attend school for more than a few days because of the pregnancy you will need a note from your doctor or midwife.

In some parts of the country there are education units set up specifically to assist pregnant teenagers where midwives provide antenatal care and help girls to continue their education during and after their pregnancy. Ask your midwife or doctor for more information on these. You could also contact the government-run organization Connexions, which offers advice and support to all 13–19-year-olds in their education decisions (see p.310).

MIDWIFE WISDOM

✱ Avoiding isolation
building up a support network

It is important for all pregnant women to have emotional and practical support, and this is especially important if you are in a vulnerable situation.

✱ Attend all your antenatal appointments and build a relationship with your midwife; she is an invaluable source of information.

✱ Book yourself in for antenatal classes. If you are single, daytime courses may be less populated by "couples"; this gives you a chance to build up a network of women, which will be invaluable after the birth.

✱ Don't be too proud to accept offers of help from friends and family.

ESSENTIAL INFORMATION: NOW YOU'RE PREGNANT

Young mums and older mums
Adapting to pregnancy

Pregnant women who are older or younger than average are likely to have additional concerns about how they will cope with pregnancy and impending motherhood.

How will I cope as a younger mum? There are pros and cons to being a younger mum. On the downside, you may have more concerns about how you will cope financially and how this may affect your education or career, and you may be in a less stable relationship and be concerned about the possibility of separating from your partner. On the practical and physical side, you are likely to have far greater reserves of energy to cope with childbirth and babycare, and some younger mums have good support in the form of relatively young grandparents.

What can I expect as an older mum?

There are advantages and disadvantages to giving birth later in life. If you are over 35, your pregnancy will be higher maintenance and you will be offered a greater range of screening and diagnostic tests as there is a higher risk of complications for you and the baby (see p.116). As a result, you are likely to be more anxious during pregnancy. Once the baby is born, sleepless nights and constant childcare may be more taxing than it would be for a younger mum with greater energy reserves. On the plus side, women today are fitter than ever and plenty of older women have trouble-free pregnancies. You are less likely to have financial worries, are more likely to be in a stable relationship, and be more self assured and confident in your abilities.

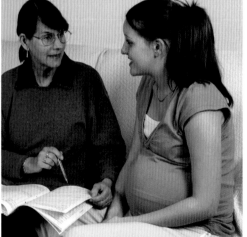

TEENAGE PREGNANCIES: Being a pregnant teenager can be very stressful as you worry about how you will cope with the responsibility.

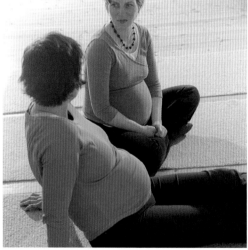

OLDER FIRST-TIME MUMS: Having a first baby late in life can be a far bigger adjustment as you will have established routines.

Q I've just started university and now I'm pregnant – my parents will be furious. What can I do?

Most young women feel a strong mixture of emotions when they find out they are pregnant, with many feeling terrified of telling their parents and worrying that they are somehow letting them down. However, it's important to talk to someone, and probably the best people to talk to are your parents. When you feel able, sit down and explain the situation to them. It may help to have someone else with you to help break the news. Although your parents' initial reaction may be one of disappointment and shock, they may feel guilty too, thinking that they have failed you in some way. Try to remind yourself that ultimately your parents love you and will most likely support you, although you may need to give them some time to adjust to the pregnancy.

If you feel you really cannot talk to your parents and discuss your options, try to find a trusted and supportive adult friend to talk to. Alternatively, talk to a midwife or doctor, or a tutor from university whom you trust. Any of these people will have had previous experience of situations like yours and be able to offer impartial advice.

You should be able to continue with your studies and many educational institutions have childcare facilities, such as a nursery or crèche – pregnancy need not mean an end to your education plans. Being able to reassure your parents on this point will help them come to terms with your pregnancy.

Q My boyfriend said it was safe, but now I think I'm pregnant – who can I talk to?

Although there are times during your menstrual cycle when you are less likely to conceive, it's important to understand that there are no guarantees and, if you are not planning a pregnancy, then it is always wise to use a form of contraception.

It is frightening to find out that you are unexpectedly pregnant, but confiding in someone can help enormously. First, it is important to establish that you definitely are pregnant. Home pregnancy

Even if you don't wish to follow in your mother's path, you may find that she does provide some helpful words of wisdom!

tests, purchased across the counter in any chemist or supermarket, are very accurate (see p.34), or you can get one free from a family planning clinic.

If you are pregnant, talking to a close friend or trusted relative who you believe would give you support at this emotional time may be extremely reassuring. You could also talk to your doctor or, if you are not registered with one, there are "drop-in" health centres where you can talk to a health professional in confidence. Although telling your parents may seem like a frightening prospect, you may find their support invaluable, and of course you need to talk to your boyfriend, who actually may be a great source of support too.

Q I know my mum cares but she wants to come everywhere with me – how can I tell her to back off?

Pick the right time, over a coffee perhaps, and try to explain sensitively to your mother that you need and want to do some things on your own. Let her know that although you value her support, you also need your own space and time to reflect and bond with your baby, even during the pregnancy. If you state how you feel now, this will also help to set some boundaries for after the birth.

Although your mother may be upset at first and possibly feel excluded, with time she will most likely come to appreciate your point of view. Ask her how her own mother reacted to her pregnancy when she was carrying you. You may well discover that she was overprotective too.

Q I thought I was menopausal, but I'm pregnant. Our youngest child is 10. How will we adapt?

It is a shock to discover that you are pregnant when you thought your childbearing years were finished. Although fertility does decline fairly rapidly in your 40s, a pregnancy is still possible, and it is not unusual for women in this age group to believe they are entering the menopause when in fact they are pregnant, as symptoms for both are fairly similar. Couples may also become more relaxed about contraception, believing that a pregnancy is unlikely. So a late pregnancy is not uncommon.

The pregnancy affects not only you and your partner, but the whole family; it will take a while for all of you to adjust to the news, and many different emotions may be felt during this time. The most important thing is to keep talking so that any concerns can be ironed out rather than left unresolved. Involve the whole family in your pregnancy plans to reduce jealousy and make everyone feel involved and needed.

It is important too that you give your children time to adapt to the news. Some children are delighted with a new pregnancy, while others are embarrassed and may need time to adjust. Your partner may experience a mixture of emotions too, ranging from full-on excitement at being a new dad again to shock and disbelief, and maybe even disappointment. Take heart, these will be temporary feelings, and no doubt as time goes on, and as your family adjusts, you will feel more supported.

You are probably aware that there may be some additional risks associated with your pregnancy, such as an increased risk of Down's syndrome (see p.116). When planning your care, your midwife or doctor will take into account your age and explain the appropriate tests and care available.

Q It's 12 years since my last pregnancy. Have benefits and care changed much in this time?

A lot has changed since your last pregnancy. You should take time to find out about current pregnancy

---

MIDWIFE WISDOM

Preparing older siblings
helping your older children to adapt

If you become pregnant when your other children are grown up, you may need to take more time preparing them for the arrival of their sibling.

* Don't be cross or impatient if they seem less than enthusiastic about the baby; they may be worried about the impact a baby will have on family life.

* Reassure teenage children that you will still have time for them and that you won't just expect them to be an unpaid babysitter.

* Allow older children to express their concerns and take time to reassure them.

---

care as there may be tests and scans available now that you were not offered in your last pregnancy (see p.116). Also, childcare provisions and maternity benefits have improved considerably over the last few years so, even if this baby was unexpected, it may not be such a bombshell after all.

Q My daughter is eight years old. Will she get on with the new baby or is it too big an age gap?

There is no right or wrong age gap between siblings and, often, how siblings get on together is more to do with their personalities rather than the age difference. Although they are likely to have independent interests, she is probably very excited at the prospect of a new baby.

Q Our first baby is only 10 months old – how can I be pregnant again?

Usually, periods begin again between two and four months after the birth, but if you are breastfeeding, your periods may not return until your baby starts on solids, or even later. Some women use breastfeeding as a form of contraception and although it reduces the likelihood of pregnancy, it is not reliable. If you are breastfeeding, the time it takes for the return of ovulation depends on the frequency, intensity, and duration of feeding, the maintenance of night feeds, and the introduction of supplementary feeding. The absence of periods does not guarantee that you are not ovulating, so there is a risk of pregnancy.

It is quite possible to ovulate within a month or two of giving birth, and not unknown to ovulate as early as two or three weeks following the birth. This is why midwives always discuss contraception in the days following the birth, even though some new mothers find this an inappropriate time to discuss family planning. Although you may feel daunted at the prospect of having two very young children, there are advantages to having a close age gap. Your children are likely to grow up as playmates and the period of sleepless nights, nappy changes, and of having very dependent young children can be dealt with altogether in a shorter space of time.

Q I've left it too late for an abortion – is it wicked to let my baby be adopted?

Adoption is often dismissed as an option, but sometimes it is the best choice for you and your baby. The nine months of pregnancy provide you with time to explore all options available to you, including temporary voluntary foster care. During this time you will be able to talk to adoption agencies and social workers who can inform you of the process and support you. View this as a positive process, in that you care enough about your baby to find the best care at a time when you feel unable to be the one to provide this.

When it comes to making a final decision, bear in mind that it should not be made during pregnancy, since you are subject to a range of emotions and feelings and you have not yet met your baby or know how you will feel in the longer term. Talk to your doctor to find out more about the process, your rights, and your right to change your mind.

Q My boyfriend doesn't want to know about my pregnancy – will he have rights after the birth?

Your boyfriend is quite possibly shocked by the news that you are pregnant but, given time, he may come round to the idea and be more supportive. Although it is a difficult and hurtful time for you, try not to overreact by denying access to the father after the birth, unless you are certain this is what you want. Once your boyfriend sees your baby, his attitude and feelings may change, so it could be worth giving him time to adjust. It can help to seek support from trusted family members and friends.

A biological father does not have automatic rights to be involved in the upbringing of his baby if he is not legally married to the mother and he is not named on the birth registration forms. (If the parents aren't married, the father has to accompany the mother to register the birth if he wants to be named on the birth certificate.) If he is named on the birth certificate, he has some basic rights in terms of access and has some financial responsibility for his child. If you do not wish your boyfriend to have access then you do not need to name him on the birth forms. If he has been named on the forms and you decide later that you don't want him to have access, you will need to go to court to seek a formal injunction and be able to justify why you require this. You should bear in mind the financial implications of your decision if you do not include him on the forms and whether this means that he would not be obliged to provide financial support for you and the baby.

Whatever your situation, it's important that you don't feel isolated. Never feel afraid to seek additional support and advice

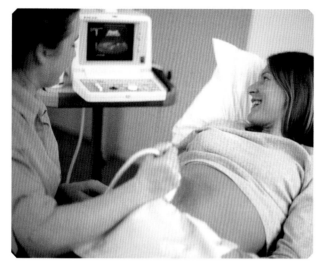

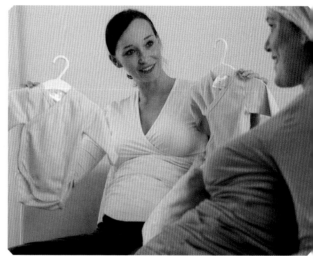

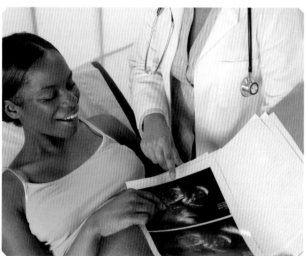

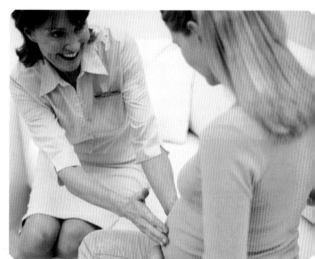

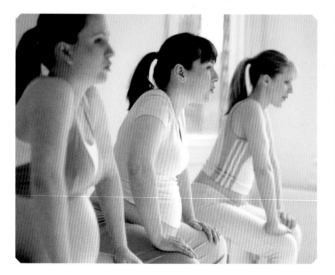

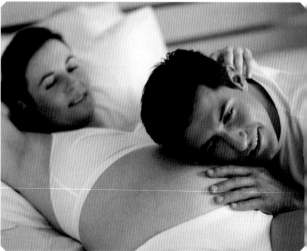

Your 40-week journey

Who will handle my care?
a guide to antenatal care

Q What types of antenatal care are available to me?

The options for antenatal care in the UK vary from one region to another, and sometimes according to the hospital you choose, so it's worth asking your doctor or midwife early on about your choices. There are four main types of care (see p.76). The most common is shared care, where you are cared for by your doctor and community midwife, with visits to the hospital limited to scans or investigations. In some areas, midwifery care is offered where you are looked after by a midwife or a team of midwives, sometimes called one-to-one care or team midwifery care. Women with pre-existing medical problems, or a more complicated pregnancy, such as a multiple pregnancy, may have consultant-led care with visits to a hospital-based consultant. If you opt for private care, you will be cared for by an independent midwife. Appointments will be timed to suit you and scans may be with a private obstetrician. The midwife will be on call for the birth, which may be at home, in a birth centre, or at the local hospital.

Q How many antenatal appointments will I need?

The exact number of appointments and how often you have them depends on your individual situation. Usually, if this is your first pregnancy, you will have up to 10 appointments, whereas if you have had a baby before, you should have around 7 appointments.

Q When will I have my first antenatal appointment?

Your first "booking" appointment should be between 8 and 12 weeks, depending on the midwives' preferences in your area. This is often the first time you will meet the midwife who will be organizing, and in most cases providing most of, your care.

Q I'm going for my first appointment next week – what will happen there?

The purpose of your first appointment with your local midwife is for her to obtain your medical history and exchange information so that your future care during the pregnancy and birth can be planned. This is also an opportunity for you and your midwife to get to know each other and for you to ask any questions you may have and discuss the schedule for appointments, blood tests, scans, and antenatal classes. You will also be given booklets, information leaflets, and important contact telephone numbers.

Your midwife will ask you about your medical history; your family's medical history; your partner and your partner's family's medical history; about any previous pregnancies you have had; and how this pregnancy has been so far. Your answers to these questions will help your midwife to build up a picture of your current state of health, and will also help identify any factors that may affect your pregnancy, for example if there is a family history of pre-eclampsia (see p.89).

Your midwife will also take your blood pressure, weigh you, test your urine (see below), and listen to the baby's heartbeat if you are 12 or more weeks

The meaning of "midwife" is "with woman". As you get to know your midwives, you will also find out more about your body and baby pregnant. She may also take some blood tests (see opposite). These observations provide a useful baseline for future antenatal checks.

Q Why do I have to bring a urine sample to the clinic each time?

Your midwife is looking for the presence of protein in your urine. If protein is present, this could indicate that you have a urine infection that may need a course of antibiotics. After around 24 weeks of pregnancy, protein in the urine is an indication of pre-eclampsia (see p.89), a potentially serious condition that needs close monitoring.

If you have a body mass index (BMI) (see p.18) over 35, you will be offered a glucose tolerance test, also done by testing your urine. Glucose in the urine is a sign of gestational diabetes (see p.87). If glucose is present, you may be referred for blood tests to analyse your sugar levels. If diabetes is diagnosed, you would receive care and advice accordingly.

Q Why are some of my appointments with my doctor and others with the midwife?

The type of antenatal care you receive can vary slightly between different areas. If your pregnancy is straightforward, your care is usually shared between your doctor and midwife, or in some areas all your appointments are with your midwife. If you feel more comfortable with your midwife, you should be able to arrange to have the majority of your appointments with her, and the same applies if you feel happier seeing your doctor. Whichever way, it is important that you feel able to ask any questions or discuss any issues, which may be personal or sensitive.

Q Will I have to have an internal examination at my first antenatal appointment?

It is unlikely that you will have an internal examination at your first antenatal appointment. Twenty years or so ago, when home pregnancy tests weren't as reliable and ultrasound scans were not so accurate or widely available, an internal examination was the

Blood tests
How these contribute to your antenatal care

You will be offered quite a few blood tests during pregnancy and the results provide vital information that may affect your pregnancy and help your caregivers to plan your care.

At your booking appointment, you will be offered blood tests to check for the following:

* Anaemia (low iron levels).
* Your blood group.
* Your Rhesus status (see p.79).
* Hepatitis B.
* Your rubella (German measles) immunity.
* HIV and syphilis.

These are usually taken at the same time, so you won't need a separate test for each!

best way to confirm and "date" a pregnancy. The midwife or doctor placed two fingers into the vagina, and pressed on the lower abdomen with the other hand to judge the size of the uterus.

Nowadays, there are a few instances when an internal examination may be recommended during early pregnancy. If you have an infection, such as thrush, an internal examination enables the vagina to be visualized to check for any signs of infection and for a tissue sample to be taken with a swab (like a long cotton wool bud). The swab is sent to the hospital for testing so that the appropriate treatment can be offered.

If you have vaginal bleeding, you may have an internal examination with a speculum (an instrument shaped like a duck's bill, used for smear tests) to allow the cervix to be seen: a small erosion on the surface is a common cause of bleeding in pregnancy. Although internal examinations are not enjoyable, it is important to try and relax to help the muscles of the vagina to relax and loosen, which may prevent discomfort. Many women find it helpful to breathe slowly and steadily during the examination.

ESSENTIAL INFORMATION: YOUR 40-WEEK JOURNEY

Antenatal care options
Who provides your care

The options for antenatal care in the UK vary from area to area, so this section will provide a general overview. You will find out more when you go for your booking-in appointment, usually around 8–12 weeks. Midwives are specialists in providing maternity care where there are no complications and they provide the majority of antenatal care to women. As they are specially trained to look after normal births, women should only have to see a doctor if a problem arises, or if they are at a higher risk of complications. Within the NHS there are three main types of care: shared care, midwifery care, and consultant-led care. The Association for Improvements in Maternity Services (AIMS), has a useful website that provides plenty of support, advice, and information on maternity choices in the UK (see p. 310).

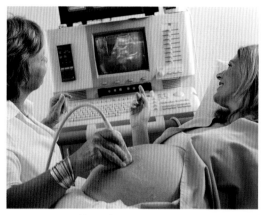

HOSPITAL SCAN: Part of your antenatal care will take place at the hospital where you will receive ultrasound scans to check your baby's development.

What is shared care? Most women have their antenatal appointments with their doctor or community midwife during pregnancy, with visits to the hospital only for routine scans or for investigating problems. Care is then transferred to the hospital midwives and obstetrician, if required, for the birth and postnatal stay.

How does midwifery care work? In some areas, teams of community midwives provide continuous care throughout pregnancy, birth, and the postnatal period, and when this type of care is available it tends to be a popular choice in low-risk pregnancies as it enables women to build up a relationship with their midwives. The community midwives are responsible for your antenatal care, your care in hospital during the labour and birth, and then for home visits after the delivery. It is not guaranteed that you will have the same midwife all the way through your pregnancy and birth. For this reason, it's a good idea to request antenatal appointments with different midwives within the team, so that you meet as many members of the team as possible during your pregnancy, and it will therefore be more likely that you will know the midwife who is with you for the actual labour and delivery of your baby.

When might you have consultant-led care? Women with pre-existing medical conditions, such as hypertension, or those with more complex pregnancy issues, such as twins or multiple births, may have the majority of antenatal care with an obstetrician. Most of their appointments may be carried out in hospital. There are other conditions, such as diabetes or epilepsy, which may require the care of two specialists: an expert in the medical condition as well as an obstetrician. A hospital midwife will usually participate in this care too.

What about independent midwives? Outside the NHS, there is also the option of independent midwives. Independent midwives are midwives who have chosen to work in the private healthcare sector. They charge a fee to provide antenatal care, care during labour and the delivery, and postnatal care. Because they only look after small numbers of women, independent midwives can provide a continuity of care that is not always available on the NHS and they will also tailor care to suit your individual needs, for example timing antenatal appointments when most convenient for you. You can find out more details by visiting the wesbite of the Independent Midwives Association (see p.310).

Does my care change if I'm having a home birth? As well as hospital delivery in a birthing or delivery unit, there is also the option of having a home birth within the NHS framework (see p.153). When a pregnancy is straightforward, research hasn't found any difference in the safety of having a baby at home or in hospital. If you are having a home birth, your antenatal care will be provided by community midwives who are attached to a maternity unit. Once in labour, your midwife will stay with you until your baby is born, and she will visit regularly for between 10 and 28 days after your baby has been born, or you can attend a postnatal drop-in centre in your local area.

How will I choose my antenatal care? This may be partly dictated by the type of care that is available in your area. It's worth talking to other local mothers with young children to see if they have any advice or recommendations. The type of care you receive may also depend on where you choose to give birth. If you have a low-risk pregnancy and decide to have a homebirth or to deliver in a birthing unit, then you will probably just see midwives and your doctor in your own home or the doctor's surgery. If there are complications, your care may be shared between your midwives and doctor and a hospital obstetrician.

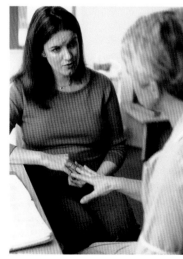
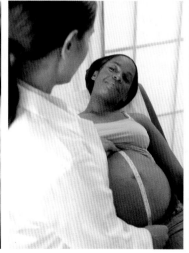
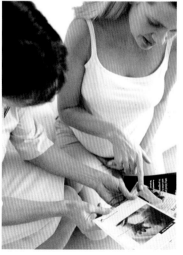

AT THE DOCTOR'S SURGERY: If you have shared care, some of your antenatal appointments will be with your doctor at your local surgery.

HOSPITAL CARE: A hospital-based obstetrician will be involved in the care of women with complications or a multiple pregnancy.

MIDWIFE HOME VISIT: If your care is midwife-based, a midwife may visit you at home for some of your antenatal appointments.

Q I'm very small and have tiny feet – will that be a problem when I give birth?

In the past, doctors used to measure a pregnant woman's feet to assess her likelihood of needing a Caesarean section, as small feet were thought to indicate a narrow pelvis. Although there is some truth in the fact that small feet generally indicate that a woman is small-framed and therefore likely to have a small pelvis, small women also tend to grow small babies in proportion to their pelvic size. True cephalo-pelvic disproportion (CPD), where the baby's head is too large to fit through the pelvis and be born vaginally, is relatively rare.

During labour there are other factors that help you to deliver your baby. The pelvis is not a fixed structure and the hormone relaxin helps to soften the ligaments that hold the pelvic bones together to help the pelvis to stretch and accommodate the baby.

Preparing for visits
Getting ready for your antenatal appointments

Knowing what to expect at your antenatal appointments and having the necessary information to hand for the midwife will mean the allotted time is used efficiently.

At your first antenatal appointment, your midwife is gathering as much information about you as possible to build up a picture of your health and consider the most appropriate type of care for you. Make sure you have the date of your last menstrual period, as well as the dates of any previous pregnancies, including ones that ended in miscarriage. You will also need to be clued up on your family's medical history and your partner's medical history, including any inherited abnormalities, so check before the appointment if you are unsure about anything. Read any information sent by the hospital and make a list of any questions so that you don't forget them.

Also, your baby's head is designed to mould into shape. The skull is made up from separate bones that are able to overlap each other slightly in order to reduce the overall size of the head as it travels through the pelvis during labour. This is a normal part of the birth process. Labour positions also affect the dimensions of the pelvis. For example, squatting can increase the internal measurements of the pelvis by around 30 per cent. Sitting, or lying on your back can actually reduce these measurements by restricting the natural backwards movement of the tailbone (coccyx) during birth.

Q My midwife is lovely but she's always in a hurry – how can I get her to answer my questions?

This is a common problem. Antenatal clinics are often very busy, with lots of women for the midwife to see. As a result, most clinics allow only a 10- to 15-minute appointment for each woman – barely enough time to go through the basic physical checks. However, it is important that your questions are addressed and it may be helpful to write them down so that you remember what you want to ask. If your midwife doesn't have time to discuss the issues during your appointment, ask her to arrange to talk to you at a mutually convenient time. This could be in the form of a phone call, or another appointment at the clinic. Or she may be able to direct you to other sources of information such as books, leaflets, websites, or other healthcare professionals.

It is a crucial part of your antenatal care that you feel comfortable with your caregivers and are given the opportunity to discuss any questions you have or issues that arise, and this is recognized by the National Institute for Clinical Excellence (NICE) in their guidelines for antenatal care (see p.310).

Q I'm four months' pregnant and haven't had many appointments. Will they get more frequent?

Yes, you will find that your antenatal appointments become more frequent as the pregnancy progresses. With your first pregnancy, you can expect a total of

Rhesus negative

Each person's blood carries a Rhesus factor (Rh-factor), which is positive or negative. Problems arise if a Rh-negative woman carries a Rh-positive baby who has inherited the status from the father. If the mother's blood comes into contact with the baby's blood during delivery, she may produce antibodies against the baby. This does not usually affect a first baby, but may cause problems in subsequent pregnancies when a mother's antibodies attack the cells of another Rh-positive baby.

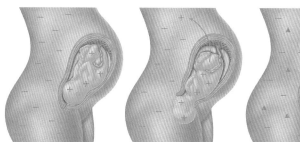

FIRST PREGNANCY: At delivery, the mother may be exposed to her baby's blood. The baby's and mother's blood mix and she develops antibodies against the baby.

KEY

━ mother's blood   ✚ baby's blood   ▲ antibodies

SUBSEQUENT PREGNANCY: Anti-D antibodies attack the next baby's blood and can cause heart trouble and anaemia. Rh-negative women are given anti-D injections to combat this.

---

about 10 appointments but if you have had a baby before, you may only have 7. If you develop any complications, additional appointments would be arranged according to your needs. The schedule of antenatal appointments differs slightly from area to area, but as a general rule you can expect an appointment at the following stages of pregnancy: one to two appointments by 12 weeks of pregnancy, and then appointments at 16 weeks, 25 weeks, 28 weeks, 31 weeks, 34 weeks, 36 weeks, 38 weeks, 40 weeks, and if, your baby is overdue, 41 weeks. If you are expecting your second or subsequent baby and the pregnancy is straightforward, you may miss out appointments at 25 weeks, 31 weeks, and 40 weeks.

I want a home birth. Will this make a difference to my antenatal appointments?

Usually, women planning a home birth will have the same type of antenatal care as any another healthy pregnant woman in regards to frequency and location of antenatal appointments. Midwives in some areas may provide a home visit towards the end of

the pregnancy if a woman is planning a home birth. This is helpful as it offers an opportunity to discuss the preparations for labour and birth, such as what equipment to have ready and the intended place for the actual delivery. If your midwife cannot offer a home visit to discuss the arrangements for your home birth, you should be given an opportunity to talk about it together during one of your usual antenatal appointments.

Is it OK to bring my partner with me to the antenatal appointments?

It is absolutely fine to bring your partner with you to some or all of your antenatal appointments. It is a good way for him to feel involved in the pregnancy, and also gives him an opportunity to ask questions that he may have. It is a legal requirement that you are allowed paid time off work to attend antenatal appointments, but your partner does not have this right, which may pose a problem as most antenatal clinics are during the day. Another way to involve your partner in the pregnancy is to attend birth preparation classes together. Classes are often held at the weekends or in the evenings to make it easier for partners to attend. This gives you both a chance to find out more about labour and birth and about babycare after the birth.

When will I hear my baby's heart beat?

Your baby's heart starts beating around 20 days after conception, and can be seen on an ultrasound scan at about six weeks of pregnancy. It is usually not until around 12 weeks of pregnancy that it is possible to hear the heartbeat with a hand-held monitor, known as a sonicaid, as it is around this time that the uterus starts to grow upwards out of the pelvis, making it easier to detect the heartbeat. When the heartbeat can be heard also depends a bit on your build; if you are very slim, it is usually easier to find the baby's heartbeat than if you are overweight.

Antenatal jargon
Understanding your notes

Once your midwife has compiled your notes, you will be in charge of these and will need to take them to appointments. Abbreviations will be used for much of the medical information.

* **BP** Blood pressure.
* **Hb** Haemoglobin levels.
* **Primagravida** A first pregnancy.
* **Multigravida** A subsequent pregnancy.
* **NAD** Nothing abnormal detected (usually referring to urine sample).
* **FHHR** Fetal heart heard and regular.
* **FHNH** Fetal heart not heard.
* **FMF** Fetal movements felt.
* **EDD** Estimated date of delivery.
* **Ceph or Vx** Baby head down.
* **Br** Baby is breech – feet down.
* **Eng/E** Baby's head is engaged for delivery.
* **NE** Baby's head is not engaged.
* **SFH** Symphysis fundal height: size of the womb.

Will I have my own midwife?

Midwives realize that it is important for a woman to develop a relationship with them so that they feel supported and able to ask questions, and continuity of care is provided if possible. However, how many midwives you meet in pregnancy, labour, and birth and the postnatal period depends on how services are arranged in your area. Generally, the midwife linked to your doctor's surgery provides the majority of care. Depending on your situation and common practice in your area, you may also meet other midwives if some of your appointments are at the hospital. When you go into labour, you are usually cared for by hospital-based midwives who you may not have met. In some areas, community midwives look after women in hospital. If this is the case, you may be familiar with the midwife caring for you in labour. Midwives working on a labour ward work shifts, so it is likely that you will meet more than one midwife during your labour and birth. Your postnatal care is usually carried out by community-based midwives. This may include the midwife you saw for antenatal appointments at the surgery.

I've only just found out I'm pregnant and I must be at least four months. What should I do?

One of the first things you need to do is to contact your local maternity unit and inform them of your pregnancy. Women can refer themselves, although many still approach their doctor first. If you inform your doctor, he or she will send a referral to the hospital or to a midwife to arrange a booking appointment as soon as possible. You should also review your diet (see p.50). Depending on the number of weeks of your pregnancy, you may be due a scan, which may need to be done before the booking appointment. Most units offer a scan around 10–14 weeks, and a second one around 20 weeks. You will be offered a range of blood tests (see p.117) and should be aware of their purpose before consenting. Each unit may have a slightly different schedule for care. The earlier you book in the better, so that you do not miss out on any aspects of antenatal care.

Sick and tired
the side effects of pregnancy

Q Why does pregnancy make you feel so sick?

Although no one is really clear about the cause of sickness in pregnancy, it is thought to be due partly to the hormone human chorionic gonadotrophin (hCG), released early in pregnancy. For most women, symptoms are mild and begin to ease at 12 weeks. For some, the sickness may last throughout the day and continue beyond this time. A small percentage of women experience severe nausea and vomiting, known as hyperemesis gravidarum (see p.92).

There are practical measures you can take to relieve nausea and sickness (see p.82).

Q I'm two months' pregnant and feel incredibly tired all the time. Is this normal?

Yes, tiredness is a common complaint in pregnancy with most women feeling a sudden loss of energy in the early stages as their body gets used to the changes caused by pregnancy. This often lasts throughout the first trimester, but after about week 13 you should start to feel a bit more energized. When you're not resting, try to stay active and take some gentle exercise.

Another cause of tiredness is anaemia, a common condition in pregnancy that needs to be monitored. Although it's more likely that your tiredness is due to the pregnancy itself, when you see your midwife you will be offered a blood test to check your iron levels, and if these are found to be low you will be offered supplements. To avoid anaemia, eat iron-rich foods, such as dark green leafy vegetables, red meat, wholegrain cereals, pulses, and prune juice. Vitamin C helps your body to absorb more iron from your diet, so try drinking fresh orange juice with meals, and limit your tea and coffee intake, as caffeine inhibits iron absorption.

Q I often feel faint – what could be causing this?

Feeling faint or having a dizzy spell is quite common in pregnancy as pregnancy hormones cause your blood vessels to relax and widen. Although this improves the blood flow to the baby, it also has the effect of slowing down the flow of blood around your body, which can lead to low blood pressure, known as hypotension. Although this is unlikely to be a risk in itself, it can cause feelings of faintness, most commonly when you stand up too fast from a sitting or lying position.

Other causes of faintness include lying on your back (as this can put pressure on several large blood vessels involved in returning blood back to your heart, which can cause low blood pressure and in turn make you feel dizzy and faint); a lack of food or drink; getting overheated; and fast breathing (hyperventilating).

Sometimes, feeling faint can be more serious. If the feeling does not pass by eating, drinking water, cooling down, or taking things slowly as you stand up, it may need investigating further and you should seek the advice of your midwife or doctor as this could be due to anaemia (see above) and you may need treatment in the form of iron tablets.

Try to think of your pregnancy as a season that will pass. If you feel overwhelmed, visualize your baby in your arms

Coping with morning sickness

To alleviate feelings of nausea and sickness in pregnancy, try eating little and often, and sip water continually during the day. Some women find ginger helps, so you could try nibbling ginger biscuits, perhaps before you get out of bed. Acupressure bands worn on the wrists and available from most chemists are also thought to relieve the symptoms.

TOP LEFT: Sipping peppermint tea can help relieve feelings of nausea. **BOTTOM LEFT:** Snacking on ginger biscuits can reduce nausea. **RIGHT:** Activating acupressure points may ease symptoms.

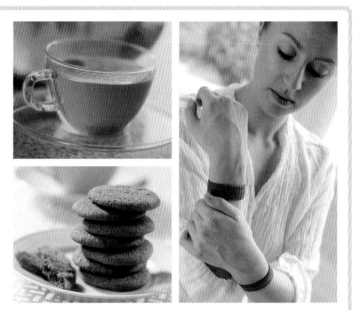

Is it normal to have pelvic pain in early pregnancy?

Pelvic pain is associated with the soft area supporting your pelvis, the symphysis pubic joint. This can swell or separate causing considerable pain, termed symphysis pubis dysfunction, or SPD. This is thought to be caused by pregnancy hormones and is quite common in late pregnancy, but can occur earlier. Many women feel most pain when walking or lying. Wear comfortable shoes; use pillows to support the hips and legs in bed; keep your legs together when getting out of bed; avoid breast stroke; and get lots of rest. Some women find sitting on a birthing ball helps. You may be referred to an obstetric physiotherapist and advised to wear a support belt. In severe cases, crutches may be needed. Most cases resolve after the birth.

I'm embarrassed because I think I've got piles. I don't want to go to the doctor – what can I do?

Haemorrhoids (piles) are swollen veins at or near the anus that can be very uncomfortable, especially during pregnancy. Piles are a common feature in pregnancy, with many women experiencing them at some stage, so your doctor will not be at all surprised. You could also speak to your midwife about the problem if this is easier. Your doctor or midwife will be able to recommend a treatment, such as a cream or a cooling maternity gel pad.

As piles often develop as a result of straining due to constipation, increasing your fibre and fluid intake may help you to have regular bowel motions, which in turn may help to relieve the problem. Eat fresh fruit and vegetables and drink lots of water. If you are very constipated, you could ask your doctor to prescribe suppositories. I know you may feel embarrassed, but it is best to approach someone rather than to suffer alone.

I've been getting regular headaches since becoming pregnant – should I be worried?

Headaches in the early stages of pregnancy are quite normal and are thought to be related to the effects of pregnancy hormones. Headaches can also be caused by other factors such as dehydration, low blood sugar, a stuffy environment, tiredness, and lack of sleep. Try increasing your intake of water, aiming to drink at least eight glasses of water a day, and have small regular meals to maintain your blood sugar. If you feel a headache coming on, drink two glasses of water and have a rest for 30 minutes. Taking a lose dose of paracetamol is considered safe, although it is best to avoid this if possible.

If you are suffering with headaches at around 28 weeks or more, you should inform your doctor or midwife of these, especially if your headaches are accompanied by blurred vision, an inability to focus, or flashing lights, as this may be a sign of pregnancy-induced hypertension (high blood pressure), which could indicate pre-eclampsia (see p.89). Try not to worry, as even though many women complain of headaches and some will have high blood pressure in pregnancy, few go on to develop pre-eclampsia. It is thought that the incidence is somewhere between two and five per cent of all pregnancies.

Q My gums have started bleeding since I've been pregnant – why is this?

It is very common for gums to bleed in pregnancy. The pregnancy hormone progesterone causes areas of tissue that connect muscles and ligaments to soften and become stretchier so that your body can make room for the growing baby. However, this can affect tissue in other parts of the body, such as in the gums, making them softer and more prone to bleed.

Also, some women crave sweet foods in pregnancy, an excess of which can affect the gums, causing them to become tender, swollen, and more likely to bleed, and increasing the chances of developing gingivitis, a gum infection. Pregnant woman are encouraged to see a dentist early in pregnancy for a checkup (dental care is free up until the baby's first birthday).

It is important to brush your teeth more than usual and floss regularly when pregnant to minimize the risk of an infection. Unlikely as it may sound, it has been suggested that there is a link between premature birth and gum disease.

Q Whenever I sneeze, I leak – is that going to last for ever?

Many women suffer from stress incontinence during pregnancy, which means a leakage of urine when you cough or sneeze. The leaks are caused by the loosening of muscles in the pelvic floor – a group of muscles and ligaments that support the pelvic organs – due to pregnancy hormones. Also, as the growing baby puts more pressure on the bladder, stress incontinence becomes more likely.

It is recommended that you carry out pelvic floor exercises (see p.57) to reduce the likelihood of leakage. These can be started at any stage of pregnancy, but the earlier you begin the better; once you get the technique right they are simple. As these are such discreet exercises, it is easy to practise without anyone else realizing what you are doing.

Stress incontinence should improve following the birth, although it can take up to six weeks. There is some suggestion that the problem can persist longer depending on the type of birth you have, with a natural vaginal birth more likely to cause ongoing problems than a Caesarean delivery.

MIDWIFE WISDOM

Fatigue
coping with tiredness in pregnancy

One of the most cited complaints in pregnancy, particularly in the first trimester, is extreme tiredness as your body deals with its extra workload. Accepting this and adapting your routine accordingly can help you cope.

✳ Slow down and take a break, or even a catnap, whenever possible.

✳ Eat small, healthy snacks throughout the day and drink plenty of fluids to maintain energy levels.

✳ Whenever possible, go to bed earlier.

✳ Take regular, gentle exercise to relieve stress and improve your fitness and stamina.

Q I've been getting nosebleeds for the first time in my life. Why is this?

It's not unusual for nosebleeds to occur in pregnancy due to the increased blood supply in the body. Nosebleeds are not serious, but if the bleeds are severe, you can ask your doctor for a spray to help the blood to clot. If your nosebleeds are frequent, a simple surgical procedure can cauterize the vessel.

When you have a nosebleed, sit for a few minutes with your head upright and apply pressure to the bridge of the nose. To avoid further nosebleeds, make sure you blow your nose gently, drink plenty of fluids to avoid dehydration, use vaseline on dry nostrils, avoid smoky environments, and open your mouth when you sneeze to relieve nasal pressure.

Q I'm 30 weeks' pregnant and have persistent backache – is there anything that can help?

The weight of your baby and the fact that joints and ligaments soften in pregnancy can cause backache. Sometimes sciatica occurs, a sharp pain that travels down the back and leg when the sciatic nerve is trapped in a joint in the lower back.

For lower backache, warm baths and a warm compress can help, and gentle massage done by an experienced practitioner. Exercise, such as yoga, pilates, or aquanatal classes (see p.55), strengthens back muscles, but check with your doctor before embarking on a new exercise regime. Watch your posture, making sure that you sit upright – you could try using a birthing ball – and wear flat shoes.

If you have sciatica, ask your doctor or midwife to refer you to a physiotherapist to assess your condition and teach you exercises to help relieve the pain and minimize a reoccurrence. Some women have a maternity girdle or back brace fitted.

Q Little moles are appearing on my skin. Why is this happening?

Skin changes occur frequently in pregnancy due to the effect of pregnancy hormones. However, some changes, such as new moles and freckles appearing,

When pregnancy symptoms get you down, book a massage, or ask a close friend to give you a relaxing shoulder rub

although not usually serious, should be discussed with your midwife or doctor, particularly if new or existing moles seem to change shape, are red or tender, or start to bleed.

In general, skin either becomes quite oily in pregnancy, due to an increase in the production of the skin's natural oil, sebum or, if skin is prone to dryness, it may become even drier and more sensitive. Many women experience a darkening of the skin, while others notice a pattern on their face that looks like a patchy sun tan, called chloasma (see p.105). If your skin is sensitive, avoid scented creams and oils, and perfume. Regular cleansing of the skin and avoiding oil-based products may also help.

Q My mum had varicose veins – am I likely to get them in pregnancy?

Around a third of women suffer from varicose veins in pregnancy to some degree (see p.86). These occur because increased levels of the hormone progesterone cause the walls of the veins to become more relaxed; there is also increased pressure within the veins as a result of the enlarged uterus pressing on major veins in the pelvis. A family history of varicose veins does increase the possibility of them occurring, but there are several things that you can do to reduce the risk or severity of varicose veins.

If varicose veins do appear during pregnancy, they usually improve within three months of giving birth, although unfortunately in subsequent pregnancies they are likely to recur.

Q My feet are swollen and tight; can I do anything about it?

Swollen feet and ankles, known as oedema, are due to excessive fluid seeping into the tissues because of the increased volume of blood. By late pregnancy, as blood volume continues to rise, this is a common problem. The swelling is usually worse later in the day and when the weather is warmer. There are steps you can to take to help reduce the swelling, such as elevating your legs when sitting, rotating your feet, and lying on the floor with your feet up the wall. Wearing support tights or stockings also improves circulation in the legs. Make sure that you drink plenty of fluids, particularly water, as this improves the kidney function and reduces water retention. Gentle exercise, such as swimming or aquanatal exercises, also increases the efficiency of the circulatory system. There is evidence that reflexology from a registered practitioner may help.

If you also have swelling in your hands or face, it is worth having a blood pressure check to rule out pre-eclampsia (see p.89). Most women find that the swelling gradually disappears after they give birth.

Q My fingers are tingling and my midwife said it might be carpal tunnel syndrome – what is this?

Carpal tunnel syndrome occurs when swollen tissues in the wrist compress the nerves and cause pins and needles and numbness. Other symptoms include difficulty grasping with fingers and thumb and a general weakness in the hands. This is common in pregnancy due to the increased volume of blood, which can cause fluid retention.

There are ways to reduce the symptoms, such as circling and stretching exercises to improve circulation and increase wrist mobility. Wearing wrist splints and elevating your hands on a pillow at night can also help. There is some inconclusive evidence that ultrasound treatment may help in mild cases.

Q I'm 35 weeks and get terrible leg cramp. What can I do?

Leg cramp, where the leg muscles go into a painful spasm, is common in pregnancy, particularly at night, which may be due to the pressure of the uterus on pelvic nerves. This usually resolves itself once you

Sleeplessness

You are often very sleepy at the beginning and end of pregnancy, and towards the end of pregnancy you may find it increasingly difficult to sleep restfully in the night as your bump makes it hard to find a comfortable position, pressure on your bladder causes you to get up frequently to use the toilet, and your baby may not share the same sleeping pattern as you and wakes you frequently with his kicking. Coupled with the fact that your body is working extremely hard, a poor night's sleep adds to your general levels of fatigue. If possible, try to compensate for broken night-time sleep by catnapping in the day, or find time to sit down and put your feet up.

RIGHT: Don't feel guilty about grabbing a quick nap after lunch or falling asleep on the sofa early, as this helps you to cope with disrupted sleep during the night. Learning to take a rest when possible is also good practice for after the birth!

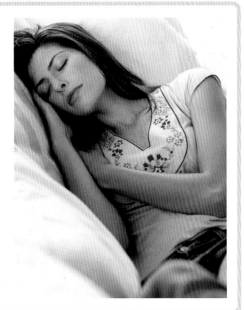

are out of bed and using the muscle. However, if the pain doesn't recede and there is any reddening or swelling in one leg, you should seek medical advice urgently to eliminate the possibility of a clot.

To reduce the incidence of cramp or its severity, drink lots of water to prevent dehydration and try leg stretches and ankle exercises, circling your heel first and then wiggling your toes, before going to bed. Gentle exercise, such as walking or swimming, can also help and getting your partner, friend, or relative to massage your legs, particularly the calf muscle, can improve circulation. Some research suggests that taking magnesium supplements reduces the incidence of cramps, but further studies are needed.

I'm itching to the point where I'm bleeding. What can I do?

Most itching in pregnancy, especially on your tummy, is due to stretching of the skin, hormonal changes, and heat. However, if you have significant itching, see your midwife or doctor to determine whether you have a condition called obstetric cholestasis, a serious but rare condition that affects the liver and occurs in about one per cent of pregnancies (see p.90) – a blood test can rule out this condition.

Using a non-perfumed moisturizing lotion or emoillient cream daily after washing may help, and avoid bathing in very hot water. Try not to scratch, as broken skin is vulnerable to infection; wearing cotton gloves at night may stop you scratching in your sleep. After 28 weeks, five drops of essential lavender oil in a bath helps to soothe the skin. Antihistamine creams or tablets may be prescribed by your doctor if the itching is severe and other measures aren't working.

My breasts keep "leaking". Should this be happening now?

In pregnancy, your body prepares for breastfeeding and some women find that they leak colostrum, the first watery, yellowish milk, as early as 16 weeks. Some leak large amounts, some small amounts, and some not at all. The amount you leak has no bearing on the amount of milk produced after the birth or your ability to breastfeed. If you are self-conscious,

MIDWIFE WISDOM

Varicose veins
how can I avoid them?

Self-help measures to avoid the risk of varicose veins include:

* Wearing support hosiery – this is one of the best ways to avoid varicose veins. All pregnant women are entitled to two free pairs of compression tights.
* Doing regular ankle and foot exercises to reduce swelling and cramp.
* Avoiding standing for long periods.
* Raising your legs when sitting down.
* Getting up to take regular walks if you have to sit for long periods.
* Avoiding high-heeled shoes, which reduce the work done by the calf muscles, to maintain blood flow in the legs.

wear breast pads to protect clothing. You may leak more when sexually aroused as oxytocin, one of the hormones responsible for the "let-down" reflex in the breasts, is released at this time.

I've got terrible indigestion – why is this?

Progesterone, the hormone that relaxes smooth muscle (muscle that controls unconscious actions) in pregnancy, has the unfortunate side effect of relaxing all smooth muscle in the body, including the whole of the digestive tract. This slows digestion and the ring of muscles called a sphincter at each end of the stomach become less effective, which can cause heartburn and indigestion as acidic juices from the stomach leak back into the oesophagus. In addition, your growing baby is squashing your stomach so that you have a smaller space to digest food.

To relieve indigestion, eat little and often, eat slowly, don't eat late at night, and cut down on fatty or spicy foods. Rather than lie flat, prop yourself up with pillows. Talk to your midwife, doctor, or pharmacist about remedies that are safe to use in pregnancy.

What's a high-risk pregnancy?
complications in pregnancy

Q The midwife says I'm "high risk" because of my blood pressure. What does this mean?

Blood pressure is monitored in pregnancy as raised blood pressure can be a sign of pre-eclampsia (see p.89). At your first antenatal visit, your midwife will record your blood pressure and assess your risk of pre-eclampsia based on the blood pressure reading, your medical history, and family medical history. Certain factors increase your risk. These include:

* **High blood pressure**.
* **Pre-eclampsia or raised blood pressure** in previous pregnancies, or having a mother or sister who had pre-eclampsia.
* **Being aged over 40 years** and this being your first pregnancy.
* **Being significantly over- or underweight**.
* **Having a multiple pregnancy**.

If your midwife thinks you are "high risk", she will refer you to a consultant obstetrician and discuss a plan of care for your pregnancy. Many women who are assessed as high risk have pregnancies that progress without complications, but they are monitored a little more closely.

Q I've been told that because of my diabetes I have to go to the hospital clinic – why is this?

Whether you develop diabetes in pregnancy (known as gestational diabetes), or have pre-existing diabetes, you will require special care with support from a diabetic health care team and a consultant obstetrician. This is because diabetes poses risks in pregnancy if there is poor control of blood glucose levels. In the mother, these include hypertension (high blood pressure), thrombosis (blood clots), pre-eclampsia, diabetic kidney disease, and diabetic retinopathy, a condition that affects the retina in the eye. For the baby, there is an increased risk of congenital abnormalities and growth may be too fast or too slow. It is important that your care is tailored to you, taking into account any other complications you may already have from diabetes.

The key to a healthy pregnancy and baby when you have diabetes is good blood glucose control as your insulin requirements will change throughout pregnancy. Controlling blood glucose levels reduces the risk of birth defects and stillbirth, or a larger than expected baby, which can present problems during birth. If you have gestational diabetes, you will need to adapt your diet to include carbohydrates and fibre and reduce fats and sugar; you may also need insulin injections to help control blood sugar levels.

Q I have epilepsy – will I need special care in pregnancy?

Ideally, women with epilepsy should discuss their situation with their doctor prior to conception. Epilepsy and the medication used to control it do carry some risks in pregnancy, but there are ways to minimize these. Some anti-epileptic drugs (AEDs) are thought to be more harmful to a developing baby than others, so your doctor may wish to change your medication before you become pregnant. Although

Pregnancy can be challenging. Staying focused on the arrival of your baby can help you to stay positive most women taking AEDs have healthy babies, taking any type of AED increases the risk of birth defects, so you will probably be offered extra scans. The aim is to control your seizures on the minimum dose. AEDs also restrict your body's absorption of folic acid, which reduces the risk of an unborn baby developing neural tube defects such as spina bifida, so your doctor will probably discuss taking a higher dose of folic acid. Once your baby is born, you will generally be advised to breastfeed if at all possible, as any risk to the baby from AEDs is outweighed by the many health benefits of breast milk.

Q I'm 28 weeks and have been having contractions. Is my baby going to come early?

From early pregnancy, the uterus "practises" contracting in preparation for labour. A mother is usually unaware of these practice contractions, known as "Braxton Hicks", until later in pregnancy, when they can be felt as a hardening of the "bump". Each contraction lasts from a few seconds to a few minutes before the uterus relaxes and becomes soft

again. These contractions are painless (although they can feel quite uncomfortable!), follow no regular pattern, and having them does not necessarily mean that your baby is going to be born early.

However, if you experience painful contractions – described as being like strong "period-type" pains – and they seem to increase in strength and frequency, you should contact your hospital as you could be going into labour. You should also seek medical advice if you leak any fluid or blood from the vagina.

Q My last baby was premature – is this likely to happen again?

Having one premature baby, born before 37 weeks of pregnancy, means that you have about a 15 per cent chance of having a second preterm birth, although this also depends on why you had a premature birth originally. Reasons why babies are born prematurely include:

* **Infection in the mother**.
* **Early rupture of the membranes** ("waters breaking").
* **Multiple pregnancy**.
* **Weak, shortened cervix** (neck of the womb).
* **Unusual shaped womb,** for example, a bicornuate uterus (heart-shaped womb).
* **A medical condition in the baby,** for example if the baby is not growing as expected, which means that labour has to be induced early.
* **A medical condition in the mother,** such as pre-eclampsia (see opposite), which also means that labour has to be induced early.

Although most of the causes of premature birth cannot be prevented, there are steps you can take to reduce the risk of premature labour. These include not smoking, avoiding being under- or overweight, and avoiding extreme stress. In addition, it is essential that you attend all your antenatal appointments so that the wellbeing of both you and your baby is constantly assessed. You should discuss whether there was an obvious reason for your last baby being premature, and if there are any specific preventative measures you can take to help avoid a reoccurrence this time round.

MIDWIFE WISDOM

Prescribed bedrest
when you may need to rest in pregnancy

Towards the end of pregnancy, there are some circumstances when you may need to be admitted into hospital for bedrest and monitoring.

* If you have contractions, but your waters haven't broken; you may also be given a drug to slow contractions.
* If you develop pre-eclampsia in pregnancy you may have to stay in hospital and measures will be taken to reduce your blood pressure.
* If you have placental abruption (see p.91), you will be monitored in hospital and early delivery may be needed.

ESSENTIAL INFORMATION: YOUR 40-WEEK JOURNEY

Pre-eclampsia
Pregnancy-induced hypertension

Pre-eclampsia is a condition that affects around 10 per cent of women during their pregnancy (or, rarely, in the first 72 hours after the delivery). The cause is still unknown, although it is thought that it may be caused by a malfunction of the placenta.

What are the symptoms? There are varying degrees of pre-eclampsia, from your blood pressure rising a little bit towards the end of your pregnancy and a small amount of protein detected in your urine (which affects about 1 in 10 pregnant women), to a large rise in your blood pressure and a considerable amount of protein found in your urine (affecting about 1 in 50 pregnant women). Your blood pressure and urine will be checked (and the size of your baby measured) at your antenatal appointments to look for signs of pre-eclampsia and you will be referred to the hospital if necessary. Sudden swelling, headaches, pain under your ribs, and visual disturbances also indicate pre-eclampsia and you should contact your midwife or doctor straight away if you experience any of these.

What can be done? If you have the milder form of pre-eclampsia, this will only require your blood pressure and urine being tested a little more frequently – perhaps weekly. However, the more serious form will require you to go into hospital, where you and your baby will be monitored and given medication to lower your blood pressure. This is because if you are left untreated, it could develop into eclampsia, which is a very serious condition in which you may suffer convulsions, and your and your baby's lives could be in danger. However, with both types of pre-eclampsia, you will generally need

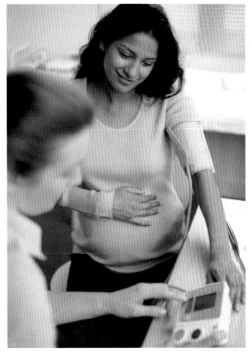

ANTENATAL MONITORING: Regular monitoring of blood pressure at antenatal appointments helps to detect women at risk of pre-eclampsia.

to be induced early (see p.190) as once your baby is born and the pregnancy is over, this will end the pre-eclampsia.

Who is at risk? Women are at a greater risk of pre-eclampsia if they have had the condition before; are over 40 years old; have a body mass index (BMI) over 35; have a family history of pre-eclampsia (mother or sister); had high blood pressure, diabetes, or kidney disease before the pregnancy; or are carrying more than one baby.

Q I'm expecting triplets. Will I be treated as "high risk"?

Yes, you will be classed as having a high-risk pregnancy as all the usual risks are increased for women with twins and multiple pregnancies. This is partly because hormone levels are higher when there is more than one baby, and partly because it is hard work for your body to carry and nourish three little lives! There will be an increased risk of miscarriage; severe pregnancy sickness (hyperemesis gravidarum); raised blood pressure/pre-eclampsia; anaemia (iron deficiency); diabetes; and premature and/or low birth weight babies. There is also an increased, although small, risk that one or more of the babies will die during the pregnancy. With triplets, you will almost certainly need to give birth by Caesarean section. Although considered a very safe operation, this is still major surgery and carries the associated risks.

You can expect to be referred to an obstetrician, who will plan your antenatal care with you and you will probably have more frequent checkups and scans. If you attend all your appointments and look after your health, it is likely that you will have three healthy babies at the end of your pregnancy. For more information about multiple pregnancy and details of local support groups, contact the Twins and Multiple Births Association (TAMBA) (see p.310).

Q I have lupus – how will this alter my care during pregnancy?

Lupus is an autoimmune disease that causes inflammation in the bone joints, blood, kidneys, and skin and sufferers often find that symptoms flare up due to certain triggers. The condition is more common in women than men, especially women of childbearing age. Some women find that pregnancy aggravates lupus, causing a flare-up, probably due to the hormonal changes that occur, while others find that pregnancy eases the symptoms. As lupus can affect an unborn baby, increasing the risk of stillbirth, miscarriage, premature labour, and slow growth, your pregnancy will be monitored very closely, especially when checking your blood pressure and

---

Obstetric cholestasis
A rare liver condition in pregnancy that causes intense itching

Cholestasis is a condition in which bile does not flow freely down the bile ducts in the liver, causing bile to leak into the bloodstream. This condition poses serious risks for both the mother and the baby, and so it is important that it is diagnosed with a blood test and managed as soon as possible. Medication will be given to relieve the itching and improve the liver function. The aim of the medication is to stabilize the condition until it is safe for the baby to be delivered. Usually labour is induced between 35 and 38 weeks of pregnancy.

urine. However, the likelihood is that you will have a completely healthy pregnancy resulting in a healthy baby. You can contact Lupus UK for support and information (see p.310).

Q I've had a few small bleeds during pregnancy – will my baby be OK?

Bleeding in early pregnancy is not uncommon. Usually, the reason is unknown, but there is a theory that although the hormones of the menstrual cycle are suppressed, variations in the cycle continue. This could explain why some women have light "spotting" around the time a period would be due. If the bleeding is light, and not accompanied by abdominal cramping or pain, then it is unlikely that there is anything wrong.

Bleeding after early pregnancy can be due to a cervical ectropian, when the surface of the cervix becomes "raw". This results from hormonal changes and is not harmful to the baby. Sexual intercourse can aggravate a cervical ectropian, stimulating bleeding.

Bleeding in late pregnancy may be more serious as it can be due to the placenta partially, or totally, detaching from the wall of the uterus, known as placental abruption, or to a low-lying placenta, known as placenta praevia (see below and p.92).

If you have a mucus discharge tinged with blood in late pregnancy, this may be a "show", when the plug of mucus sealing the cervix comes away. This is normal and can indicate that labour isn't far away.

It is important that you seek advice for any type of bleeding at any stage of pregnancy, as serious causes for bleeding must always be ruled out.

We know our baby has Down's syndrome. How can we best prepare ourselves?

On a practical level, you can prepare in much the same way as every parent, thinking about your preferences for labour, attending antenatal classes, and buying baby equipment. Knowing in advance that your baby is going to be born with a condition such as Down's gives you time to adjust and find out as much as possible about what to expect. You may wish to tell family and friends too, to give them time to prepare. Ask your health visitor for details of local support groups and contact the Down's Syndrome Association for more information (see p.310).

I had an emergency Caesarean last time. Now the doctor says I'll have a trial of labour, what is this?

This means labour after a Caesarean section. Another term is VBAC (Vaginal Birth After Caesarean section). Until relatively recently, most doctors

advised women who had had a Caesarean to have a planned Caesarean for the next baby to avoid uterine rupture, where the Caesarean scar tears in pregnancy or labour. Although serious this is rare, and it is now thought to be preferable for both the mother and baby to have a natural vaginal delivery if possible. Even so, if you want a vaginal delivery, it would be wise to opt for a unit that has fetal heart monitoring and that can carry out Caesareans if one turns out to be required.

Your chances of having a successful labour depend partly on why you had a Caesarean section. If it was because the baby was breech or you had a low-lying placenta, your chances of a natural labour this time are higher. If it was due to complications in labour, such as slow cervical dilatation, then the problem may recur. Overall, about half of women have natural deliveries after a Caesarean. You can contact the Caesarean organization for more information (see p.310).

My friend had placental abruption. Is this serious?

Placental abruption means that the placenta has started to come away from the wall of the uterus before the pregnancy has reached full term. This is a potentially serious condition that may mean the baby needs to be delivered as soon as posssible by Caesarean section. If there is persistent pain in the abdomen during pregnancy, which may be accompanied by fresh, bright red, bleeding and/or a change in the baby's movements, then medical help should be sought straight away.

I have had three miscarriages – will my antenatal care be different because of this?

While one or even two miscarriages are relatively common, three is less so. If you have had recurrent miscarriages, you will be offered extra antenatal care. You may be advised to take low-dose aspirin if there is evidence that you have a blood-clotting condition called anti-phospholipid syndrome (aPL). A vaginal scan may also be offered to check if you

Advances in antenatal care over the past few decades mean that even the most serious conditions can be dealt with successfully

Placenta praevia

Placenta praevia means a low-lying placenta, which occurs when the placenta is either partially covering (minor), or completely covering (major), the cervix. In major placenta praevia, the baby cannot be born vaginally. Major placenta praevia poses a high risk of heavy bleeding, either in the later stages of pregnancy or during the actual labour, which is treated as an emergency. If a low-lying placenta is detected at your 20-week scan, you may be offered a scan in late pregnancy; this is because the placenta may "move up" as the uterus grows, and by about 34 weeks may no longer be low. If you have placenta praevia, particularly major placenta praevia, most hospitals admit you for bedrest in the last weeks of pregnancy until the birth so that if you bleed heavily, you can be treated immediately.

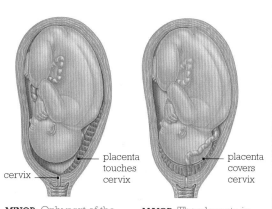

cervix — placenta touches cervix   placenta covers cervix

MINOR: Only part of the placenta is covering the cervix, which means that a natural vaginal delivery may be possible.

MAJOR: The placenta is directly above the cervix, which means the baby will need to be delivered by Caesarean section.

have a "weak cervix", where the cervix is unable to support the growing baby. If a weak cervix is diagnosed, you may be given a stitch during pregnancy to hold the cervix shut. There is some evidence that taking the hormones progesterone or human chorionic gonadotrophin in early pregnancy can reduce the risk of miscarriage.

My baby is very small for her dates – can anything be done about this?

From 25 weeks, your midwife will measure and palpate your tummy to estimate the fetal size. If she thinks you are "small for dates" she may refer you for a scan for a more accurate assessment of the baby's size and of the efficiency of the placenta. You may be offered a repeat scan in a week or so to measure growth over time. If babies do not grow as they should, this is called intra-uterine growth restriction (IUGR). This can be due to a problem with the baby or the placenta, affecting the amount of oxygen and nutrients reaching the baby. Pre-eclampsia can cause IUGR, as can smoking, drinking alcohol, and

recreational drugs. If your baby is very small and the rate of growth drops off considerably, it may be necessary to deliver the baby early.

My friend had hyperemisis gravidarum in her pregnancy – can you tell me more about this?

Hyperemesis gravidarum (HG) is severe pregnancy sickness, a debilitating condition affecting around one per cent of women. The woman is unable to keep down food or fluids without vomiting and becomes clinically dehydrated. This can begin at around week 6 of pregnancy and may last until 16–20 weeks (although some women suffer throughout pregnancy). Sufferers may need hospital treatment with intravenous fluids, and medications to control the vomiting may be given, but their success varies. No-one is sure what causes the condition, but it is thought that high levels of the hormone hCG, fluctuations in thyroid levels, and changes in liver function may all be involved. Sometimes the condition runs in families. There is a support group that provides information and tips (see p.310).

MYTHS AND MISCONCEPTIONS

Is it true that...

✳ All women love being pregnant?

That pregnancy makes women completely happy is a myth. While being pregnant and starting a family can cause tremendous joy, it is also quite an exhausting and overwhelming experience, with biological, psychological, and social changes to cope with. Everyone's pregnancy is different – you'll probably find that it's a great experience but may have its challenges.

✳ My vivid baby dreams are a bad sign?

Pregnant women often have strange, vivid dreams, but this is completely normal. Experts attribute the vividness of these dreams to hormones, as well as all the emotional and physical changes you're going through. The vivid dreams may be a way for your subconscious to deal with all the hopes and fears you may have about pregnancy and impending motherhood.

✳ Morning sickness will starve my baby?

Morning sickness is one of the most common pregnancy symptoms, and is believed to be caused by pregnancy hormones. It's easy to panic if you're throwing up every morning and you don't seem to be gaining weight, but try not to worry – you won't really start to gain weight until later in your pregnancy. As long as you were healthy before you became pregnant, your baby will be more than adequately nourished. However, it is possible that severe pregnancy sickness (hyperemesis gravidarum) can compromise your baby, so tell your obstetrician or midwife if you aren't able to keep any liquids or foods down.

What's happening to my baby?
fetal development

Is it true that much of the really important brain development happens in the first trimester?

Your baby's brain starts to develop soon after conception when brain cells begin to form at the tip of the embryo. After about three weeks, a structure called the "neural tube" begins to change in order to form the spinal cord, and the brain and brain cells (neurons) start to develop and send messages to each other. In the early weeks, brain cells multiply at a rate of about 250,000 per minute.

After about 20 weeks of pregnancy, the rate at which brain cells multiply begins to slow down and the brain starts to organize itself into over 40 systems to direct vision, language, movement, hearing, and other functions. By the time you are half way through your pregnancy, almost all the brain cells your baby needs for life are present.

During the third trimester, the connections between the brain cells start to mature and the baby's nervous system becomes more developed. Brain development is not totally complete by the time the baby is born and many important brain connections that help your baby develop skills and personality are made after the birth.

So, although fetal brain development occurs throughout pregnancy, and after, crucial foundations are certainly laid during the first three months.

Is there anything I can do to help the development of my baby's brain?

You can ensure that your diet includes good sources of omega-3 fatty acids, as these are thought to play an important part in the development of the brain. They can be found in oily fish such as mackerel and salmon (limit to one or two portions a week); omega-3 supplements designed to take in pregnancy are available.

When will my baby's face be formed?

The development of the face starts as early as the sixth week of pregnancy, when grooves that will form the structures of the face and neck start to grow. A week later, the eye starts to develop and a primitive mouth and nose are evident. By the end of the first trimester, the face is well formed and has a definite human appearance, although the skin is still transparent. By the 24th week of pregnancy, the eye is fully developed, the eyebrows and lashes have formed, and the skin becomes less transparent, but the eye remains fused shut and does not open until around the 28th week of pregnancy.

During the last trimester, your baby's hair begins to grow on the head and fatty deposits give your baby rounded cheeks.

I would like to communicate and bond with my baby before the birth. Is there anything I can do?

As your pregnancy progresses, there are many ways to focus on your baby and communicate with him, and these occasions are a chance for you to relax and take time out, too.

* **Relax in a warm bath** and concentrate on feeling your baby's movements, imagining what he is doing inside you.
* **Talk to your baby.** Your baby can detect sounds from outside the womb by the second trimester and is especially likely to tune in to your voice. You can give a running commentary on your activities, or even read to your baby. Get your partner to chat too!
* **Rub or massage your bump.** You may find that your baby responds by kicking; it's almost like having a conversation!
* **Spend some time** making plans for your baby's arrival, for example, choosing colours for the nursery

or even just buying a few sleepsuits.

* **Sign up for birth preparation classes** for you and your partner. This will give you both a chance to think about labour, birth, and your baby.

* **Start reading** through a book of baby names and make a list of those you and your partner like.

* **Some couples enjoy** taking regular photographs of their growing bump.

Q I've got a full-on career and have hardly thought about the baby. Will this stop us bonding?

Even if you work full time during pregnancy, this doesn't have to have a negative effect on your relationship with your baby. As your baby grows, you will probably find that you start to develop a relationship with your "bump" as you anticipate your baby's movements and perhaps talk to your baby. Make sure you plan enough maternity leave before your due date as this gives you time for practical and emotional preparations, as well as time to rest. There is some evidence to suggest that too much stress in a mother can affect her unborn baby's brain development, although this is not conclusive. However, it does highlight the importance of regular opportunities to relax during pregnancy.

Q I'm trying to get my partner involved; I keep letting him feel the baby move, what else can I do?

This is a common concern. Feeling the baby move inside you is a great way for your partner to begin to connect with the baby as a separate person and seeing the baby on an ultrasound scan can help too, as can hearing the heartbeat.

It is often difficult for partners to feel involved with a pregnancy since it is not physically happening to them and can feel quite an unreal experience. Try to spend time together finding out about pregnancy, labour, and birth as this will help your partner to feel as informed as you and discover ways to help you during the labour and birth and care for the baby after the birth. Some of the suggestions in the box above may also help.

MIDWIFE WISDOM

Partner bonding
getting your partner involved in pregnancy

Many men feel rather left out during their partner's pregnancy since all the attention is focused on the woman. Here are some ways to involve your partner.

* Encourage him to attend at least some of your antenatal appointments, where he can ask questions and listen to the heartbeat.

* Attend birth preparation classes together.

* Spend time at home reading about birth and babycare and share opinions.

* Write a birth plan together (see p.149).

* Share practical arrangements, such as planning and decorating the nursery and choosing baby equipment.

Q My husband didn't talk about the baby before the scan. Now he is over-protective. Is this normal?

Many fathers-to-be find it difficult to come to terms with the fact that their partner is carrying their baby, and that the baby will eventually be born and bring all the joys, trials, and responsibilities of parenthood. This is all even harder to envisage when they are not physically experiencing the changes that pregnancy brings – not feeling the symptoms or feeling the movements. The ultrasound scan is often a pivotal point for partners – suddenly they are "face to face" with their baby, and it becomes more real. Perhaps your partner is now realizing his responsibilities and affection for the baby, and is showing these feelings by taking care of you. If you are finding that his cosseting of you is a little too much, you might want to discuss other ways he can feel involved with the pregnancy and prepare for the baby (see box, above)! Try to embrace his involvement and enthusiasm for the pregnancy – it is a great way for you to strengthen your relationship as a couple and prepare to face parenthood together.

Baby's development
How your baby grows

From the moment of conception, the minute cluster of cells that is your baby starts to develop rapidly into a fully formed human being. Your baby takes all the nourishment from you that he needs to bring about this miracle of new life.

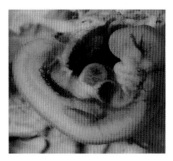

What is happening in the first two trimesters? In the first 12 weeks of life, the first trimester, your baby is changing rapidly from an indistinct bundle of cells into an identifiable human. During this time, the body starts to form and all the major organs are developing. By eight weeks, the four chambers of the heart have formed and it can be seen beating on an ultrasound. Your baby, now called a fetus, loses its tail and limbs start to form. By the end of the first trimester, your baby is fully formed; facial features are developing, and the major organs are beginning to function. The second trimester, from weeks 13–27, is a period of rapid growth as your baby grows around 6cm (2in) each month. Your baby starts to move and he can swallow and hear sounds outside the womb. By 24 weeks, most body systems are formed and, apart from the lungs, the major organs are working.

FIRST TRIMESTER: In the first trimester of pregnancy, your baby develops from a tiny bundle of cells into a fetus measuring around 10–12cm (4–5in). In this trimester, all the major organs are forming and developing along with the bones and muscles. The placenta is also developing and will eventually become the baby's life-support system, taking over from the maternal hormones.

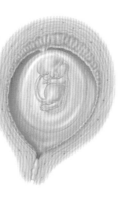

Weeks 6–7

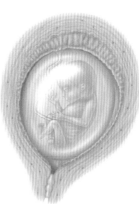

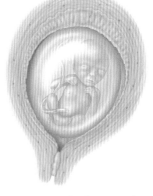

AT 8 WEEKS: Your baby measures just 2½cm (1in). His skin is translucent, but facial features and limbs are starting to form and he is becoming recognizably human.

AT 12 WEEKS: Your baby is 7cm (2½in). His face now has a chin, forehead, eyes (shut), nose, and ears high on the head. The fingers and toes have separated.

AT 16 WEEKS: By the second trimester, your baby has doubled in length. The limbs are more developed, but the skin is still translucent.

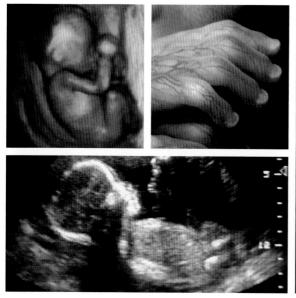

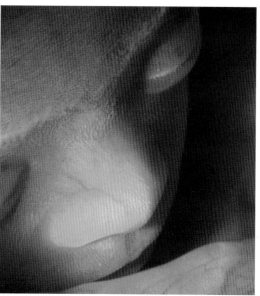

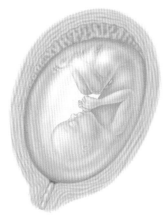

SECOND TRIMESTER: Your baby's weight increases significantly as he lays down fat supplies, and his body begins to look more in proportion. The skin is still thin and transparent, with blood vessels visible.

All the facial features are now in place and a view of the face shows a developed nose and lips. Eyelids have formed and cover the eyes and the eyebrows are beginning to develop.

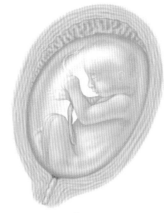

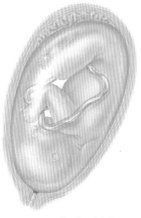

AT 20 WEEKS: Your baby is 15cm (6in) crown to rump and is laying down fat deposits. Fine hair called lanugo covers him. His eyes are still tight shut.

AT 24 WEEKS: Your baby is 20cm (8in) and starts to fill out and the skin is no longer translucent. His eyes can now open and his facial features are fully formed.

AT 28 WEEKS: By the third trimester, your baby is now much more in proportion. A greasy, protective substance called vernix covers the skin.

Baby's development continued
How your baby grows

By the third trimester, at 28 weeks, your baby has put on considerable weight and, if born now, would possibly be able to survive out of the womb with special medical care.

What is happening in the third trimester? In the last trimester, from 28–40 weeks, your baby becomes much more active and is likely to have some sort of sleeping and waking routine; he starts to fill out and resemble a newborn as fat deposits are laid down. The organs continue to mature and body systems become more and more complex. The brain and nervous system develop rapidly (the brain continues to develop after birth) and by 36 weeks, the liver and kidneys are fully developed and the liver is starting to process waste products. The digestive system has formed and the intestines are filled with meconium, a dark green substance made up of waste products. The lungs are among the last organs to fully develop, but by 40 weeks these are fully functioning and your baby starts to practise small breaths.

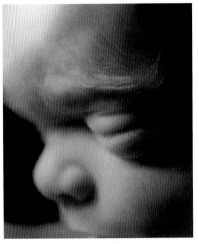

THIRD TRIMESTER: Your baby's skin loses its transparency and he begins to resemble a newborn baby.

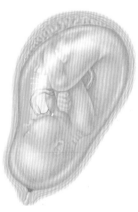

AT 32 WEEKS: Your baby now measures about 30cm (12in) crown to rump. The skin is now flesh-coloured and the wrinkles on the face are disappearing.

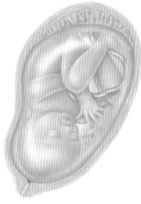

AT 36 WEEKS: Your baby now resembles a newborn. Hair is growing on the head and the fine body hair, lanugo, is beginning to disappear.

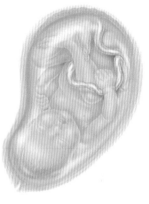

AT 40 WEEKS: At 36cm (14in) crown to rump, your baby is quite plump as he has laid down plenty of fat deposits in the last four weeks.

When can a baby first suck its thumb?

Ultrasound scans have shown unborn babies sucking their thumbs from as early as 12 to 14 weeks of pregnancy. However, this is likely to be a reflex at this stage as the brain does not have any conscious control over movement until the fetus is much more developed later on in pregnancy.

Some research has suggested that if an unborn baby shows a preference for sucking, for example, its right thumb, then it will prefer to lie with its head turned to the right after the birth. The same research also suggested that this preference in the womb could be used to predict right or left handedness in the baby as it grew older.

When will the midwife be able to hear my baby's heartbeat?

Your midwife should be able to hear your baby's heartbeat by the time you are around 12 weeks pregnant using a hand-held device called a "sonicaid". The heartbeat sounds rather like a galloping horse, and the rate is usually somewhere between 120 and 140 beats per minute – around double the rate of your own pulse.

There are factors that can influence whether or not the baby's heartbeat can be picked up. For example, if you are overweight, or the baby is in an awkward position, it may be harder to hear the heart. If your midwife is unable to locate the baby's heartbeat at 12 weeks, try not to worry. At this stage, the baby is only about 5cm (2in) long, so it's still very tiny! Your midwife will try again in a few weeks. Certainly, by 16 weeks it should be easier to pick up and listen to the heartbeat.

When will I first feel my baby move?

Although ultrasound scans have shown that babies may start to move slightly from around 6 weeks, it is not usually until the second trimester (13–26 weeks) that the fetus will make active movements. The sensation known as "quickening" is described as a fluttering type of feeling usually felt by mums

The very first sound your baby hears is your heart beating, and the first sound you will hear from your baby is his heartbeat

between 16 and 20 weeks, although exactly when a movement is felt can vary from woman to woman and may be affected by various factors. If it is your first baby, you may not notice any movement until later as you won't know what to expect. Also, if you are an active person, these slight flutters may be missed. Women with an anterior placenta (lying at the front of the womb) may feel movements later, as may larger women, as there is more flesh for the movement to be felt through.

It is not until around 28 weeks that it becomes more important to monitor the pattern of movements. From this stage, the amount your baby moves, as well as the type of movement and the time it happens, are relevant as these indicate that the placenta is sustaining the pregnancy and your baby's muscles are developing. If you are concerned about lack of movement, contact your midwife or hospital.

What sounds can my baby hear in the uterus?

The baby's outer ear is visible at around eight weeks and the first reaction to loud noises has been recorded at nine weeks. This has been measured in studies by playing a range of sounds through the mother's abdomen and recording any responses, such as movement, through ultrasound scans. It is thought that babies start off hearing low tones and then higher tones are heard later on as the hearing system continues to develop.

Studies also suggest that a fetus can determine its mother's voice and the voices of close friends and

MYTHS AND MISCONCEPTIONS

Is it true that...

 ### A fast heartbeat means it's a girl?

Even midwives and obstetricians have been known to say this, but there's no evidence to back it up. In any case, your baby's heartbeat is likely to vary, depending on how active he or she is when being monitored.

You can tangle the umbilical cord by raising your arms above your head?

Don't worry about this one! Nothing you do has any bearing on your baby's umbilical cord. How tangled the cord becomes is due to your baby's activity in the uterus when very small. If your baby's activity has caused the cord to become a little tangled, the midwife will be able to unwind it gently at birth.

I'm carrying low so it must be a boy?

This is unlikely! The general story goes that if you're carrying low, you're having a boy, if you're carrying high, then you're having a girl. The truth is, the way you carry is probably determined by your muscle and uterine tone as well as the position of your baby. There are lots of other girl-boy myths: if you have soft hands you're having a girl, rough hands you're having a boy; if the father-to-be is nervous it's a girl, if he's relaxed it's a boy; if the mother picks up her coffee cup with two hands it's a girl, if she picks it up by the handle it's a boy; if you have a sensitive belly button it's a girl, if you have cold feet it's a boy... the list is endless!

family significantly during pregnancy. One study revealed that not only did the fetus hear its mother's voice, but its heart rate decreased, indicating that her voice had a calming effect. By 16–20 weeks, hearing is considerably developed. Premature babies born at this time react to sounds, so they are living proof that babies inside the womb at that gestation can hear. Research also suggests that babies respond to stories read to them or music played during pregnancy after the birth.

Q I'm 25 weeks' pregnant, and my baby seems to "jump" when it hears loud noises – is this likely?

Babies born prematurely react to sounds, and loud sounds will produce a "startle reflex", so this provides strong evidence that babies inside the womb at that gestation will hear and react to loud sounds too, possibly with sudden movements.

As mentioned above, studies have shown that a baby can react to sounds in the womb from as early as nine weeks' gestation. As the fetus grows, the hearing develops, with babies responding to a greater range of sounds.

Q My tummy measurement has been the same for three weeks. Why isn't my baby growing?

In pregnancy, your abdomen is measured to establish the height of the top of the womb, which indicates how the baby is growing. It is important to know whether the same person is measuring you, as there is an element of subjectivity depending on techniques. In early pregnancy, it is not necessary to measure you as this doesn't give an indication of fetal growth, but from 26–28 weeks, growth can be assessed this way. However, even with your own personalized growth chart and with the same person measuring you at the correct time, on their own these are not an accurate means of estimating your baby's growth. If there are any concerns, you will probably be referred to a consultant to decide whether you need further investigations, for example ultrasound scans. If you are at the end of your

Try putting on some of your favourite music and see whether your baby responds – enjoy a dance together!

pregnancy, one possible explanation may be that your baby's head is engaging into the pelvis, so although your baby is still growing, some of his head has not been measured due to its position. If you are worried, talk to your midwife and, if necessary, she can refer you for a "growth scan".

Q Do babies have hiccups in the womb? I'm sure I can feel them.

Babies hiccup from early in the third trimester. This is a normal phenomenon that is usually short-lived but often recurs at similar times each day. It feels like a quick, spasmodic sensation in your abdomen. Hiccups are not harmful to the baby and in fact are a sign that your baby is healthy, in the same way that your baby's movements are a positive sign.

It is thought that the hiccups may be caused when, occasionally, babies take a deep breath in and ingest the amniotic fluid that surrounds them. The sudden change in chest cavity pressure when they take in fluid can cause the hiccups, just as when we drink something fast. These deep breaths help to exercise breathing muscles and stimulate their lungs to produce "surfactant", which is essential for the lungs to function. The baby cannot drown, as it receives its oxygen supply from the placenta.

Q When will my baby grow fingernails?

Babies begin growing fingernails from the end of the first trimester and the nails reach the fingertips between 34 and 36 weeks of pregnancy. It is possible for babies to scratch themselves inside the womb and when they are newly born, even though their nails are soft in comparison to ours. The function of fingernails is to protect the pads of the fingers, particularly, when gripping; as babies have a grip reflex from birth, this protection is necessary straight away.

After birth, cutting a baby's nails can be a cause of concern for parents. Newborn nails grow rapidly and the best time to shorten them is after a bath, when they are at their softest and the baby is more relaxed. There is some controversy over whether to use scissors, clippers, or simply bite them off. Scissors and clippers may easily cut the skin, but biting carries a higher risk of infection if the skin is broken. Pressing the nail helps to distinguish nail from skin. Using emery boards or simply peeling them off can be slightly safer options, or put your baby in scratch mittens.

At what stage could my baby survive outside of the womb?

Until relatively recently, babies born under 28 weeks' gestation often did not survive. Today, with medical advances in special care baby units, babies of 22 weeks' gestation have survived outside the womb, although this is still very rare. The guidelines for most hospitals is that 24 weeks is the earliest point at which they will resuscitate a baby, unless the baby shows signs of life at birth.

Extremely premature babies have an increased risk of disability, even with the best medical care, and often the delivery itself can put an enormous strain on the baby.

Very experienced doctors, midwives, and nurses will be involved in the care of extremely premature births. If possible, the delivery should take place in a hospital with a dedicated special care baby unit (SCBU). If this is not possible, babies are often transferred to a specialist centre when they are stable enough to be moved.

As each day and week is a milestone for your baby, the nearer to your due date you deliver, the better the chances for your baby.

Talking to your unborn baby helps you to feel connected, and as his hearing develops he will recognize your voice

I like to rub my tummy and talk to my baby as even now I feel like my baby is here – is this daft?

No, this is perfectly normal and may be soothing for him as babies can determine their mother's voice in the womb and sometimes their heart rate decreases in response. However, I wouldn't recommend that you rub your tummy too vigorously or too often as, in some cases, this can cause contractions and may trigger a premature labour if you are around 37 weeks' gestation.

Many women feel that the mother-child bond is there before the baby is born. It is good that you are having these positive thoughts during your pregnancy, as this is an excellent foundation for your future relationship with your baby.

Can my baby see bright lights? I'm 32 weeks' pregnant.

A baby's eye structures begin to develop from as early as 4–5 weeks, with the eyelids forming at around 8 weeks and closing between 9 and 12 weeks. By 24 weeks, all of the eye structures are fully developed and at around 28 weeks, the eyelids start to open and shut. Although we tend to presume the uterus is dark, this is not so. Between 30 and 32 weeks, the baby experiences light and dark environments, depending on where the mother is and the time of day. It has even been reported in studies that not only do babies react to light, but have been seen on ultrasound scans trying to grasp at the light source. When a baby is born, he reacts to lights by frowning or blinking and can see to a distance of around 15–20cm (6–8in) (the same distance to mum's face from the breast!).

Q Is it normal for babies to stop moving around so much towards the end of pregnancy?

Towards the end of pregnancy, your baby's range of movements may change as there is less room for him to extend his limbs and trunk. However, you should still be aware of a regular pattern of movement. Over the last 30 years, women have been actively encouraged to count how much their babies kick. However, in 2003, the National Institute for Clinical Excellence (NICE) recommended that this practice of counting movements stopped, as counting how many kicks a baby makes is not an accurate indication of whether the baby is well and each baby makes a different number of kicks. Nowadays, women are encouraged instead to tune in to their babies' pattern of activity, including the type of movement they make and the periods when they are most active. Studies have shown that over 50 per cent of women who had a stillbirth noticed a change in the pattern of movement. The general advice is, if you are worried about your baby's movement pattern you should speak to your midwife or hospital.

Q When will my baby's head engage?

Engagement, when your baby's head moves from higher in your abdomen down into your pelvis in preparation for the birth, can happen at any time from 36 weeks until the onset of labour (see p.148). The head tends to engage earlier in a first pregnancy.

Q Can my baby's position in the womb affect when his head engages?

A baby's position can affect how it engages into the pelvis. For example, if the baby is lying in a "back-to-back" position, with his back lying along the mother's back, this can make it more difficult for the baby's head to move through the pelvis. Similarly, if the baby is in a breech, feet first, position or a transverse position (see p.145), then engagement will not be

First kick

The moment when you feel your baby's first movements is a truly emotional experience, as you start to become completely aware of, and connect with, the baby growing inside you. Usually, the first movements are felt as a fluttering sensation, or a "quickening", as your baby starts to stretch and turn. This can be felt from around 18 weeks, although for some women it is much later; if you have had a baby before you are likely to be aware of these movements earlier, but for a first baby, awareness of the baby's movements is usually later, around 22 weeks. It is not until about 24 weeks that you will really start to feel regular, more definite movements and you will soon become accustomed to your baby's activities.

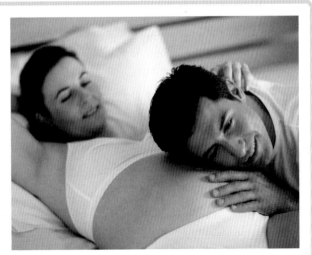

YOUR BABY'S MOVEMENTS: As your bump grows, your baby is increasingly active and you will feel unmistakable movements. Sharing this with your partner is an exciting prospect.

possible unless the baby moves and a Caesarean delivery may be necessary.

It is thought that the mother's level of activity and the positions she adopts can influence the position of the baby in the womb. Nowadays, it is more common for babies to lie in a back-to-back position and it is thought that this may be due to people leading a more sedentary lifestyle. In the past, when women were possibly more active, perhaps performing tasks such as scrubbing the floor on their hands and knees, there was less incidence of this position.

Q Will my baby develop much in the last month of pregnancy?

During the final month of pregnancy, your baby is busy preparing for birth. He will be practising breathing movements and sucking, and will start to turn towards light. You may notice that there are fewer vigorous movements now – this is natural as there is less space within the uterus. However, you should still be noticing plenty of nudges and wriggles. The downy hair that covered your baby's body starts to disappear and the hair on the head and your baby's nails continue to grow. Meconium, the waste product that will be your baby's first poo, starts to form in the bowels at this time. During this last month, most of your baby's organs are fully mature and the lungs will continue to develop. "Full term" is considered to be from 37 weeks.

Q I feel very emotional at times and am scared that I won't love my baby – is this normal?

The feelings you have are not uncommon. An increase in hormones during pregnancy can cause some extreme and deep feelings, some of which are irrational. Pregnancy is a major life event and, as well as the physical changes that are going on in your body, the emotional pressures are vast. There may be a range of pressures that are adding to how you are feeling, such as relationship problems, financial pressures, caring for other children, lack of space in your house, or returning to work after the birth. It is fine if these are occasional feelings, but if you find

that you are constantly snapping or crying, tired, having difficulty sleeping and eating, or sleeping and eating too much, are unable to concentrate, feel reluctant to leave the house, feel sad and anxious most of the time, or have developed obsessive compulsive disorder (OCD), then you need to speak to your midwife or doctor for help and advice as these are all symptoms of depression.

Q I've recently lost a parent and am very traumatized. Can stress affect my baby's development?

This is a major life-changing event and with the additional fluctuation in hormone levels and the physical changes that are occurring in pregnancy, you are obviously under a great deal of stress. However, it may be helpful to bear in mind that your body is designed to deal with episodes of stress.

There are studies that have suggested that women experiencing long-term stress may have an increased risk of pre-eclampsia (see p.89) and premature birth, although how reliable this evidence is has been questioned. It has also been suggested that there may be a link between extreme stress in pregnancy and children becoming hyperactive, but again this is inconclusive. The most important thing to do, now that you have recognized you may be at risk of long-term stress, is to speak to your doctor or midwife, particularly as there has been a recent increase in levels of support and treatment offered to pregnant and new mothers in your situation, which may help to limit any adverse effects of stress.

Try not to fret about how you might feel towards your baby. Love is not always instant – it can take time to grow and develop

What's happening to my body?
how your body changes

Q **I'm feeling like a beached whale and I'm only 16 weeks, what can I do?**

Weight gain during pregnancy is not only due to the baby, placenta, and amniotic fluid, but to a number of factors. Changes in your metabolism, the development of certain organs, such as the uterus and breasts, and an increase in your blood supply causing more fluid retention and swelling, all contribute to your weight. In addition, extra stores of fat are laid down as pregnancy requires more energy for the work involved in developing the fetus and coping with the demands of labour. Although most of this fat is stored in the first 30 weeks, weight gain is usually slower at the beginning of pregnancy and suddenly increases in the second half.

The average weight gain is 12.5kg (27lb), 4.5kg (10lb) of which is gained in the first 20 weeks, and the remainder thereafter. If you feel you have put on more than this, my advice is to eat healthy, smaller, more regular meals and take some gentle exercise.

Q **People keep telling me I'm too small, but the midwife says everything is fine. Can you explain?**

Tell them to mind their own business! If your midwife says she is not worried, then I would feel reassured – some women just hide a pregnancy very well! Your midwife starts to measure your tummy at around 26–28 weeks, as by then the major organs are more or less developed and your baby is concerned with growing and laying down fat supplies. Most units use personalized growth charts that are designed to take into account your individual traits, such as your race and height, which influence how big your baby is likely to be. By taking these factors into account, your midwife can predict more accurately the expected weight and measurements of your baby.

Q **I'm 17 weeks and my breasts have changed – they're painful and look different. Is that normal?**

It's perfectly normal and very common to experience breast changes in pregnancy. These are caused by both an increased blood supply and a rise in pregnancy hormones, particularly in the first 12 weeks. Before your pregnancy was confirmed you may have felt tingling sensations (especially in the nipple area) as the blood supply increased. As early as 6–8 weeks, breasts can get larger and more tender and may begin to look different on the surface, with threadlike veins starting to appear. At around 8–12 weeks, the nipples darken and can become more erect, and as early as 16 weeks, colostrum, the first milk, may be expressed.

Q **Why am I getting more vaginal discharge since becoming pregnant?**

In pregnancy, the layer of muscle in the vagina thickens and this, combined with an increase in the pregnancy hormone oestrogen, causes the cells in the vagina to multiply in preparation for childbirth. As a side effect, the extra cells mean that there is an increase in vaginal discharge, known as leucorrhoea.

If you feel sore or itchy and the discharge is anything other than cream or white, or smells, see your midwife or doctor so that a swab can be taken to rule out infection. Some infections, such as thrush, cause an abnormal discharge. They are common in pregnancy and are easily treated.

Q **Dark patches have appeared on my face. What could they be?**

The dark patches on your face are called "chloasma" or "pregnancy mask" and these patches affect around half of pregnant women. Nearly all pregnant women notice some changes in skin colouring, with skin usually darkening from 12 weeks. This is due to an increase in the hormones that stimulate skin pigmentation, with darker-skinned women affected more. This darkening may be more apparent on certain areas, such as the nipples, perineum (skin between the vagina and anus), and naval, or areas that experience "friction rubbing", such as the inner thighs and armpits. You can reduce or prevent dark patches on your face by minimizing your exposure to the sun and using high-factor sun creams.

I'm a model and I'm worried I'll get stretch marks. Is there anything I can do to avoid them?

I appreciate your concern, especially as looking good affects your work. Stretch marks, also called *striae gravidarum*, are thought to be connected to the collagen and elastin content of your skin rather than to how much your stomach expands. They occur as the collagen layer of the skin stretches over areas of fat deposits on the breasts, abdomen, and thighs. Unfortunately, there are no pills, creams, or magic lotions that can influence whether or not you will get stretch marks or, if you do, how badly you will get them, although taking regular exercise can help you to maintain an ideal weight during pregnancy and so minimize your chances of developing stretch marks.

Take comfort from the fact that although the marks may be red and livid in pregnancy, in the months following the delivery they lose their colour, usually becoming silvery-white and less obvious.

Stay positive by looking beyond the stretch marks and thinking about how incredible it is that you are carrying a tiny baby

My tummy is really itchy. Is it safe to use moisturizers on my skin in pregnancy?

As your abdomen grows it can become itchy as the skin stretches. You can use moisturizers on your body in pregnancy, and these may relieve the discomfort. Choose non-perfumed lotions, oils, or creams to avoid further irritation. Rubbing almond oil, vitamin E, or wheatgerm oil over the abdomen may also help.

Eating a healthy diet with fruit and vegetables and drinking plenty of clear fluids to keep you well hydrated will also help the condition of your skin.

I can't look in the mirror as I'm feeling so depressed about my size. Will things get better?

You are not alone in battling with your self-image in pregnancy. For many women, their changing body shape can create very negative feelings. Eating a healthy diet and taking some exercise helps to keep weight gain to a minimum, and exercise will help to lift your spirits and improve your sense of wellbeing. There is no set emotional response to pregnancy, but as well as coming to terms with a momentous life and body change, you are also under the influence of fluctuating hormones, all of which affect your moods and add to feelings of negativity.

Mild depression in pregnancy is often helped by reassurance and support from your partner, family, or friends. Talking over your fears and concerns with your partner, or with other pregnant women at antenatal classes, may help to relieve your anxieties – you will probably find that other pregnant women are experiencing the same feelings.

If your depression is very severe and you feel desperate, consult your midwife or doctor as antenatal depression is now recognized as having an effect on pregnancy and birth outcomes, with studies showing a possible link between medication given to treat depression in pregnancy and a lower birth weight and increased risk of premature birth. Your doctor or midwife may refer you for counselling, and some areas hold group classes for pregnant women suffering from antenatal depression.

Weight gain in pregnancy
Monitoring your weight

The recommended weight gain in pregnancy depends on your pre-pregnancy weight. If your BMI was less than 19.8 you should aim for a gain of between 12.5–18kg (28–40lb); between 19.8 and 26 you should aim for 11.5–16kg (25–35lb); above 26 you should aim for 7–11kg (15–25lb).

What if I gain too much or too little? There is a link between not putting on enough weight in pregnancy and low birth weight babies. If you gain too much weight, you are more likely to suffer from pre-eclampsia, high blood pressure, diabetes, backache, varicose veins, tiredness, shortness of breath, and to have a large baby.

How do I maintain a healthy weight? Take moderate exercise, eat healthily (see p.50), and follow a weight-reducing diet only under supervision. You need only 200–300 calories more per day, so "eating for two" is not a healthy option.

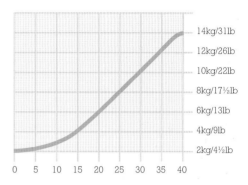

14kg/31lb
12kg/26lb
10kg/22lb
8kg/17½lb
6kg/13lb
4kg/9lb
2kg/4½lb

0   5   10   15   20   25   30   35   40

WEIGHT GAIN OVER 40 WEEKS: Weight gain is slow in the first trimester, then rises to around 0.7–1kg (1½–2lb) a week, increasing in the final weeks.

Where does the weight go? It is distributed between your baby and you. About 6kg (13lb) is the baby, placenta, and water around the baby. The rest is the fat deposits, extra blood, and fluid that you need. Additional weight is made up of fat.

Your changing shape

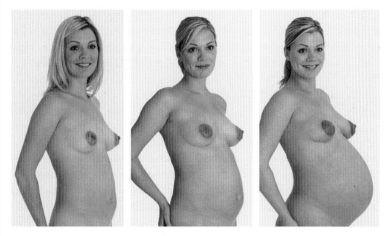

FAR LEFT: At 16 weeks you have gained up to 4.5kg (10lb) and your pregnany tummy starts to show. **MIDDLE:** By 24 weeks you are clearly pregnant and will have gained almost 8kg (17½lb). **LEFT:** By the end of pregnancy at 40 weeks, you will have gained a total of around 14kg (31lb); weight gain now slows.

Q Why do people talk about the second trimester as the time when pregnant women "bloom"?

For many women, the second trimester is the most enjoyable part of pregnancy. As women find themselves released from the draining symptoms of early pregnancy, this can lead to an upsurge of energy, and many find it easier to eat, sleep, and work. Many women also notice that their skin is glowing and their hair is glossier than usual. It is also around this time when you first feel your baby move and, as your baby grows, you start to notice a definite bump and begin to look pregnant – changes that can help you feel more positive and excited.

However, not all women feel this way. A sizeable minority of women don't feel any better as the second trimester progresses, with nausea, tiredness, and other symptoms continuing unabated. Some may find it hard to come to terms with physical changes such as weight gain, or skin and hair changes. If this is the case, it's important to remind yourself that almost all of pregnancy's downsides clear up as soon as the baby is born. If you're feeling particularly down or low on energy, it may be a sign of other problems, such as anaemia (see p.81). Speak to your midwife or doctor for further advice.

Q I'm worried that my husband doesn't find me attractive any more. Am I being paranoid?

Self-image can be a big problem with pregnant women and many worry that they are unattractive to their partners in the latter stages of pregnancy. This worry is usually unfounded and more to do with their own feelings about their increased size. Keeping anxieties bottled up can make them seem bigger than they actually are, so talk to your husband about your worries and explain how you are feeling. He may be completely unaware of what you are thinking.

As your husband isn't carrying the baby, he cannot truly understand the physical demands of pregnancy. Informing him about the changes your body is going through can help him to understand the process of pregnancy and be better equipped to

provide support when you need it most. Some men actually find their partners more attractive during pregnancy, but you won't know this unless you talk to each other about your changing shape.

If you are worried about gaining too much weight in pregnancy, focus on eating a healthy, balanced diet (see p.50) and take some light, daily exercise. Even if this is only a short walk or swim, it will help to keep you toned and supple, which will help your confidence as well as prepare you for childbirth.

Q Can I wear high heels?

Although lots of pregnant women continue to wear the same footwear during pregnancy, it is advisable to avoid heels and opt for a flatter shoe, particularly as your pregnancy progresses.

Later in pregnancy, your posture and centre of balance changes, as your increased weight is now mainly at the front of your body. In addition to this, increased levels of hormones secreted during pregnancy, such as relaxin, make the joints and muscles of the body more lax. So wearing high heels can increase the strain on the lower back and pelvic joints, giving rise to aches and pains in those areas. However, it's alright once in a while to wear high heels, for example at a party, but it might be wise to take flat shoes to change into for walking home.

What shall I do about my pierced belly button?

If you are pregnant and your navel is pierced, your midwife will probably recommend that you remove any metal jewellery from your navel for the duration of your pregnancy. Some women are happy with this advice, but a lot of women do not want to risk letting their piercing heal up, and then having to have it re-pierced after their baby is born, so they try to wear jewellery in their navel through their pregnancy.

You can use something called a "pregnancy retainer". Due to the popularity of body piercing, these have been manufactured to help pregnant women maintain their piercing as their body shape changes. They are made up of a soft, flexible substance called PTFE (polytetrafluoroethylene) in the shape of a "banana" bar that has two acrylic screw-on end balls. There is a wide range of sizes and styles for women to choose from. As a general rule, you should choose a retainer that is at least 4mm longer than the size of the jewellery you are currently wearing, although, as you can imagine, every tummy is different and will obviously change in size as your pregnancy progresses. The important factor is that your pregnancy retainer should not pinch into your skin at any time – if you feel your retainer is causing you discomfort, then buy a larger size.

Even if you look and feel fabulous on the outside, it's important not to forget to keep looking after yourself on the inside too

I don't have much to spend on maternity clothes, any ideas?

Lots of women are faced with this predicament when they become pregnant, but you don't need to spend a lot of money. Most women's clothes shops now stock selections of maternity wear at very reasonable prices. Invest in a couple of pairs of trousers or skirts that you will be able to adapt as your pregnancy progresses and then mix and match colours and styles with a few tops. The tops don't have to be maternity wear – you could just buy ones a couple of sizes up from your normal size.

You could look in charity shops too, or loan maternity clothes from friends and family, as women wear maternity clothing for such a short period that it is often in good condition. Ebay is a good place to pick up a bargain, and local NCT (National Childbirth Trust) sales have plenty of items in excellent condition. Lastly, don't forget your partner's tops and jeans, which may be the perfect fit!

I'm 20 weeks' pregnant and have noticed that I get short of breath very easily. Is this normal?

When you're pregnant, your lungs have to work much harder to meet your body's increased oxygen needs. To help you take in more air, your ribs flare out and your lung capacity increases dramatically. This can make you feel breathless, particularly from mid-pregnancy onwards. In the last three months, most women find they get breathless even during mild exertion, which happens as the expanding uterus pushes up against the lungs. However, being breathless can also be a sign of anaemia, which may need to be treated (see below). Your breathing may start to get easier when your baby engages – moves down into your pelvis ready to be born.

My midwife has told me I'm anaemic. Can I improve my iron levels through my diet?

All pregnant women should be offered screening for anaemia, which is done early in pregnancy (at the first appointment), and again at 28 weeks. Generally, an iron-rich diet is advised in pregnancy and this is enough to prevent or improve anaemia. Eat plenty of lean red meat, beans, dried fruits, dark green vegetables, fortified cereals, and bread. Try including a vitamin C-enriched food or drink in your diet, as vitamin C helps the body to absorb iron more efficiently. Vegetarians need to eat plenty of eggs, pulses, beans, and nuts to boost iron supplies. Iron tablets may be recommended depending on how low your iron levels have become.

I have developed a dark vertical line down the middle of my tummy. What is this?

A brown line down the centre of your stomach is known as the linea nigra. This occurs due to changes in skin pigmentation, which are extremely common in pregnancy, affecting 90 per cent of all women in some way or another, and is often more noticeable if you are darker skinned. As well as the line on your tummy, you may also notice a darkening of the skin around your nipples and a darkening of freckles, moles, or birthmarks. A few women may also experience brown patches on their face called chloasma or "pregnancy mask" (see p.105). These changes are caused by the extra amounts of the hormone oestrogen in pregnancy, which affects the melanin-producing cells of the skin – the cells that produce the pigment that darkens the skin. These colour changes are normal and will usually fade once the baby is born.

I'm 32 weeks and my pelvis is really aching now – what are the reasons for this?

Mild pelvic discomfort is a common symptom in pregnancy as your ligaments loosen, due to the increased levels of the hormones relaxin and progesterone in pregnancy. These changes in your pelvis prepare your body for the birth. This feeling is quite normal and happens to most pregnant women. If your pelvis continues to give you discomfort, you can try to adapt your day-to-day living to relieve the symptoms. Keep your legs together and swing them

round when getting in and out of a car or bed. Think about your activities for the day and plan your movements ahead so as not to exacerbate any discomfort you have. Avoid wearing high-heeled shoes and take a rest whenever the discomfort becomes more noticeable.

If your pelvis is more than just uncomfortable, seek medical advice. More extreme discomfort that causes chronic pain is a sign that there's a dysfunction in the pelvic area, which may require treatment and support as pregnancy progresses. The most common form of pelvic dysfunction is symphysis pubis dysfunction (SPD), which is caused by the pubic joint not working as it should (see p.82).

I've never looked better – why is that?

Hormone levels in early pregnancy can make for a miserable time for many women as they battle against morning sickness, tiredness, and sore breasts. However, at around 12–16 weeks, when pregnancy hormones begin to settle and these symptoms start to subside, many women feel that their skin and hair are in great condition and their energy levels are at a high. This is sometimes called "blooming" (see p.108) and you may be lucky and find that this continues throughout your pregnancy.

If you are feeling particularly well, you may feel tempted to do too much, but you should exercise some caution as there will still be times when your body needs additional rest and you need to store up energy in preparation for labour and birth.

Although your body is steadily preparing for the labour and birth, try to enjoy the moment and not focus on the labour ahead

Safe sleep positions in the third trimester

It can be hard to find positions that are comfortable and safe in the third trimester. By this stage, you should avoid lying on your back because your baby's weight may press on your major blood vessels, compromising the blood supply to the baby and making you feel dizzy and faint. Most women find the best position is lying on their side with the upper leg bent and with pillows supporting the knee to make room for your abdomen. This takes the weight off your back and doesn't restrict your circulation. You could also place a pillow under your bump.

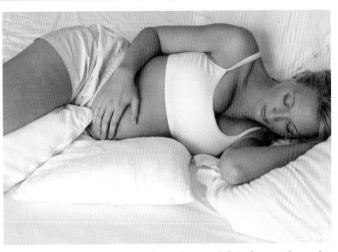

GETTING COMFORTABLE: Achieving a decent night's sleep at the end of pregnancy can be challenging as your bump limits your options. Lying on one side with supporting pillows is often most comfortable.

I'm 36 weeks and have noticed that I'm more comfortable and breathing more easily. Why is this?

It sounds like your baby has moved down into the pelvis. The baby's head is "engaged" when the widest part of the head has passed down into the pelvis. This means that when the midwife feels your abdomen, less than half of the head can be felt abdominally. Engagement is normally recorded in your antenatal notes in fifths, ranging from 1/5 to 5/5, so if the midwife has written "1/5 palpable" your baby's head is deeply engaged in the pelvis, as this means that 4/5 of your baby is down within the pelvis. The timing and significance of engagement depends on several factors. Women expecting their first baby tend to have firmer abdominal muscles, which gently ease the baby down into the pelvis during the last four weeks of pregnancy. This appears to be what your baby has done, and that is why you suddenly feel you can breathe a little easier as your lungs and rib cage are not so squashed. A second or third baby may not become engaged until labour starts, as the abdominal muscles tend to be more lax.

What is perineal massage?

Perineal massage is the practice of massaging the perineum, the stretch of skin between the vagina and anus, to make it more flexible in preparation for childbirth. The intention is to prevent tearing of the perineum during birth, and the need for an episiotomy or an assisted (forceps or vacuum extraction) delivery, as the skin in this area may become more stretchy as a result of massage. Clinical trials indicate that perineal and vaginal massage can reduce the seriousness of tears and so some consider it beneficial.

Use a lubricant such as KY jelly, cocoa butter, olive oil, vitamin E oil, or pure vegetable oil on your thumbs and massage around the perineum. Place your thumbs about 3–4cm (1–1½in) inside your vagina and press downwards and to the sides at the same time. Gently and firmly keep stretching until you feel a slight burning, tingling, or stinging sensation. With your thumbs, hold the pressure steady for about two minutes, or until the area becomes a little numb and you don't feel the tingling as much. As you keep pressing with your thumbs, slowly and gently massage back and forth over the lower half of your vagina, avoiding the urinary opening, and along your perineum, working the lubricant into the tissues for three to four minutes. This helps stretch the skin in much the same way that the baby's head will stretch it during birth. Do this massage once or twice a day, starting around the 34th week of pregnancy. After about a week, you should notice an increase in flexibility.

I'm 35 weeks and feeling as tired as I did in the first trimester. Is that normal?

Tiredness can cause real problems for women in the first and last trimesters and is often worse for women who are overweight or who have a multiple pregnancy. In the early stages, you may feel tired and lethargic due to hormonal changes, while later in pregnancy, tiredness is caused by the extra demands on your body. Rest is the best cure, though this may be difficult if you're working or looking after children.

Boost your energy levels with regular, balanced meals. Late pregnancy is also the time to get your partner, family, and friends to help out with things like shopping, chores around the house, and cooking.

Severe tiredness in the last trimester may indicate that your iron levels are low, so it may be worth getting your iron levels checked.

I've gone from an A cup to a size D – my husband hopes this will last forever, but it won't will it?

Many women notice an increase in the size of their breasts in the second trimester and some maintain a bigger size after the birth, especially if they breastfeed. This is due to the effects of oestrogen, which causes fat to be deposited in the breasts. As your breasts enlarge, the veins become noticeable under the skin, the nipples and area around the nipples (areolae) become darker and larger, and bumps may appear on the areolae. Some women get stretch marks on their breasts, but these fade in time. After the birth, your breasts may get even bigger when the milk comes in! They do reduce in size once you finish breastfeeding, although the majority of women report a permanent increase of some degree.

Maternity bras

Breast changes are one of the first signs of pregnancy, as from around 3–4 weeks' gestation there is an increased blood flow, which increases tenderness. Some women notice a change in breast size early in pregnancy, while others may not notice any change until they breastfeed. Nevertheless, it's a good idea to get advice from a shop that stocks maternity bras with staff trained to measure and advise on what size you need. If your current bra fits well, wait until later in pregnancy to get measured when changes in cup size are more likely. In the early days of feeding, you may experience some engorgement of your breasts, but don't panic and send your partner out for a bigger size as this settles in a few days.

CHOOSING A SUPPORTIVE BRA: Wearing a properly fitted bra will increase your comfort and offer adequate support to your enlarged breasts during pregnancy and breastfeeding.

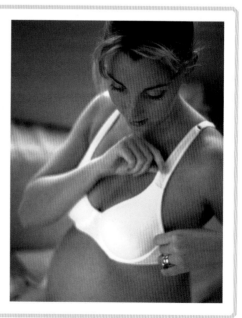

Sex in pregnancy
a fulfilling relationship

Q Can having sex in pregnancy harm the baby in any way?

Unless you have been told by your midwife or doctor to avoid intercourse because of specific problems, such as a history of miscarriage or unexplained bleeding, then sex is perfectly safe as your baby is cushioned in fluid in the amniotic sac inside your womb and protected by a cervical plug, and even deep penetration isn't harmful. Enjoying intimacy with your partner will also be beneficial for your relationship.

Q I'm either uncomfortable when we make love or not in the mood. Should I fake it?

Levels of sexual desire in pregnancy vary greatly, with some women finding their sex drive is heightened, while others feel too ill, anxious, hormonal, or just too uncomfortable to attempt sex at all. If you really don't want sex, be as honest and open as you can about your lack of sex drive. Don't be pressurized into doing something you really don't want to do, as this could complicate your relationship. Communication is very important at this time, so talk to your partner about how you are feeling – you may find that he is completely unaware of your feelings, anxieties, and worries.

You could use the presence of your "bump" as an ideal excuse to experiment with different positions, as most couples find the missionary position very uncomfortable in late pregnancy. Some couples prefer it if the woman is on top as this allows her more control over the amount of penetration and there is less weight on her bump. A "spooning" position, with your partner behind you, also allows for shallower penetration and removes pressure on your bump totally. Having a baby is all about adapting to new experiences, and most couples find they need to adapt their sex life too.

Q Since we hit the second trimester I've wanted sex more than ever – why is this?

Often, in the second trimester, women find that once early pregnancy symptoms wear off they feel far more energetic and sexier than ever! However, this may not be the case for everyone as each woman is affected differently by the physical and psychological changes that occur in pregnancy, and women have different views about their changing bodies, which can affect their libido.

From a physiological point of view, an increased blood flow to the pelvic area combined with an increased lubrication of the vagina means that, in theory, having sex can be better than ever. So if you and your partner are quite happy with your increased sex drive, this is not a problem.

Q My placenta is low and I've been told to avoid sex. Why is this? I'm only 30 weeks' pregnant.

As the baby develops and grows so does the womb, with the result that the placenta is carried upwards away from the opening of the womb. However, in 10 per cent of women, the placenta remains low-lying during late pregnancy and then poses a risk because of potential bleeding (see p.92). A low-lying placenta is often first detected at an early scan and, if this is the case, it is usual for a repeat scan to be carried out at around 34 weeks of pregnancy to determine if the placenta is still low and exactly where it is situated in respect of the opening of the cervix (neck of the womb).

The biggest risk from a low-lying placenta is bleeding and if you have already experienced any bleeding, it is usual to recommend that you avoid sexual intercourse, as agitation of the cervix, which happens during sex, can encourage more bleeding.

If in doubt, it's probably best to discuss your particular circumstances with your midwife or consultant obstetrician.

Q My partner hasn't wanted sex at all since I've become pregnant. Will he ever fancy me again?

It isn't uncommon for either partner to experience a reduced sexual desire in pregnancy for a variety of reasons. It is important that you talk to your partner and ask about his feelings while also explaining your own thoughts and feelings.

Some partners find pregnancy a little scary, and some of these fears centre around sex and concerns about harming the baby or you. Sometimes, these worries may be based on real concerns, for example if there have been any problems in early pregnancy such as threatened miscarriage, bleeding, pain, or excessive morning sickness. Equally they can be based on misunderstanding, and this is where discussion between the two of you will help. Although you may feel more attractive and sexy, perhaps your partner is feeling clumsy and

uncomfortable. Each couple is different and you will need to talk to each other to find your way through this. You may also feel that you want to talk to someone who isn't so closely involved, such as your midwife, doctor, a trusted friend, or a relative.

Q Is it best to stick to oral sex during pregnancy?

Research on the benefits and risks associated with oral sex in pregnancy is limited and the findings are very often contradictory. There is nothing that indicates that oral sex is recommended in place of penetrative vaginal sex unless you have been advised to avoid sexual intercourse because of the risk of bleeding, threatened miscarriage, or premature labour, when avoiding orgasm is also advisable and so complete abstinence is the better option for a while. Apart from this, it is important to remember that some infections can still be passed on easily by oral sex.

Q Will having an orgasm cause me to go into labour?

In a pregnancy without problems, an orgasm alone will not cause premature labour, and at full term orgasm will only cause the onset of labour if your body is ready for labour anyway. If you have had any signs of premature labour, or if you have had premature rupture of your membranes (see p.167), you will be advised to avoid sexual intercourse. This is because the hormone oxytocin increases during sexual arousal and the effect from the oxytocin is to cause the muscles of the uterus to contract.

During pregnancy, the muscles of the uterus experience practice contractions, known as Braxton Hicks (see p.168), which are not harmful, and orgasm may increase these practice contractions.

If you have gone past your due date and are at a point when your body is ready to go into labour, then sexual intercourse may help things to start for two reasons: the prostaglandins in semen will help the cervix to soften at this stage of pregnancy, and the contractions stimulated by orgasm have more chance of developing into early labour contractions.

MIDWIFE WISDOM

Talking to each other
maintaining a healthy relationship

It is essential that you and your partner keep the lines of communication open during this time of change and some uncertainties.

* If you have gone off sex completely, reassure your partner that this is a temporary situation and explain how the pregnancy is making you feel mentally and physically.

* Likewise, if your partner seems reluctant to initiate lovemaking, don't take it personally. Try to find out how he is feeling.

* Don't allow a quieter sex life to stop you being affectionate at other times.

Comfortable lovemaking

You and your partner may need to experiment more during pregnancy to find lovemaking positions that are comfortable for you and your rapidly growing bump. As pregnancy progresses, most women find that lying on their back in the missionary position becomes increasingly uncomfortable as your partner presses on your bump. You may find being on top an enjoyable position, which allows you to control penetration and does not put pressure on your tummy. Lying in the spoons position, with your partner behind you, can be pleasurable and puts no pressure on your abdomen. Other positions that don't restrict your pleasure and are comfortable include sitting together, kneeling while your partner enters from behind, and lying side by side with your legs bent over your partner's legs.

TIME TO EXPLORE: As your body changes, you and your partner may have to use your imagination during lovemaking to find comfortable positions. You may both find you enjoy this time of discovery.

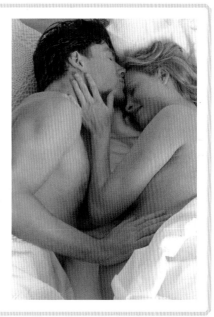

Q I've got problems with my pelvis – is there a comfortable way for us to have sex?

Problems with the pelvis, particularly symphysis pubis dysfunction or SPD (see p.82), tend to be made worse by moving your legs too far apart, so it is a matter of finding a position that you feel comfortable in that doesn't involve too much stress on the pubic area. Many women find the "missionary position" the most difficult as it involves significant parting of the legs, plus there is the weight of a partner to consider. Some, although not all, women find an all-fours position for intercourse more comfortable, both for sexual intercourse and for giving birth. If intercourse is really proving difficult, then it could be that while you are experiencing significant problems you will need to find alternative ways for you and your partner to be intimate that don't involve penetrative sex.

Many women find that pelvic discomfort improves significantly once they have had the baby. A very useful organization that has a lot of information and advice on pelvic pain during pregnancy is the Pelvic Partnership (see p.310). You can also talk to your midwife or doctor for a referral to a physiotherapist, which may be beneficial and help you to achieve a greater degree of comfort during pregnancy.

Q I'm 36 weeks. My boyfriend insists on regular sex and has been a bit abusive. Is this normal?

It is not normal for someone to be abusive to another person or to force them to have sexual intercourse when they don't want to. You should never be forced to do something that is against your will. In almost 30 per cent of all domestic abuse cases, the first incidence occurs in pregnancy. It is very important that you talk to someone about how your boyfriend is treating you, perhaps to a close friend or relative. There are also organizations that offer confidential advice and help you if you really feel there is no one you can talk to or trust (see p.310). You could also try talking to your midwife, who will treat everything you say in the strictest confidence and will have details of local organizations that can help and advise you.

Testing, testing
investigations in pregnancy

Q What is the difference between diagnostic and screening tests?

Screening tests identify your baby's "risk factor" for a particular condition, but do not confirm that your baby definitely has a condition. For example, a screening test for Down's syndrome may give your baby a risk factor of 1:200. This means that your baby has a 1 in 200 chance of being affected by Down's syndrome. Another way to view this result could be that the baby is most likely to be healthy. If your baby has a high risk factor, you may then decide to have a diagnostic test, such as amniocentesis or chorionic villus sampling (see pp.122–123), which gives a definite yes or no as to whether or not a condition is present. These tests are more invasive, as they require a sample of amniotic fluid or blood from the fetus or placenta, and they carry a slight risk of miscarriage.

Certain screening tests, such as first- or second-trimester screening for Down's syndrome, are offered routinely to all women regardless of any factor other than they are pregnant. These tests, in the form of scans or blood tests, identify who would benefit from further diagnostic tests. This avoids subjecting all pregnant women to diagnostic tests, which carry some risks (see p.125). Any benefit from a test should outweigh the potential risk.

Q What do these tests look for?

Screening and diagnostic tests aim to identify abnormalities in the unborn baby, which may be congenital, genetic, or chromosomal. Congenital abnormalities are often detected in the 18–22 week scan (see p.121) and these include conditions such as heart abnormalities or extra digits. These abnormalities can sometimes be treated after, or sometimes even before, the birth and are not inherited. Some conditions, such as spina bifida, are thought to be due to a combination of genetic and environmental factors; a dietary deficiency of folic acid may also contribute to this condition. Other congenital abnormalities may be caused by infections caught in pregnancy.

Diagnostic tests are usually carried out to identify genetic or chromosomal abnormalities, such as Down's syndrome, cystic fibrosis, sickle-cell anaemia, and muscular dystrophy. (Cystic fibrosis and muscular dystrophy are screened for if there is a family history.) These conditions occur either because there is a problem with the inherited genetic material, for example a gene has mutated, or because there is a chromosomal problem, for example there may be an incorrect number of chromosomes, as in Down's.

Down's syndrome, or "trisomy 21", is a chromosomal abnormality in which there is an extra copy of the chromosome 21. It is the most common "trisomy" disorder. Babies born with this condition have physical anomalies, such as slanting eyes and a protruding tongue, and there is a high incidence of heart, intestinal, hearing, and sight problems. Down's is the biggest single cause of learning difficulties. The majority of Down's syndrome conceptions are lost through spontaneous miscarriage early on in pregnancy, although over 600 babies are born with Down's syndrome in the UK each year.

Despite the concerns that often accompany screening tests, try not to let these overshadow the joy of being pregnant

I'm 38 – will I have more tests because I'm older?

Although the risk of Down's syndrome increases as you get older (see p.118), currently many women regardless of age are offered one of two types of screening test for Down's. This is either a first trimester screening that involves a blood test and a scan to measure nuchal translucency (see p.118), or second trimester screening, which is a blood test only, called the triple, or Bart's, test (see below). Both tests give the result as a risk or a percentage risk. If the test indicates there is a high risk of Down's, then all women are offered a diagnostic test such as amniocentesis (see p.123). However, if you are over 35, amniocentesis is offered routinely in the UK.

Your midwife should discuss with you in detail all the tests that are available and give you written information about them. Ideally, you should have this information several weeks before you are asked to decide if you wish to go ahead with any screening or diagnostic tests so that you have plenty of time to consider the possible outcomes and whether these tests are something you wish to undergo.

Depending on your past medical history and other factors, such as your blood pressure during your pregnancy or problems you had in previous pregnancies, you may be offered additional scans to check your baby's growth after 26–28 weeks.

We don't want invasive tests as we will love the baby whatever. Can we refuse diagnostic tests?

Whether or not you have a diagnostic test is your choice and you can refuse at any time to have any test offered. As well as the question of whether you are prepared to have a Down's baby, there is also the risk of miscarriage to consider (see p.125). On the other hand, you might decide you want a definite diagnosis to be able to prepare for your child.

What blood tests will I be having, and when?

There are various blood tests offered during pregnancy. As well as routine blood tests taken

The triple test
Blood screening for Down's and other conditions

Also known as "Bart's test", this is commonly used to screen for abnormalities.

The triple, or Bart's test, carried out around 16–18 weeks, measures alpha-fetoprotein (AFP), human chorionic gonadotrophin (hCG), and oestriol. If the levels of AFP are unusually low and levels of hCG high, this indicates a higher risk for Down's and you may be offered further tests to confirm whether your baby has this condition.

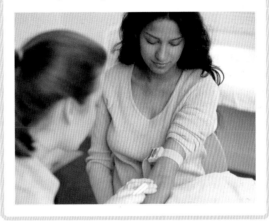

during antenatal checks to assess your health, there are also blood tests to screen for problems with the baby. Within the first 12 weeks you will be given a routine blood test to check your levels of haemoglobin, the oxygen-carrying part of blood. Although these fall slightly in pregnancy as the blood becomes more diluted, a significantly low haemoglobin level indicates iron-deficiency anaemia (see p.81). You will also have tests to identify your blood group, Rhesus factor, and rubella immunity (see p.15), and to screen for infectious diseases including syphilis, HIV, and hepatitis B. You may also be tested for sickle cell and thalassaemia, inherited blood conditions more commonly found in people of African, Caribbean, Indian, or southern Mediterranean origin.

Nuchal fold and dating scans
Ultrasound examinations

A dating scan at 10–14 weeks measures fetal growth so that a gestational age can be given. The nuchal fold scan, or nuchal translucency scan, is offered between weeks 11 and 14 and assesses the risk of Down's syndrome. Only some hospitals offer this scan at the moment. The risk of Down's syndrome rises with age. At 20 the risk is 1:1527; at 25 it is 1:1352; at 30 it is 1:1895; at 35 it is 1: 356; and at 40 it is 1:97.

What does the dating scan look for? The distance is measured from the top of the baby's head to its bottom (crown–rump measurement), and the diameter of the head is recorded, known as the biparietal diameter – the distance between the parietal bones either side of the head.

How is the nuchal fold scan done? The sonographer will measure the width of the fold of skin behind your baby's neck to see if any excess fluid has collected there. This measurement is calculated into a risk ratio based on your age. The ratio is considered high if it is above 1:300. You will be given the results of the scan immediately. If your baby has a high risk, you will be offered further tests and, depending on the results and after counselling, the choice of continuing your pregnancy with support or having a termination.

Is it reliable? The nuchal fold scan is considered to be 80 per cent accurate, which means there is a 20 per cent (1:5) chance of it being inaccurate. If your hospital offers you a blood test (PAPP-A, see p.119) with the scan, it becomes 85 to 90 per cent accurate. When the nasal bone is also measured, the accuracy rises to 95 per cent. Your local maternity unit should be able to provide you with information as to how accurate their scans are.

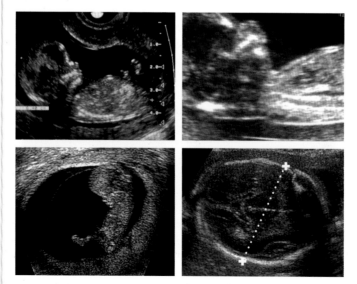

TOP FAR LEFT: In this 2-D scan taken at 12 weeks, the fetus is taking on a recognizable shape and a tiny heart is visible. **TOP RIGHT:** This fetus has a small amount of fluid behind the neck (seen as the black area at the back of the neck), which suggests a low risk of Down's. **BOTTOM FAR LEFT :** At 12 weeks, the fetus has a clearly defined profile with a prominent nasal bone. **BOTTOM RIGHT:** One of the measurements taken to plot fetal growth is the biparietal head diameter: the distance between the two head bones.

Other blood tests may be offered to screen for congenital abnormalities in the baby. Between 10 and 14 weeks, a blood test that measures the levels of the substance known as pregnancy associated plasma protein (PAPP-A) may be offered that is combined with the nuchal translucency scan (see opposite) to calculate a risk of Down's syndrome.

If first trimester Down's syndrome screening isn't available, then second trimester blood screening tests are offered, which also include screening for neural tube defects, such as spina bifida. These tests, carried out between 16 and 18 weeks, include the triple, or Bart's, test, which measures the levels of the hormones AFP, hCG, and oestriol; and the quadruple test, which, in addition to the other three hormones, measures inhibin A and PAPP-A.

Will I have a test for HIV?

All screening and diagnostic tests recommended in pregnancy are optional, so it is up to you and your partner to decide whether to have them. One of these is a blood test to check if you have the human immuno-deficiency virus, or HIV, and, indeed, some women only find out about their HIV status in pregnancy. It is worthwhile to test for HIV in pregnancy as, if the result is positive, anti-retroviral medication, careful monitoring of maternal blood levels, and careful, safe delivery of the baby can reduce the chance of transferring the infection to the baby from 40 per cent to 2 per cent.

For pregnant women with HIV, a blood test is taken around the time of delivery to measure the levels of the virus. Depending on the results of the blood test, the obstetrician will either recommend a planned Caesarean section or decide that the levels are low enough to have a normal delivery.

After the delivery, HIV-positive mothers are advised to bottlefeed, again to reduce the risk of transferring the virus to the baby.

How do ultrasound scans work?

Ultrasound scans use high-frequency sound waves – so high we can't hear them – that bounce off solid objects and create a picture, visible on a computer screen, of your baby, the placenta, and your organs in the surrounding area.

How many scans will I have and when?

All women should routinely be offered two scans: a dating scan between 10 and 14 weeks and an anomaly scan between 18 and 22 weeks. Some units routinely offer a screening scan for Down's syndrome between 11 and 14 weeks, known as the nuchal scan (see opposite), although this isn't available nationwide. You can also arrange to have private scans that may be 3D/4D (see p.124) and which you have to pay for.

I'm quite scared about my first scan. What happens during the scan and what does it feel like?

Although not painful, early scans can cause discomfort as you need a full bladder (see p.124). Ultrasound scans can be carried out by a doctor, a midwife, or a sonographer. You will lie on a couch and need to wear something that makes it easy to expose your tummy. The person doing the scan puts cold gel on the lower part of your tummy, which improves contact with the skin, making it easier to view the baby. You will feel a little pressure as a transducer is pressed against your skin and moved around to look at the baby from different angles and to take measurements. The image produced by the scan is viewed on a screen similar to a computer monitor. The person carrying out the scan may spend some time first studying the image and taking measurements before talking to you about what they can see. Although this can be unnerving, it does not mean that anything is wrong.

Some units offer a transvaginal scan in early pregnancy, which can give an improved image at this stage. This internal scan is done using a probe that is covered by a condom and gently inserted into your vagina. The image is viewed on the screen in the same way as an abdominal scan. This may be offered before 10 weeks if there is bleeding or pain.

Many units offer to print an image from the scan for you to take home. Although ultrasound scans primarily are a clinical screening tool to determine if your baby is growing and developing as expected, they are also an opportunity to see your baby for the first time and often see your baby moving even before you feel the first flutters inside your uterus. So scans become part of the developing relationship between you and your partner and the baby. In recognition of this, most units offer the facility of providing photos of the scan for a small charge to cover printing costs. Ask your community midwife whether the maternity unit where you are having your scan has this facility.

How long do scans last?

The length of time an ultrasound scan takes varies depending on the reason for the scan and the experience of the ultrasonographer.

During the dating scan, performed at around 10–14 weeks, the sonographer takes some basic measurements. This includes the measurement from the top of the head to the end of the bottom, known as the "crown–rump" measurement, used to calculate how many weeks old your baby is and

therefore your due date. This scan can take around 20–30 minutes. The nuchal fold scan (see p.118), during which the sonographer measures the fluid at the back of the baby's neck, takes around 20 minutes. Anomaly scans, performed between 18 and 22 weeks, are detailed scans that take approximately 40 minutes (see opposite). At this scan, the sonographer measures the baby and looks at physical and structural development. The size and position of the placenta are examined and the amniotic fluid around the baby is measured.

If, during your pregnancy, your midwife has any concerns about your baby's growth or wellbeing, she may refer you to an obstetrician who may recommend another scan. As this will be to identify a specific problem, such as whether there is a concern about your baby's growth, it may take a bit longer. This may be in the form of a Doppler scan, which measures the blood flow in the uterus, placenta, and umbilical cord and can help to identify growth problems in the baby. This procedure usually takes around 30 minutes.

Do I have to have scans in pregnancy?

Official guidelines are that all women should be offered two routine scans during their pregnancy, but the choice to have one is yours. As scans are screening tests to look for anything out of the ordinary, some women choose not to have any as they prefer not to know about any problems until the baby is born, or are confident that they will continue with the pregnancy regardless. You need to decide whether you fall into this category.

Can my partner come along for the scans?

There is no reason why your partner should be excluded from attending these appointments if you want him to be there and, indeed, it's very common for partners to attend ultrasound scans. For many couples, the scan is a special moment as it's the first time they get to see their baby and begin to think of themselves as parents.

MIDWIFE WISDOM

Should I have a scan?
is ultrasound safe in pregnancy?

Ultrasound scans in pregnancy, first introduced 40 years ago, have become a routine part of antenatal care.

✳ Most research indicates that they are a safe way to view the baby, even when extra scans are needed for medical reasons.

✳ Suggested links between additional scans and growth problems and dyslexia are tentative as babies scanned more often are more likely to have problems linked to other factors.

✳ Recommendations are that scans are carried out only for clinical reasons and the number done is kept to a minimum.

The 18–22 week anomaly scan
Your baby's physical examination

Also known as the fetal anomaly or anatomy scan, this detailed scan is offered to all women between the 18th and 22nd week of pregnancy. At this stage of gestation, your baby has well-developed limbs and facial features and all its major organs and body systems are in place and can be checked.

How is it done? The scan involves transmitting high-frequency sound waves through the uterus that bounce off the baby, and the returning sounds are converted into an image (see p.119). The biggest echoes are from hard tissues, such as bones, which appear white in the image on the screen, while soft tissues are grey-flecked. Fluid-filled spaces, such as the stomach, bladder, blood vessels, and amniotic fluid surrounding the baby, do not return sound waves so appear black. It is the difference between echoes and colours that enables the ultrasonographer to interpret images.

What will be checked? The ultrasonographer starts by checking the fetal heartbeat and then counts the babies – rarely, twins are not revealed until 20 weeks! She will measure the head circumference and diameter (biparietal diameter), and the abdominal circumference and the femur (thigh bone) to date the pregnancy and ensure your baby is growing well. She will check for abnormalities in the brain, face and lips, spine, abdomen, heart, stomach, kidneys, bladder, and hands and feet. Lastly, the placenta, umbilical cord, and amniotic fluid are examined. You may be able to find out the sex of your baby, although you can ask not to be given this information (see p.124).

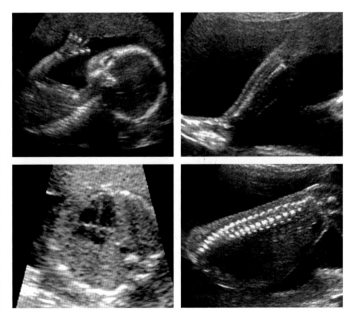

TOP FAR LEFT: This profile of a fetus at 20 weeks shows its well-developed skull and spine and clearly defined arm and hand. **TOP RIGHT:** The length of the leg bones are a good indicator of normal growth. **BOTTOM FAR LEFT:** At this stage of pregnancy, the four chambers of the heart are clearly visible in the black area on the scan. **BOTTOM RIGHT:** The spine has straightened and each vertebra is counted and checked for evidence of spina bifida.

ESSENTIAL INFORMATION: YOUR 40-WEEK JOURNEY

Diagnostic tests
Identifying fetal abnormalities

Diagnostic tests give a definitive answer as to whether or not your baby has an abnormality such as Down's syndrome. These tests are not carried out routinely and you will be offered one only if a screening test indicated that your baby had a higher risk for Down's syndrome, if you are over 35, or you have a family history that puts you at a higher risk of having a baby with an abnormality. All diagnostic tests also carry a small risk of miscarriage and you will need to weigh up the pros and cons before deciding to go ahead with one.

Chorionic villus sampling (CVS) This is a diagnostic test that involves taking a tissue sample from the placenta to identify for certain whether your baby has Down's syndrome or a genetic

abnormality. This can be done as the placenta contains the same genetic information as the baby. The test is carried out between 11 and 13 weeks. The advantage of this test is that it can be performed earlier in pregnancy than amniocentesis, so if an abnormality is found and you decide to terminate, it is early enough to have a suction termination.

How is it done? There are two procedures for CVS; one method extracts a sample of the placenta via the abdomen, and the other method carries out the procedure vaginally. With the abdominal method, a fine needle is inserted through your abdomen and, using an ultrasound scan for guidance, the doctor removes a very small sample of tissue from the placenta. You have to wait about

Chorionic villus sampling

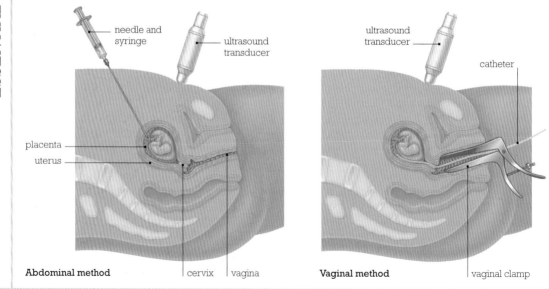

needle and syringe

ultrasound transducer

ultrasound transducer

catheter

placenta

uterus

Abdominal method   cervix   vagina

Vaginal method   vaginal clamp

10 days for the results, which means that if your baby has an abnormality and you want to terminate your pregnancy, you can do so well before you start to feel your baby kicking.

To carry out CVS vaginally, the doctor inserts a small tube through your vagina and the cervix, which then passes through the uterine wall. As with the abdominal method, the doctor then takes a small sample of tissue from the placenta, using ultrasound for guidance. The sample is sent to a laboratory, where it is grown in a culture for around seven days. The sample is then studied under a microscope to check for chromosomal abnormalities or other defects.

Amniocentesis Amniocentesis is a diagnostic test used mainly to identify a chromosomal abnormality and it is the most commonly used test for identifying Down's syndrome. During the test, a sample of amniotic fluid containing cells from the baby's system is taken from the uterus. It is a relatively quick and painless

Amniocentesis test

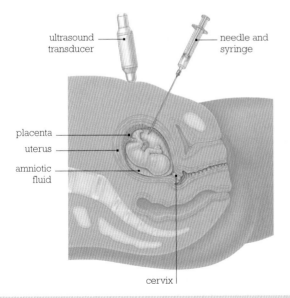

ultrasound transducer

needle and syringe

placenta

uterus

amniotic fluid

cervix

procedure and may be offered at around 16–19 weeks of pregnancy. It is offered later than CVS because there may be insufficient fetal cells in the amniotic fluid before this stage of pregnancy. The results from this procedure are usually very accurate and, although there is a slight risk of miscarriage, this is lower than the risk of miscarriage with CVS, especially in units where a large number of the tests are carried out and the doctors are particularly practised at conducting the test. Apart from the slight risk of miscarriage, the main disadvantage of amniocentesis is that it has to be carried out later in pregnancy, so if the result comes back as positive, then you will be half way or even further into your pregnancy should you decide to terminate and would need to be induced to undergo a vaginal delivery.

How is it done? Using an ultrasound scan to guide the procedure, a long, thin needle is inserted through the mother's abdomen into the amniotic sac and a small sample of amniotic fluid is extracted. This contains fetal cells, which are then grown in a culture in a laboratory to be analysed. As there is a small risk of miscarriage, you may be advised to rest for a day or two afterwards to minimize this risk. Depending on the maternity unit and the laboratories used, there may be a chance that the result could be back before the end of one week, but the majority of units still have to wait two or even three weeks. It usually takes 2–3 weeks for the fetal cells to grow. Very occasionally this does not happen and you may need to have another amniocentesis test.

Cordocentesis This diagnostic test is also known as "fetal blood sampling" or "umbilical vein sampling". In this test, blood is taken from the baby's umbilical cord to diagnose Down's syndrome when earlier screening tests have shown a possible problem. Since this is an extremely specialized procedure, it can only be carried out at a regional specialist fetal medicine centre in certain parts of the country.

Q Do you have to drink pints of water before a scan? I'm scared I'll have an accident.

For the 10–14 week dating scan, it's important to have a full bladder to make it possible to view the baby. This is because until 12 weeks the uterus stays in the pelvis and the bowel obscures the view; a full bladder raises the uterus and pushes the bowel out of the way. You may need a full bladder for a nuchal scan, between 11 and 14 weeks, depending on when it is done. Some units do transvaginal scans (a small ultrasound probe placed inside your vagina) before 10 weeks if the image from an abdominal scan is poor. In this case, you won't need a full bladder and research indicates that transvaginal scans are more comfortable in early pregnancy compared to abdominal scans. You don't need a full bladder for the 18–20-week scan, as the position of the uterus has changed.

Q I'm pregnant through IVF. Will I have more scans than normal?

It's usual to have one extra scan in an IVF pregnancy, usually carried out by the centre where you had the procedure. This scan is usually done around two weeks after the embryo has been transferred to confirm the pregnancy and make sure that the pregnancy is within the uterus rather than in a Fallopian tube (see ectopic pregnancy, p.25). Although the main purpose is to reassure you that all is well, the centre also has to inform the Human Fertilisation and Embryology Authority (HFEA) of the outcome of the IVF treatment. Once your pregnancy is confirmed, you will continue with routine antenatal care like any other pregnancy.

Q Can they really tell the sex of the baby early on? I'm 18 weeks and not sure if I want to know.

It is possible to identify the sex of a baby on routine ultrasound scans from around 20 weeks, but this is dependent on a number of factors, including the expertise of the person performing the ultrasound, the quality of the equipment being used, the position the baby is lying in, and the position of his or her legs. Even if all of these factors are favourable and the genitalia can be seen, there is an error factor, so

3D and 4D ultrasounds

Many companies now offer special scans that reveal your baby in three dimensions or moving on film or video. These 26–32 week scans can be quite expensive and are carried out for curiosity value and not for medical reasons. The quality of the pictures is usually amazing and parents are sometimes able to spot genetic similarities between themselves and their baby. However, the scan is often lengthy, which means the baby is exposed to ultrasound for longer than is normal. Also, if the baby is in the wrong position, it may be difficult to get a clear picture. The position of the placenta, the amount of amniotic fluid, and the size of the mother can also affect the quality of the pictures obtained.

MOVING PICTURES: These detailed scans offer incredible clarity, often revealing family resemblances and sometimes enabling parents to see their baby moving around, perhaps sucking its thumb, rubbing its eyes, or yawning.

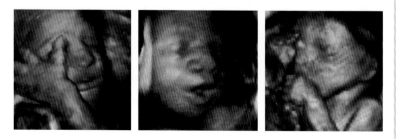

the information given about gender from a scan is never seen as 100 per cent accurate. Some research has been carried out to try and determine gender at an earlier stage, but this was even less accurate. Sometimes when you are watching the scan you may be able to see the genitalia yourself and may decide you know the sex of your baby without being told. But remember you may be wrong. If you have an amniocentesis, the sex of the baby can be definitely identified during the procedure.

Most units have a written policy only to reveal the baby's sex if this information is requested. Some units have a policy of not telling anyone the sex of the baby from scans alone, partly because they cannot be 100 per cent accurate and also because, in a small number of cases, the information about gender may lead to a request for termination. If you want to know the policy in your area, ask your community midwife.

Q I've seen lots of companies advertising scans and videos of scans – are these safe?

Many companies offer 3D scans (still pictures) and 4D scans (moving pictures copied onto video or DVD) (see opposite), and the detail in these can be very good. If you have a private scan, you should check the expertise of the person carrying out the scan, and check if the company has a referral policy to an appropriate consultant obstetrician if anything untoward is discovered, as not all companies employ the services of obstetricians or midwives.

Q There are twins in our family. When will they be able to check whether I'm having twins?

Most women find out that they are having twins at their ultrasound dating scan between 10 and 14 weeks. Very occasionally, one twin is hidden on the first scan and is seen at the second ultrasound scan, but nowadays this is less likely due to advances in scanning. Family history also gives a clue to the possibility of twins, but only if they are fraternal, or non-identical (see p.129).

Q Is everyone offered amniocentesis?

Amniocentesis is a diagnostic test (see p.123) that is routinely offered if you are over 35 and so have a higher risk of having a baby with Down's syndrome. Alternatively, you may be offered the test if your family history suggests there may be a risk of your baby having muscular dystrophy, haemophilia, cystic fibrosis, or another genetic disorder. Also, if you have had a screening test that suggests your baby has a high risk for a congenital condition, you will be offered a diagnostic test to confirm or rule it out. For example, if the nuchal scan (see p.118) showed a high risk of Down's, amniocentesis may be offered.

Q I've heard that amniocentesis carries a risk. Is this true?

Amniocentesis does carry a small risk of miscarriage. It is thought that the risk of miscarriage is increased above the normal risk by 1 per cent immediately following an amniocentesis, but after two days the risk returns to normal. You need to balance the risk against the value of the test to you and also be aware that a normal test result is not a guarantee that there will not be any other problems, but is nonetheless reassuring.

Q Can chorionic villus sampling cause miscarriage?

Chorionic villus sampling (CVS) is another diagnostic test used to establish whether a baby has Down's syndrome (see p.122). Unfortunately, as with other invasive tests, this carries a risk of miscarriage, of around 1.5–2 per cent, with the risk reducing each day. Larger hospitals carrying out more than 100 CVS tests a year may have lower miscarriage rates due to the opportunity for the doctors to fine tune their ability to carry out the procedure.

Q When is cordocentesis used?

Cordocentesis is a diagnostic test used to diagnose Down's syndrome and other problems in a baby. It can also detect infection from diseases such as toxoplasmosis (see p.45). Additionally, cordocentesis is used to detect rubella infection (see p.15), as well as to perform a blood count on a baby that is suspected of having anaemia. From 18 weeks, the baby's blood is examined using a sample of blood carefully extracted from the umbilical cord. The test is carried out in a similar way to that of amniocentesis, though results are available within 72 hours. The risk of miscarriage is 1–2 per cent.

Will I get weighed at my antenatal appointments?

In 1941, routine weighing of all pregnant women at each antenatal appointment began. Although it was thought that there was a connection between a mother's weight gain and a baby's birth weight, it was decided more recently that this is not a good indicator of when a baby is not growing, and so over the last 10 years routine weighing at each appointment has been abandoned. Furthermore, weight gain can vary from woman to woman in normal healthy pregnancies as widely as 3–18 kg (7–40lb).

Nowadays, all women are weighed once at the beginning of pregnancy and then, together with a height measurement, their BMI (body mass index) is calculated (see p.18), which helps to predict certain risk factors, for example in women who have a very high or very low BMI. The only time that you might be weighed on successive visits is if there is a medical reason to do so, for example if you had significant weight gain in a short space of time that could indicate excessive fluid retention (oedema), a sign of pre-eclampsia (see p.89).

Knowing that you are receiving such thorough antenatal care throughout your pregnancy can be deeply reassuring

My friend is 27 and has had a Down's baby – is that unusual?

Although the risk or chance of having a baby with Down's syndrome increases with age, particularly over 35, the majority of Down's babies are born to younger mothers. This is probably due to the fact that more women have their babies younger, and also because women over 35 are likely to have more tests. The risk of having a baby with Down's at the age of 20 years is 1 in 1,700. This risk increases to 1 in 1,400 by the age of 25 and by the time the mother reaches 35, the risk has increased to about 1 in 400.

My partner wants to hire a Doppler so we can listen to the baby's heartbeat. Is this a good idea?

During pregnancy, your midwife listens to the baby's heartbeat with an instrument called a Doppler sonicaid or pinard (ear trumpet). Most midwives use a sonicaid so the parents can hear the heartbeat too. This passes sound waves through the abdomen, which pick up movement and bounce it back to the machine, where it is converted into sound.

Being able to hear your baby's heartbeat during pregnancy is reassuring, especially when the earlier symptoms wear off but the baby's movements have yet to be felt. However, your baby's heart beats at a rate approximately double the rate of your heart. If the closest moving thing to the "beam" is your blood pulsating through your aorta, the sonicaid will pick this up, and if you pick up your heart rate, this might cause you anxiety. Also, depending on your gestation and the position of your baby, the heartbeat will be found in different areas on the abdomen. If you can't pick up a heartbeat, you may be unduly worried.

Midwives undergo specialist training to find the heartbeat and many won't try to find the heartbeat until the baby is around 16 weeks, and even then may have difficulty. Occasionally, due to the baby's position, they may need to call another midwife or doctor to help them locate the heartbeat.

It is up to you and your partner if you decide to hire a sonicaid, but it would be wise to be aware of the anxieties that may accompany this decision.

MYTHS AND MISCONCEPTIONS

Is it true that...

✳ You shouldn't take baths?

This isn't true. Excessive heat (above 38°C/101°F) isn't good for babies, but taking a warm bath or shower shouldn't increase your core body temperature too much. Just make sure the water isn't too hot, and avoid jacuzzis and saunas. Bathing shouldn't cause a vaginal infection either, although if your water has broken you shouldn't sit in standing water without consulting your midwife.

✳ It's not safe to exercise while pregnant?

Quite the opposite – gentle exercise throughout your pregnancy will boost your energy, keep you mobile, and relieve stress. You shouldn't start any new, vigorous activities, and avoid high-impact exercise, but walking, swimming, or antenatal yoga are ideal. Also, if you're taking an exercise class or going to the gym, make sure your instructor knows you're pregnant.

✳ Pregnant women have that "glow"... ?

Many people believe that pregnancy causes a woman's skin to glow. All the hormones produced by your body at this time may have beauty benefits, such as thicker hair and faster-growing nails. But while some may bask in a rosy glow from the increased blood volume churning through their bodies, others endure broken blood vessels and spider veins.

Twins and multiple births
we're having more than one!

We are expecting twins following IVF treatment. How will we cope?

Although finding out that you will be the parent of two babies rather than one can be a shock, the initial surprise will settle and you will soon start to get used to the idea. There are many associations that offer information and support to parents of twins, as well as companies that make products for parents of two or more children (see p.310). Your midwife and obstetrician will offer information and support and may put you in touch with local multiple birth support groups. You will also be invited for more regular antenatal appointments and scans than if you were having just one baby to keep an eye on the growth of your babies.

As with all multiple births, there are no additional financial benefits if you are having twins, although you may receive more of certain benefits that are dependent on income (see below).

We're having triplets. Help! My wife is over the moon, but I feel numb. Where can we get advice?

As having triplets is relatively rare – only 149 sets of triplets were born in the UK in 2006 – the majority of information and support for couples does relate to having twins. However, more and more research is being carried out into how to help and support parents having more than two children.

Your midwife and obstetrician will be great sources of information and will be able to put you in touch with other parents of multiple-birth children. There are also several organizations that offer support and information for parents having a multiple birth (see p.310). As you and your wife learn more about having triplets, your anxiety will hopefully start to ease.

Will we receive any additional financial or practical support as we're having more than one baby?

Unfortunately, there are no financial benefits available to all parents having twins or multiple births. However, there are some benefits that are dependent on your income, some of which you may be able to claim per baby. One of these is the Child Tax Credit, made up of three elements: a family element; an amount payable per child dependent on your joint income; and a baby element of £545 if you have one or more children under a year old. This credit is the focus of the Twins and Multiple Birth Association's current campaign, as they feel strongly that the baby element should be paid per baby, so that a family with newborn triplets would be entitled to £1635. The Sure Start Maternity Grant, a payment of £500, is payable per baby, so if you are entitled you would be able to claim £1500 for triplets. This must be claimed within three months of the birth so it is important to apply as soon as possible. For practical support, it is worth finding out about Home Start schemes in your area. Home Start is a charity that provides trained volunteers to lend support at home. Each scheme is locally based, managed, and run by individual communities, supporting families in that community.

> Being pregnant with twins means even more work for your body – so looking after yourself is more important than ever

How are twins conceived?

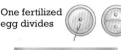

One fertilized egg divides

Two separate eggs are fertilized

Identical "monozygotic" twins are produced when a single egg is fertilized by a single sperm, and the egg then splits into two. The babies may share the membranous, or amniotic, sac that surrounds them in the uterus. Depending on when the egg splits, they may also share a placenta. Identical twins, therefore, are the same sex and look almost completely alike as they share the same genetic makeup. Non-identical, or "dizygotic", twins result when two eggs are fertilized by separate sperm at the same time and each therefore has its own individual genetic makeup. Each fetus also has its own amniotic sac and placenta.

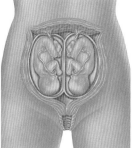

IDENTICAL TWINS: Twins conceived when one fertilized egg divides may share the same placenta in the uterus.

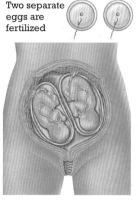

NON-IDENTICAL TWINS: Two eggs fertilized by different sperm results in non-identical twins that each have their own placenta.

Q Does taking folic acid increase the incidence of twins?

There has been some debate and conflicting studies about whether taking folic acid pre-conceptually could increase the chance of having twins. A study in Sweden in the 1990s found a higher incidence of multiple births among women taking folic acid. However, this could be attributed to other factors, such as a greater number of women undergoing fertility treatment, which carries an increased probability of twins. Also, subsequent studies have refuted these findings; in 2003, the medical journal *The Lancet* reported on a large-scale study in China that found there was no significant difference in the number of women who had taken folic acid carrying twins.

Q Are all same-sex twins identical?

No. Whether or not twins are identical depends on how they were conceived, not on what sex they are (see above). While identical twins are obviously the same sex, non-identical same-sex twins are as similar or different as any other non-twin siblings.

Q How likely is it that our twins will be identical?

One in 80 pregnant women carries twins and one-third of twins are identical. Although there are factors that make you more likely to have non-identical twins, such as a family history of twins or being over 35, having identical twins is not an inherited trait and there are no other factors that make this more likely.

Q Will I know before the birth if they are identical?

The term "zygosity determination" means finding out whether twins, triplets, or more are identical (monozygotic) or non-identical (dizygotic or fraternal). It is natural for parents to want to learn all about their babies, and with twins this includes their zygosity. As well as for reasons of natural curiosity, knowing whether twins are identical can help parents to determine the chance of having a multiple pregnancy again, and also has implications on care during pregnancy, as identical twins, especially if they share a placenta, are higher risk, and so the pregnancy may be more closely monitored.

In two-thirds of cases, the placenta provides the answer as to whether twins are identical. If the babies have a single amniotic sac surrounded by one outer protective membrane, known as the chorion, they are monozygotic. However, one-third of identical twins whose egg split early, before the placenta started to form, have two chorions with either a fused placenta, where two placentas grow together, or two separate placentas. These placentas are hard to distinguish from those of dizygotic twins.

We don't know if our twins are identical. Will it be obvious after the birth?

In a third of cases, twins are different sexes and therefore obviously non-identical. In same-sex twins, by the time the children are around two years old, their "zygosity" is usually quite clear from their physical features. Before this, there are many indications as to whether twins are identical, such as the colour of their hair and eyes, the shape of their ears, the eruption and formation of teeth, the shape of the hands and feet, and the pattern of growth.

If there is doubt as to whether twins are identical, the most accurate way to determine zygosity is by the DNA probe method, when tiny amounts of DNA are collected with a swab from inside each twin's mouth. A laboratory examines specific markers present in the DNA and 12 diagnostic targets are compared. Although non-identical twins may share five marker patterns by chance, monozygotic, or identical, twins will have the same pattern for all 12 markers.

Will I love one twin more than the other?

Although this can be a concern, it is more likely to be the case that rather than favour one child over the other, a parent gives more love and attention to the baby who needs it most at that particular time.

It is also possible that the strain of having two new babies in the house may increase the likelihood of delayed bonding, although this can also happen if the birth has been traumatic; if the mother or indeed the father is exhausted; or if one baby has taken time to establish feeding, or is more fractious than the other. This does not mean that bonding will not take

Am I likely to have a normal birth?

Although many women having twins have normal deliveries, the rate of Caesareans is increased with twin births. With one baby, the Caesarean rate is around 25 per cent in the UK; with twins, the rate is closer to 50–60 per cent, which also means that 40–50 per cent of twins are delivered vaginally. Triplets and above are generally delivered by Caesarean in the UK and Europe. Whether or not twins are born vaginally depends on their position in the womb: whether one or both twins is head down (see p.133). There may be an indication as to the type of birth in pregnancy, as women with twins are usually scanned to check the position of the babies near to term, at around 27–34 weeks.

YOUR TWINS' DELIVERY: Although there is a higher chance of a Caesarean delivery, many units are happy to let women try for a vaginal delivery if they are happy with the twins' position.

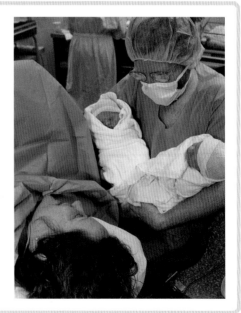

place over time, but if this is worrying you, you should mention it to your midwife or health visitor, as they may well be able to offer some helpful advice.

In every family, there are bound to be ebbs and flows of love between parents and children, which is normal and not a cause for concern. When a parent has two children born at different times, that parent may love one child differently to the other, but this does not mean that the love a parent has for one child is to the detriment of the other.

Q Will the side effects of pregnancy be much worse with a multiple pregnancy?

Although in some cases the side effects of pregnancy may be the same when you are expecting two or more babies, the likelihood is that many pregnancy symptoms will be exaggerated. Symptoms such as morning sickness, fatigue or exhaustion, disturbed sleep, and swollen hands and feet are often worse with a multiple pregnancy. Unfortunately, women with multiple pregnancies also tend to suffer more from varicose veins (see p.86). In addition to these increased side effects, weight gain is greater and more rapid for mothers carrying more than one baby and the uterus measurement is often increased for the gestational age. This extra weight and size caused by carrying two or more babies may also cause more constipation, haemorrhoids (piles), urinary tract infections, and vaginal thrush infections.

Although there may be more exaggerated symptoms with a multiple pregnancy, the majority of these problems can be monitored by your midwife or doctor, and they may be able to offer advice and treatment to ease these symptoms.

Q Will my weight gain be much greater than for someone who is having just one baby?

Mothers of twins or triplet pregnancies are likely to gain more weight than women having one baby. Indeed, in the first trimester, rapid weight gain may be an indicator of a multiple pregnancy. The increased blood volume and size of the uterus, as

---

MIDWIFE WISDOM

Getting enough rest
taking it easy with twins or more

Your whole body is under greater stress when carrying more than one baby. It's important to recognize this and take sensible measures to ensure you get plenty of rest.

✳ Try to have some time each day when you put your feet up. If you have other children, try to arrange for someone else to take them for an hour so you can relax.

✳ Get to bed earlier in the evening to give your body a break.

✳ Where possible, get someone else to help out with household chores, cooking, and shopping.

---

well as each baby's weight, possibly two placentas, and the amniotic fluid for each baby, will continue this pattern of greater weight gain during pregnancy.

Although on average a woman having a multiple pregnancy is likely to put on around 10kg (22lb) or more than a woman having one baby, this is not double the weight gain. If you are having twins, you should raise your calorie intake by only 500 calories per day in the last trimester, compared to 200 calories more for a single pregnancy.

Q I'm only 24 weeks, expecting twins, and already I've got high blood pressure. What can I do?

Unfortunately high blood pressure is more likely to start, or worsen if you already have the condition, in a twin pregnancy as the rates of pregnancy-induced hypertension (PIH) and pre-eclampsia (see p.89) are increased in multiple pregnancies.

There is little that can be done to prevent PIH. General lifestyle changes, such as reducing your salt intake, avoiding alcohol and tobacco, taking gentle, regular exercise, and getting enough rest, are thought to help. You should also ensure that you attend all your antenatal appointments and contact your midwife or doctor if you experience headaches or visual disturbances such as flashing lights or there is reduced movement from your baby.

What can go wrong if I have a vaginal delivery?

If both twins are head down, a vaginal birth is usually possible. Sometimes, the first twin may be head down and born vaginally, but the second twin may be breech. Sometimes, the second twin will turn and be head down after the birth of the first twin, and you are then more likely to deliver both twins vaginally. Studies suggest that there has been a significant increase in combined vaginal-Caesarean births of twins and a decrease in vaginal only births, which may be due to the fact that there is a greater willingness nowadays to allow women carrying twins to try for a vaginal delivery, which also increases the likelihood of this scenario. If you have a vaginal delivery, there is a greater chance of one or both twins having an assisted delivery by vacuum extraction or forceps (see p.202), either because one or both twins is positioned in a tricky way, for example facing the mother's back, or because the labour may be longer and weaker because of the amount of work involved in pushing two babies out, which means that the mother is therefore likely to be more tired and needing help at the end of labour.

Why might the doctors decide to deliver my twins by Caesarean section?

An elective Caesarean (see p.206) might be recommended for a twin delivery for several reasons, but ultimately it is your decision. The optimum time for delivering any baby is at term (37–40 weeks' gestation) and this remains the case for delivering twins as they may well be smaller than a singleton baby, having had to share your supply of nutrients. However, if one or both of the babies are compromised, possibly due to twin-to-twin transfusion syndrome (see p.134) or raised

blood pressure in pregnancy, there may be a need to deliver the babies preterm.

Many units recommend a Caesarean for a breech baby, where the baby is bottom down inside the womb, because there are more risks associated with a breech vaginal delivery. In a twin pregnancy, if the first baby is breech, this puts the second twin at risk too. Also, if the first twin is breech and the second is head first (cephalic), a Caesarean is recommended due to the rare complication of "locked" twins, when the babies' chins get locked together.

If both babies are head down and appear to be thriving, many maternity units will encourage a normal delivery. Your doctor and midwife will discuss this with you nearer the delivery time.

Will my triplets need to be delivered before 40 weeks?

Yes, it is very likely that your triplets will be delivered before 40 weeks. Although most twins are born at around 37 weeks, which is considered to be a term pregnancy, it is rare for triplets to reach term, and most are delivered at around 32–36 weeks' gestation.

As a woman's body is designed to carry one infant at a time, carrying more than one increases the risks for both mother and babies, and the decision to deliver your triplets will be taken when one or more of the babies is not coping well. To improve the chances of a good outcome, get plenty of rest and eat a healthy diet (see p.50). Although premature deliveries do carry a risk to the infant, if the baby's wellbeing is compromised an early delivery is necessary. If you go into premature labour, you may be given medication (see p.162) to try to stop labour for long enough to administer steroids, which will help to mature the babies' lungs before delivery – as long as this does not put the babies at risk.

How likely is it that my twins will have a lower than average birth weight?

Over 40 per cent of twins are born with a lower than average birth weight, which is mainly due to the fact that they are born earlier than singleton babies.

ESSENTIAL INFORMATION: YOUR 40-WEEK JOURNEY

The position of twins
How twins lie in the uterus

Twins can lie in a variety of positions in the uterus and these positions can determine how your baby will be born. One baby will always be lower than the other one, and this baby will be known as the first baby – it is closer to the birth canal and will generally be born first.

What are the possible positions? Babies can be in the head down position (cephalic) or buttocks or feet first (breech). Occasionally a baby may be lying across you diagonally, or horizontally (transverse). Twins can lie in any combination including: cephalic–cephalic, cephalic–breech, breech–breech, breech–cephalic. These positions can change throughout the pregnancy. As with a singleton pregnancy (one baby), once the presenting baby nearer to the cervix goes down into the pelvis, it will stay in that position ready for birth.

Can I have a vaginal birth? When both babies are in a cephalic position you may be offered the chance to try for a normal labour and vaginal birth. Sometimes, the first baby is cephalic and the second twin is in a breech position. If this is the case, your obstetrician may suggest that you have a Caesarean from the outset, or may suggest that you have a vaginal birth, with the doctor assisting the birth of the second twin with forceps or ventouse (see p.202) if necessary. You can certainly be party to these discussions and it's important to share your feelings about the birth and birth choices. If the first baby is breech and the second baby is cephalic, then it is highly likely that your doctor will recommend that you have a Caesarean delivery. If both your babies are in the breech position, you will almost certainly need a Caesarean, as is the case if both babies are lying across you in the transverse position.

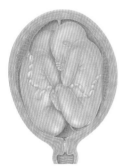 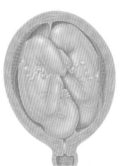 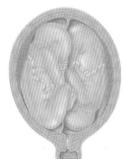

BREECH TWINS: If both babies are facing head up in a breech position, you will certainly be advised to have them delivered by an elective Caesarean.

TWINS HEAD DOWN: The most common position is for both twins to be facing head down in a cephalic position, making a vaginal birth more likely.

HEAD DOWN/BREECH: If one baby is head down and the other breech, the head down one is likely to be born first. The second baby may need an assisted birth.

A TRANSVERSE TWIN: If one baby is lying across in a transverse position, a Caesarean is likely to be recommended from the outset, especially if the babies are large.

Q Do twins run out of room to turn in the womb?

It does tend to be the case that, in the third trimester, twins find a position and settle there at an earlier stage of pregnancy than if there was just one baby. Generally, with twin pregnancies there seems to be a lot less movement in presentation from about 32–34 weeks. However, how your twins are likely to be delivered depends largely on the direction that the twin who is lowest in the pelvis is facing. If this twin is head down, then a vaginal delivery should be possible and the second twin may be able to be gently coaxed into a favourable position, or may need to have an assisted delivery (see p.202).

Q I've been told that one baby isn't developing as well as the other. What will the doctors do?

Although it is common for twins to grow at a different rate in the womb, if there is a significant difference in size, it may be that one baby is getting a greater proportion of the nutrients than the other. It is important to check that your babies are developing in line with their gestational age. It is not unusual for some babies to grow slowly and then accelerate later on, which is not a concern if it's within the accepted range of growth for their gestational age. However, if your midwife or doctor is concerned about the development of one baby, they will probably refer you to a fetal medicine specialist: an obstetrician with additional training in caring for the unborn baby. He or she may do blood tests and perform an ultrasound to assess the growth of each baby and investigate why there is a difference.

You may continue to have additional scans, known as growth scans, which will help the doctor to assess if one baby is small or growing slowly. These usually start around 26–28 weeks and continue every 2–4 weeks until your babies are due to be delivered. They look at a number of areas including the head, abdomen, and thigh bone measurements; the amount of amniotic fluid around the babies; the babies' levels of activity; the blood flow in the umbilical cord; and the position of the placentas. Your doctor should explain the findings of the scans and if there is a concern you will be closely monitored.

Q What is twin-to-twin transfusion syndrome?

This is a rare but serious condition that occurs only in identical twins who share a placenta. It is caused when there is an abnormal blood supply and a blood vessel directly connects the twins. One twin pumps blood around his own body and that of his twin and, as a result, he does not grow properly. An early delivery is usually needed to save the smaller twin.

Q Am I likely to lose one or more of my babies?

There are increased risks for both mother and babies associated with multiple pregnancies and sadly there are occasions when one or more of the babies dies in the womb. This occurs in around 2.5–5 per cent of twin pregnancies. In some circumstances, for example if there is a fetal abnormality in one twin such as a heart defect, the doctor may suggest that one or more of the babies is terminated in the very early weeks to allow the normal healthy development of the other baby or babies. However, many doctors believe that this is unnecessary as the procedure itself carries the risk of losing all the babies. Although incredibly hard, this is ultimately your decision, so you should spend time discussing the options with your doctor.

Unfortunately, the death of a baby in a twin pregnancy can sometimes cause problems for the surviving twin, although the degree and type of problem depends on whether the twins were identical or non-identical. If the twins were identical, the doctors will want to assess whether it was a monochorionic pregnancy (in which the twins share the same placenta) or a dichorionic pregnancy (in which they have a different placenta). This is because, when the placenta is shared, there is a 30 per cent risk of death or a neurological problem to the surviving twin if the other dies, whereas if there are two placentas, there is a lower risk, of 5–10 per cent, of death or disability occurring in the surviving twin.

MYTHS AND MISCONCEPTIONS

Is it true that...

 Morning sickness only happens in the morning?
Another myth is that morning sickness only lasts for the first three months. This is untrue, and morning sickness doesn't happen only in the morning; it can strike at any time of day or night. It's known as morning sickness because an empty stomach can lead to queasiness, and your stomach is usually empty when you wake up.

Having sex will hurt my baby?
It's fine to have sex in normal pregnancies. You may be advised to avoid sex if you're high risk (if you've suffered frequent miscarriages or there is a danger of early labour) but generally, sex is fine throughout. Your unborn baby is protected by the uterus, amniotic fluid, layers of muscle tissue, and pelvis, and won't be able to feel your partner's penis - so there is no need for dads to feel squeamish!

Your baby recognizes your voice?
Your developing baby can hear inside the womb, and will be very familiar with the constant background of digestive noises and maternal heartbeat. Newborn babies have been found to prefer their mother's voice to a stranger's, which suggests they recognize the mother's voice.

Do babies need all this stuff?
shopping for your baby

Q What will I need for my baby after the birth?

For hospital births, it is recommended that you pack a labour and birth bag for yourself and a bag for the newborn baby. You will need some clothes for your baby: vests and all-in-one stretchsuits, or babygrows, are easiest, especially when learning how to dress and undress your baby. If you are in hospital for several days, you will need at least three stretchsuits and vests. A baby blanket and/or a shawl can be useful and, depending on the temperature in the ward, your baby may need a hat, but be careful that she does not get too hot. Your baby needs an outdoor jumpsuit, or jacket and socks and soft booties, for when you leave hospital. Any footwear should be loose so that it does not restrict your baby's movements or circulation.

Most maternity units expect you to provide your own nappies, and one packet is usually enough. You may also need some cotton wool to clean your baby. If you choose not to breastfeed, many units provide formula milk, but this varies across units, so check what facilities are available before the birth.

You will need to have ready a baby car seat, as most hospitals won't release you without one and the law requires that your baby travels in a car seat.

Q When is the best time to buy the essentials? I'm nervous about getting anything too early.

Many parents feel superstitious about buying baby items too early, especially if it is their first baby or they have had a previous difficult experience. However, some planning is needed as you may find that by the end of your pregnancy you are too tired to shop. You should also leave enough time in case you need to exchange items. Try to buy items gradually. First, buy items that you will need for the baby after the birth; these should be ready by the 37th week of pregnancy, although many parents have these by about 34 weeks. Other essential items, such as buggies, should be in the home before the birth (see right). Once you have bought the essentials, you can purchase any additions when it suits you, which may depend on how mobile you are after the birth and your access to shops. Many parents shop online as shopping with a baby can be difficult.

Q I don't have a lot of money – do I need to buy everything new?

Having a baby does bring financial pressures and so it is sensible to acquire second-hand items, whether handed down from friends and relatives or bought. Clothes in particular are worth acquiring second-hand as babies grow out of them long before they have made full use of them and most mothers admit to buying more clothes than necessary, so quite often you can receive second-hand unused items.

One of the main items parents worry about getting second-hand is the cot mattress. Some experts believe that you should buy a new mattress with each baby to reduce the risk of cot death (see p.276), while others believe that if the mattress is clean and dry this is not necessary, so this is a matter of preference.

It's great to splash out on a couple of new items, but, equally, it's fine to opt for second-hand or handed-down baby goods

Q What do I need to consider when choosing my baby's mattress?

It is important for your baby's wellbeing that you buy a mattress that is the correct fit for your sleeping equipment. So, for example, if you are using a cot, the mattress should fit the cot properly with no gaps between the mattress and the cot sides that a baby could get stuck in. As it is also important that the mattress is clean, dry, well aired, and firm, it may be preferable to buy a new rather than second-hand mattress (see p.136).

Q My mum wants to buy us something. What can I suggest?

The gift will depend on what you need, your mother's budget, and what she would like to spend it on. You could plan a day shopping together and decide on the day, or you could browse a baby catalogue together for ideas. It also depends on whether the gift is for you and your partner, or for the baby. Good gifts for mums include underwear, nightwear, a photo frame or album, or a baby album or naming book. If your mother wishes to purchase something for the baby, this could include clothes, a baby bath, a sterilizing kit and bottles, a cot, a car seat, or a pram/buggy system.

Q Do I need a pram/travel system/buggy? Help!

Most parents are unsure about what type of transportation they will need for their baby and, as there are a number of options and types available, this can make choosing the right item difficult. You will certainly need to have some type of travel equipment for your baby and what you choose will vary depending on your circumstances. If you are mainly a car driver, you may want to consider a car seat that attaches to a pram, or a car seat and travel cot. If you intend to walk a lot, you may find a lightweight pushchair or buggy more suitable. What you choose should be practical, and within your budget, so it's worth having a look around in shops and online to compare different models.

MIDWIFE WISDOM

* Essential items
being prepared for the arrival of your baby

As well as clothes and nappies for your newborn, there are several other items that you will ideally have ready before the birth.

* A cot or Moses basket for your baby to sleep in and a clean, dry mattress.
* Suitable bedding for your newborn: either lightweight blankets and sheets or newborn baby sleeping bags.
* A pushchair or buggy to transport your baby. You may also want a sling to carry your baby around.
* A baby car seat if you are travelling with your baby in a car.

Q Is it OK to get a second-hand car seat?

Generally it is thought best not to use a second-hand car seat as you cannot be certain of its history and it may have been in an accident or damaged. Car safety experts suggest that if you must use a second-hand seat, only accept one from a family member or friend, and then only if you are absolutely certain that you know its history, that it comes with the original instructions, and it is not too old. They strongly discourage purchasing a car seat through a second-hand shop or classified advertisements.

Q Do I need to buy a cot yet, or can I start with a Moses basket?

It may help to think about the amount of space you have and where you want your baby to sleep. A Moses basket has the advantage of being small, so your baby will feel snug and may settle sooner than in a cot, and it also means that your baby can sleep beside your bed. Some models come with a rocking motion, so you can rock your baby to sleep while you are in bed. A disadvantage is that your baby will grow out of the Moses basket after a few months. Once your baby starts to sit up, there is a danger of falling out of the Moses basket as the sides are low.

At some stage you will need a cot. Although at first your baby will look small in the cot and may feel less secure, there is plenty of growing room and your baby can stay in the cot for at least a couple of years (some cots convert into beds and last even longer). Some cots are available with adjustable bases, making it easier for you to put your baby into and lift her out of the cot. You will need a bigger space for the cot, which ideally will be in the baby's bedroom.

What bedding do I need?

Most parents choose sheets and blankets. Cotton sheets can be used in layers along with a blanket, so that you can add or remove layers to keep your baby at the right temperature. If your baby sleeps in a Moses basket or carry cot, you should buy sheets designed specifically for these. It is important to get the right fit so that your baby is not too exposed or too covered up. Nowadays, many parents opt for baby sleeping bags (see below). If you use a sleeping bag, you will still need a few bottom sheets for the cot.

What are the pros and cons of baby sleeping bags?

Baby sleeping bags, also known as grow bags, baby sacks, or sleep sacks, have been around for 25 years, but recently have become more widely used (see p.280). They can be used without other bedding with the baby in a vest and sleepsuit. Many parents prefer these as they keep the baby covered, regardless of how active they are during sleep, which in turn helps the baby feel secure. However, the Foundation for the Study of Infant Deaths warns that you should avoid over-sized bags as a baby could slide down inside, and although they can be used for newborns, some manufacturers recommend waiting a few weeks or months before using one to avoid this risk.

Which baby monitor should I choose?

Baby monitors first appeared in the UK in the early 1980s and today there are over 400,000 on the

Baby clothing

When buying clothes for your newborn, bear in mind that babies grow very quickly, so buy just a few items in smaller sizes. Choose easy-to-clean, machine-washable natural fabrics and avoid fussy styles with ribbons or tricky openings, opting instead for easy-to-use poppers. Essential clothing items for your newborn include:

✻ 3 or 4 vests.
✻ 4 or 5 all-in-one sleepsuits, or babygrows, with front-opening poppers.
✻ A snowsuit or jacket for outdoors, or a cardigan for warmer months.
✻ A woolly hat in the winter months and a light hat for your baby in the summer.
✻ Loose-fitting bootees or cotton socks.
✻ A blanket or shawl for outdoors.

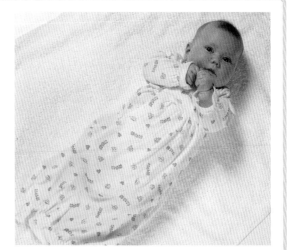

PRACTICAL CLOTHING: All-in-one sleepsuits are perfect for newborns, providing easy access for nappy changing and keeping your baby well covered.

Hold a baby shower –
invite friends over to
celebrate the forthcoming
arrival and make some
helpful gift suggestions!

market, so choosing one can be daunting. Although monitors vary, they have the same basic component – a minimum of two units: one to transmit your baby's sounds and one that stays with you so that you can monitor your baby. Additional features include dual channels, a moving lights-sound display, a sensor pad, low power and an out-of-range warning, the option to use mains or batteries, a talk-back function, and a temperature sensor. If they all have these features, it is down to personal choice and cost.

Should I buy disposable nappies?

Although many parents opt for disposable nappies as they find them more convenient, particularly when out and about, nowadays many people look for a more eco-friendly alternative, as disposable nappies, dumped in landfill sites, may take hundreds of years to decompose. Also, it is estimated that it costs parents about £2000 to use disposable nappies for each child. You may want to investigate the different options (see p.140).

What baby changing items do I need apart from nappies?

You need a waterproof changing mat that wipes clean. Some parents use warm water and cotton wool to clean their baby's genital area and bottom, or you can use baby wipes. You may also want to use a cream to prevent nappy rash. As well as the essentials, you could buy some oils (see p.219) and use changing time to massage your baby's skin.

Should we put a dimmer switch in the nursery?

The benefit of a dimmer switch is that you can control the lighting, so that your baby's eyes can adjust slowly. However, a dimmer switch is not essential, as long as you have access to a soft light, such as a lamp or mobile that can project light.

Should we buy a baby bath or can she use our big bath?

A baby bath is useful as you can use it in any room. Most parents are a bit apprehensive when they first bathe their baby, and even experienced parents say that it can be tricky to hold a wriggling baby safely while trying to wash them, so using a smaller baby bath helps you to develop confidence. For newborns, a washing-up bowl can also suffice. However, a baby outgrows a baby bath by around six months and the bath can take up a lot of storage space. Once your baby can sit up, at around four to six months, you could use a bath seat in your main bath, or enjoy a bath together as long as you keep the water tepid.

I want to breastfeed, but should I buy some bottles just in case?

The problem with having bottles to hand is that it may weaken your resolve to breastfeed, and evidence shows that women are more likely to continue breastfeeding if they do not have an alternative readily available. Having said that, if you wish to give your baby some water, or to start expressing once you are breastfeeding confidently, then you will need some bottles.

I plan to bottlefeed. What do I need to get in advance?

You will need plastic bottles (teats are included), a sterilizing unit or kit, which often has everything you need, and your preferred formula. Each comes in a range of options, so you need to decide what works best for you. As you get to know your baby, you may have to change the type of teat and/or formula, so it is not advisable to buy too many before the birth. There is a range of sterilizers available (see p.239).

Eco issues
Raising a "green" baby

An eco-aware approach to raising your children can be healthier for them, for you, and for the planet. It can even, as is the case with reusable nappies, save you money. This environmentally friendly approach need not just extend to nappies – it can also include choosing organic baby clothes, wooden toys, organic baby foods, and buying second-hand.

Why is nappy choice so important?

Disposable nappies can have an impact on the environment. This can range from the materials that are used to make the nappies to the chemicals released as they decompose. Equally, the distribution chain to retailers carries a large "carbon footprint". Disposable nappies contribute to landfill waste and one baby's nappies can account for a large proportion of the total weekly household waste. It is thought that one baby will use approximately 5,000 nappies a year, which means that up to 36 million nappies are used each year in the UK alone.

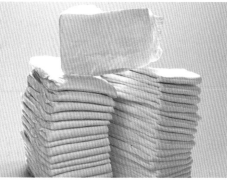

DISPOSABLE NAPPIES: Although convenient to use, disposable nappies are costly – for you and for the environment.

What happens to a used disposable nappy?

Dirty disposable nappies (or "solid waste") can contain the live Polio virus for up to six weeks, produce methane, and contribute to global warming. Nobody knows how long it takes for nappies to decompose, but it is thought that it could take up to 500 years. They can be incinerated, but this releases carcinogenic dioxins into the atmosphere. If the nappies are flushed down the toilet, the toilet can get blocked as the liquid-absorbing material in the nappy expands; if they do get through the sewerage system the sea will become polluted. This in turn has a knock-on effect on the flora and fauna of the oceans, one of the greatest buffers of our planet. Each disposable nappy uses a cup of crude oil to make and it is estimated that 41 trees are needed in total per baby, making a total of 7 million trees being used for nappies alone in the UK each year.

What is the alternative to disposables?

Reusable nappies do not contribute to the landfill problem. Although their washing can have an environmental impact, if an A-grade washing machine is used (at a temperature of lower than 60°C/140°F), and the nappies are line-dried, there is much less environmental impact. This particularly applies if non-bleached nappies and liners are used and natural products such as white vinegar and bicarbonate of soda are used to wash and soften the nappies. When cotton-based nappies are used, there are eight times fewer regenerable materials used and 90 times fewer renewable resources. They also produce 60 times less solid waste.

What other ways are there to go green? As

well as opting for a greener nappy, there are plenty of other ways to choose environmentally friendly

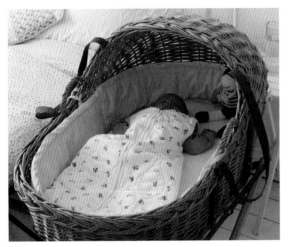

BUYING "GREEN" FOR YOUR BABY: Eco-friendly choices for your baby could include organic cotton baby clothes and a natural wicker crib.

products for your baby. Once your baby starts on solids, try to buy non-processed fresh food (ideally in season and locally produced), and consider organic products. Concern about pesticides has led to the creation of a wide range of organic baby food outlets. Organic food products have a smaller "carbon footprint", primarily because they don't use chemical fertilizers. Also consider buying second-hand or nearly-new items for your baby – clothing, pushchairs, and toys, for example. Another way to help the environment is to wash your baby's clothes at a lower temperature (30°C/86°F), which uses less electricity, and to dry them on the washing line rather than using a tumble drier. When cleaning your baby, use organic cotton wool and water or a soft flannel rather than baby wipes and, if you do use disposable nappies, avoid using perfumed nappy bags. When buying toys, opt for wooden rather than plastic.

Breast is best for the environment

Breastfeeding your baby is not only better for her, but also better for the environment. Using formula milk has an impact through everything from the packaging of the product to your use of the kettle and sterilizer every time you make up a bottle. It is even thought that, if all the women in the UK breastfed their babies, the absence of their periods would result in a saving of thousands of tonnes of paper-based sanitary products each year!

"Greener" options

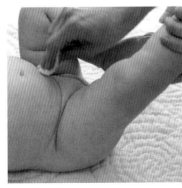

CLEANING YOUR BABY: Organic cotton wool is kind on a baby's skin and best for the environment.

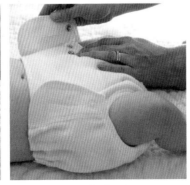

NAPPY CHOICES: Opting for reusable nappies avoids adding to non-biodegradable waste.

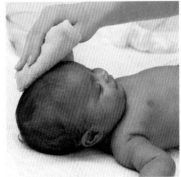

GENTLE WASHING: Using a soft flannel on your baby's skin is preferable to harsher, throwaway baby wipes.

The end of pregnancy
what to expect

Q When will I start my antenatal classes and what types are there?

Antenatal, or parent education, classes start around 32 weeks and, if you are attending classes run by your local NHS trust, are free. The classes may run for 4–6 weeks, or some trusts have a monthly afternoon session. Some hospitals provide women-only classes, evening or weekend classes, and yoga and pilates classes (see p.60). There are also private, or independent, midwives in most areas who may offer antenatal classes on a one-to-one or small group basis.

Antenatal classes are also available from the National Childbirth Trust (NCT), run by trained NCT teachers. Classes are usually held in the evenings, making them more accessible to partners and friends, and they often provide ongoing postnatal support for up to six months after the birth. There is a fee, although in some cases a reduced fee or assisted places may be offered.

Aquanatal classes are also popular. These are gentle exercises in the swimming pool along with other pregnant women, and often the teacher is a midwife who also provides antenatal information. Also many obstetric physiotherapists run relaxation and breathing technique sessions; your hospital antenatal clinic may have information on these.

Q What will I learn in my hospital antenatal classes?

Antenatal classes usually cover a different topic each week, including the physical changes that occur in pregnancy; the three stages of labour; hospital, home, and water births; pain relief, which should include breathing and relaxation techniques; breastfeeding; postnatal care of the baby; and changes in your relationships. The most popular topics tend to be the stages of labour and pain relief, along with a tour of the maternity unit.

Q Is it useful to learn and practise breathing and relaxation exercises before the birth?

Preparation before labour and delivery is beneficial for most women and their partners, and breathing and relaxation techniques in particular help you to focus on your breathing, which in turn can help you to feel less tense and increase your confidence for dealing with the contractions. Antenatal classes teach you specific techniques and antenatal yoga (see p.60) also helps you to gain control through breathing.

Q Should I practise positions for labour and birth beforehand?

Practising for labour is a good idea as you may find some positions suit you and others don't (see below). This information can be documented in a birth plan (see p.149) so that it is available for your midwife to discuss with you. It's also good for your partner to know your preferred positions during labour.

Q Do you have any suggestions for labour positions?

Some popular positions for labour are:
* **Leaning on a work surface** or the back of a chair. Putting your arms round your partner's neck or waist to lean against.
* **Leaning on to the bed** in the delivery room.
* **Kneeling on a large cushion or pillow** on the floor and leaning forwards on to the seat of a chair.
* **Sitting astride a chair** and resting on a pillow placed across the top.
* **Sitting on the toilet**, leaning forwards, or sitting astride, leaning on to the cistern.
* **Kneeling on all fours**.
* **Kneeling on one leg** with the other bent.
* **Rocking your hips backwards and forwards** or in a circle; this can also be done using a birthing ball. All of these positions can make your contractions

Breech presentation

Breech position is when your baby is bottom first instead of head first. Breech babies lie in one of three positions: a flexed, or "complete", breech, when the hips are bent, the thighs against the chest, and the knees bent with the calves against the back of the thighs and feet above the bottom; an extended, or "frank", breech when the hips are flexed, or bent, the thighs against the chest, and the feet by the ears; and a "footling" breech, like a flexed breech, but the hips aren't so bent and the feet are below the bottom. If your baby is breech at term, your doctor may recommend delivery by Caesarean section.

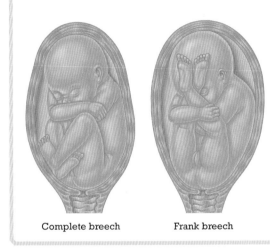

Complete breech　　　　Frank breech

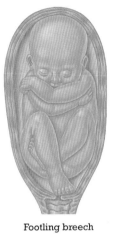

Footling breech

FAR LEFT: With a complete breech, where the knees are bent and the feet are above the bottom, a vaginal birth may be possible.
MIDDLE: A frank breech position, with the legs up in front of the body, is most favourable for a vaginal birth.
LEFT: If your baby is in a footling breech, with the feet below its bottom, you will probably be advised to deliver your baby by elective Caesarean.

more efficient and help you feel in control. When you are in strong labour, you may find that you don't want to move around much and will find a position that suits you. If possible, keep rocking, leaning forwards during contractions, and straightening up in between. If you get tired, lie down on your left-hand side, rather than propped up on your back, which stops the pelvis being able to open effectively. Lying on your left side is much better for your baby than lying on your back because he receives more oxygen, and the contractions are still effective in this position. If you feel rested after a while, push yourself up with your hands into a sitting position and get up again.

I'm 36 weeks and my baby is breech. Is this a concern?

Breech position is when your baby is bottom first instead of head first (see above). Quite a lot of babies sit in the breech position in pregnancy and there is still a chance your baby will turn. It's not until about 37 weeks that your midwife or doctor will focus on your baby's position.

Is there anything I can do to help my baby turn?

If your baby is breech towards the end of pregnancy, there are some exercises you can try in an attempt to turn your baby. A "knee-chest" position can help. To do this, kneel on your bed with your bottom in the air and your hips bent at just over 90 degrees. Try to keep your head, shoulders, and upper chest flat on the mattress. Adopt this position for 15 minutes every two waking hours for five days. If you feel nauseous or light-headed, do not continue. Positions in which the buttocks are elevated can also help, and sleeping with a pillow under your buttocks or kneeling on all fours so the weight of your pregnancy is unsupported may help. You can combine "all fours" positions with household chores, such as cleaning the floor. If these are not successful, there are other ways to try to turn your baby (see below).

Q I've heard about doctors "turning" breech babies. How does this work?

Some obstetricians may try to turn a breech baby in late pregnancy, known as external cephalic version (ECV), which has a success rate of around 50 per cent. During an ECV, an obstetrician gently moves your baby by pressing his hands on your abdomen, using an ultrasound as a guide. You may be given a drug to relax the uterine muscles. You will be scanned first and if the baby is in an awkward position the procedure may not continue. Also, if your baby is large this can affect the procedure, as can the amount of fluid around the baby, as a low amount of fluid offers less protection to the baby. If you are Rhesus negative, you will have an injection of anti-D after the ECV (see p.79) because of a small risk of a bleed around the placenta. An ECV is not recommended if you have a multiple pregnancy, have had bleeding in pregnancy, your placenta is low-lying, your membranes have ruptured, or there is a known problem with the baby.

The procedure is not without risk and some think it only works with babies who would have turned anyway. If your baby remains breech, a Caesarean may be advised, although some obstetricians are willing to try a vaginal delivery. You are not obliged to have an ECV and should discuss your options.

Finally, a form of acupuncture called "moxibustion" is sometimes used, whereby a fragrant herb is held over an acupuncture point, the aim being to relax the uterine muscles to help the baby turn. Talk to your doctor or midwife before trying this and seek advice from a qualified acupuncturist.

Q What triggers labour?

While there are many theories, no one really knows what triggers labour. One is that the mother's pituitary gland secretes oxytocin, the hormone that stimulates contractions, when the baby is ready to be born. Others now believe that the baby starts labour by sending a signal to the mother's body. One theory is that a baby's lungs secrete an enzyme when they are developed that causes a substance called prostaglandin, which triggers contractions, to be released into the mother's body. Another theory is that, when the baby is ready to be born, its adrenal glands produce hormones; these cause hormonal changes in the mother that start labour.

Q I don't want to go overdue. How can I help labour to start?

Various methods have been tried, although none is proven. Popular methods include having sex, as the prostaglandins in semen are similar to the ones used to induce labour; stimulating your breasts to trigger the release of the hormone oxytocin, which stimulates the uterus; eating spicy food to bring on a loose bowel movement, thought to stimulate labour (see p.48); and taking long walks to help the baby move down in the pelvis and put pressure on the cervix. Homeopathic remedies are also available; consult a registered practitioner for advice.

Q I've heard that raspberry leaf tea can start labour. Is this true?

Unfortunately this is a misconception as raspberry leaf tea doesn't actually help to bring on labour, but it may help to reduce the length of labour. In a study in Sydney, 192 first-time mums were given either a 1.2g raspberry leaf tablet or a placebo twice a day from 32 weeks. The tablet had no harmful effects, and the women who had taken the supplement had a shorter second stage of labour and a lower rate of assisted delivery (19.3 per cent to 30.4 per cent).

Raspberry leaf tea contains an alkaloid, "fragine", said to strengthen and tone uterine muscles, helping them to contract more efficiently. You should start taking raspberry leaf tea during the last eight weeks of pregnancy. At 32 weeks, you could have one cup of raspberry leaf tea a day, gradually increasing to four cups or tablets a day (depending on the strength of the blend). The tea can be sipped in labour, too.

ESSENTIAL INFORMATION: YOUR 40-WEEK JOURNEY

Fetal positions
Your baby in the uterus

Your baby can lie within your uterus in many different positions. Your midwife or doctor will palpate your abdomen (gently feel your tummy) to identify which way your baby is lying. There are two main positions in which your baby will lie: with his head downwards (cephalic presentation) or with his buttocks downwards (breech presentation). Occasionally your baby will lie across your uterus in a transverse position or even diagonally across you in an oblique position, particularly if there is too much fluid around the baby or you have had several babies previously. In about 17 per cent of cases, the midwives and doctors do not identify a breech presentation until the labour itself.

What is LOA and ROA? Once your midwife has identified how your baby is lying, she will also try to determine whether the baby is lying on your right or left side. The midwife will track where

your baby's back is, and you will generally feel kicks on the opposite side. The midwife will describe your baby as being LOA or ROA, which stands for left or right occipital anterior – the occiput being the back of your baby's head facing forwards, so your baby is actually facing backwards. These are the best positions for your baby to lie in for labour.

What if the baby isn't anterior? Sometimes babies lie in a posterior position, which means that their back is lying against your back and they are looking upwards. This position may prolong your labour, which can be tiring. If this is the case, you can try the same exercises for turning a breech baby (see p.143) to encourage your baby to turn to be in an anterior position towards the end of pregnancy. Sometimes your baby will only turn with the help of strong, effective contractions when you are in fully established labour.

Your baby's position

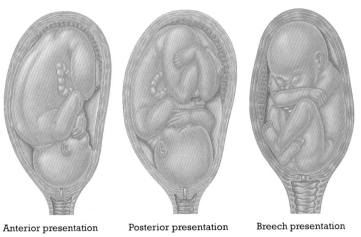

Anterior presentation   Posterior presentation   Breech presentation

FAR LEFT: An anterior position, with the head down and the back facing the mother's abdomen, is the best position for birth.
MIDDLE: A posterior position, when the baby's back faces the mother's back, can prolong labour and increase the chances of an assisted birth.
LEFT: With a breech baby, delivery by Caesarean may be suggested.

What is the "nesting instinct" and is this just a myth?

The nesting instinct is a well-documented natural phenomenon. In the final weeks of pregnancy, many women have an uncontrollable urge to clean their house and to prepare and make the "nest" safe for the new arrival. This is a primal instinct and females of the animal kingdom are all equipped with this need. Just as birds make their nests preparing for their young, mothers-to-be do exactly the same.

The act of nesting puts you in control and gives a sense of accomplishment. You may also become a homebody and want to retreat into the comfort of your home and familiar people. The nesting urge can be an indicator that labour is not too far away. If you have the energy, take advantage and get on with tasks that you won't have time for after the birth.

Is it true that first babies are often late?

Birth normally occurs at a gestational age of 37 to 42 weeks and, while it certainly isn't the case that all first babies are late, many do arrive after the predicted due date. From the point of view of waiting, if you approach the end of your pregnancy expecting your baby to be a couple of weeks late, then you may avoid feelings of frustration. It is worth considering that your body has never done this before and that your "due date" is an estimate; the majority of babies do not arrive on this date.

I'm 39 weeks and my baby's head isn't engaged. Should I be worried?

Not all babies engage into the pelvis before the beginning of labour. It is likely, from about 36 weeks onwards of your pregnancy, that you may experience your baby moving lower down in your abdomen, causing your baby's head to enter the pelvis. This process is known as "engagement" and simply means that the leading part of the baby has "engaged" the pelvic brim (see p.148). This is normal and helps to position your baby in preparation for the birth later on.

Engagement often happens earlier with first babies because the uterine muscles have not been

Your hospital bag

Although hospital visits tend to be short, with many women staying around 24 hours or less after a normal delivery, you will need a few essential items. Many mums have a bag for themselves and one for the baby, while others organize a labour bag and postnatal bag for mum and baby. It's up to you. Basic requirements include:

✳ Clothing for labour (including socks and/or footwear).
✳ Nightwear.
✳ Toiletries.
✳ A towel, sanitary pads, disposable pants, and a bra.
✳ Music, books, and magazines, as well as money, telephones, phone numbers, and cameras.
✳ A food bag with nutritious snacks to keep you going.

For your baby you will need:
✳ Clothing, cleaning materials, and some clothes for returning home.
✳ Nappies (check with your midwife if the hospital provides these or whether you need to supply your own).

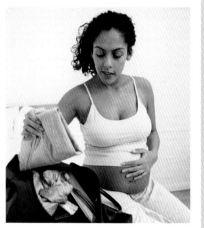

PACKING YOUR BAG: Getting your bag ready well in advance of your due date can be reassuring, helping you to feel prepared and ready for labour.

MYTHS AND MISCONCEPTIONS

Is it true that...

✳ The eighth month is the worst?

Another popular myth is that by the eighth month of pregnancy women start feeling cranky and get irritable. However, the truth is that due to high levels of oestrogen – which can rev up your libido – some women actually feel great.

✳ Men can't feel your pain?

This is untrue. The father of your baby is probably as concerned about the pregnancy as you are. Encourage him to share fully in the pregnancy – go to antenatal classes together and let him talk or sing to the baby and feel your stomach when the baby kicks!

✳ I should eat for two?

Not true! The average pregnant woman, with one baby, needs to add about 200–300 extra calories a day. Dieting is not a good idea during pregnancy, but it's also unwise to eat junk food or to put on too much weight. Just try to follow a nutritious balanced diet, and eat when you're hungry.

Engagement

Engagement is when your baby's head starts to move down into the pelvic brim in preparation for birth, and this can occur any time from around 36 weeks until the start of labour. In the last weeks of pregnancy, your midwife will palpate your abdomen to see if the head has started to engage. The degree to which a baby's head is engaged is measured in fifths. If three- or four-fifths of the head can be felt above the pubic bone, then the baby is not engaged. If only two-fifths of the head can be felt, then the baby is said to be fully engaged, and if just one-fifth is felt, the baby is recorded as being deeply engaged.

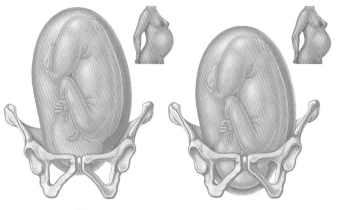

NOT ENGAGED: The baby's head has started to move down into the pelvis, but more than two-fifths of the head can be felt above the pelvic brim.

ENGAGED: The baby has dropped down into the pelvis in preparation for birth and you may notice a change in the shape of your bump.

previously stretched and so they tend to exert more pressure on the baby, moving it down into the pelvis earlier; whereas a second or third baby may not become engaged until your labour actually starts. When your baby's head engages can also depend on other factors, such as the position in which your baby is lying within the womb (see p.145) and the shape of your pelvis.

Am I likely to feel any different once my baby's head has engaged?

Many women report feeling more physically at ease following the engagement of their baby's head as there is a release of pressure within the abdomen. As a result, you may find that it feels easier to breathe, sleep, and walk around.

On the other hand, sometimes when the baby's head engages this can increase the pressure on your bladder and you may experience a sensation of fullness and pressure between your legs. Many women also report shooting vaginal pains. Engagement is also likely to affect bowel sensations.

My midwife mentioned checking the position of the placenta. Is this normal?

This is not routine, but if your 20-week scan indicated that the placenta was low-lying, known as placenta praevia (see p.92), your midwife would suggest a further scan at 34 weeks to see if the placenta had moved up and away from the cervix.

My baby isn't moving so much now – should I be worried?

There is some natural reduction in the range of your baby's movements towards the end of pregnancy as he has less room to stretch his limbs. However, you should still be familiar with your baby's pattern of movement in later pregnancy as this is a good indicator of your baby's health and is just as important as the number of movements a day (see p.103). You may find at this stage that your baby is developing a pattern for waking and sleeping, often different to yours, so your baby may be awake when you go to bed and may start kicking. Or your baby may get the hiccups and you will feel the jerk of each hiccup, a sign that your baby is preparing for life after delivery. If your baby's movements have reduced or stopped, contact your maternity unit. You could also try things like having a cold or hot drink, having a bath or shower, or massaging your tummy. A formal assessment may be recommended and if there are concerns, you will be asked to make a conscious effort to increase your awareness of when your baby moves. There should never be fewer than 10 individual groups of movements a day between 9am and 9pm. Some areas have walk-in antenatal day units (ANDU) where you can have a cardiotograph (see p.192) to record your baby's movements.

Q I'm practically incontinent. Is there anything I can do to stop this?

During pregnancy, many women find that they leak urine slightly when they cough, laugh, exercise, bend over, or lift something. This is known as stress incontinence. The pelvic floor muscles are under strain during pregnancy as they have to support the weight of your growing uterus and cope with the changes caused by pregnancy hormones. As a consequence, a sharp increase in abdominal pressure when you cough and so on may be too much for the muscles to hold back the flow of urine. Stress incontinence may happen at any time in pregnancy, but is more common towards the end.

The best treatment for incontinence is regular pelvic floor exercises to keep the muscles toned (see p.57). Taking some gentle exercise each day can also help and, although you may not make a full recovery during pregnancy, regular exercise now will minimize the problem and help you towards a full recovery after your baby is born. Stress incontinence is often worse for a few days following the birth, when the muscles of the pelvic floor and other structures are recovering. If it does not get better after this time, talk to your health visitor or doctor as you should not have to suffer long term without help.

Ask your midwife to refer you to your obstetric physiotherapist, who can review the problem and offer you advice and monitoring.

Birth plan
Stating your preferences for labour and birth

The purpose of a birth plan is to communicate your wishes for labour and birth.
Your plan can be as detailed or as brief as you like. Do bear in mind that circumstances may dictate that not all of your preferences are met. Discuss this plan with your midwife before the birth. Here are some suggestions of what to include:

✱ You may want to state who your birth partner will be, whether you want more than one birth partner, and if you want them present throughout.

✱ You could include your preferences for managing labour pain. Do you want to labour naturally (maybe using a birthing pool), or do you have a preferred type of medical pain relief?

✱ You can state which positions would you like to use in the different stages of labour? Do you want to be active in the first stage, and in which position would you prefer to deliver your baby?

✱ Do you have concerns about being strapped to a fetal monitor? If so, do you want to request that this be done intermittently only?

✱ State your preferences for after the birth. Do you want your baby delivered on to your tummy, and how soon do you want to breastfeed?

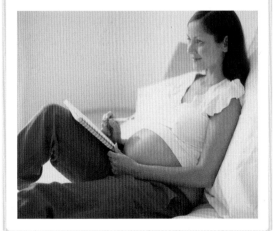

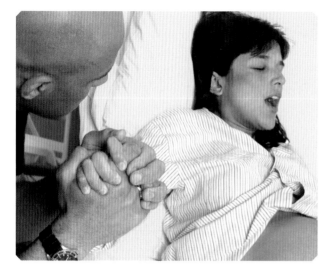
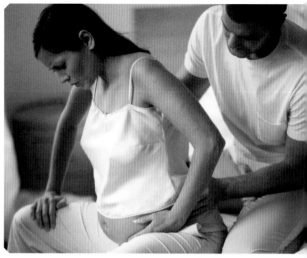
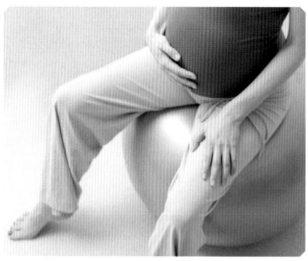
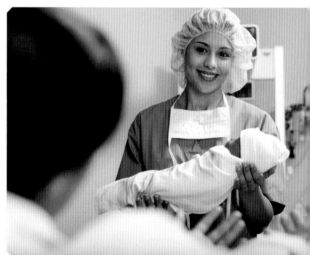
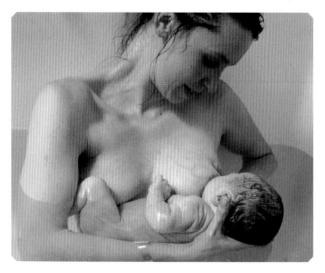
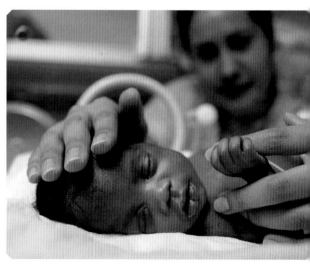

Labour
and birth

 Where should I give birth?
home or hospital?

 My baby isn't due yet!
premature births

 How will I know I'm in labour?
the signs of labour

 It's all your fault, stop the pain!
choices for pain relief

 How long will it last?
all about labour

 Why isn't the baby out yet?
assisting the birth

 They said I need a Caesarean
all about Caesarean births

Where should I give birth?
home or hospital?

Q Do I have options for where I can give birth?

Yes you do. Choosing where to have your baby is a personal choice and knowing all the relevant facts can help you to make an informed decision. You can contact an organization called BirthChoiceUK for more information (see p.310) and talk to your midwife and other mothers in your area to widen your perspective. Where you live will affect your choice, as will the decision to have NHS care, go to a private hospital, or hire an independent midwife, who can arrange to deliver your baby in the local maternity unit. If your pregnancy has been straightforward, you should be offered the option of delivering your baby at home, in a birthing centre (if one is available in the vicinity), in a hospital birthing unit (see p.154), or in the hospital obstetric unit itself.

Q Is it safe to have my baby at home?

Research has shown that for healthy women who have had a normal pregnancy, a planned home birth attended by an experienced caregiver is as safe as giving birth in hospital. There are similar findings for birth centres and GP units. Statistically, women who have home births are less likely to use drugs to cope with the pain and less likely to have an assisted delivery or Caesarean, even if they have to be transferred to hospital during labour. They are also more likely to use upright positions for giving birth compared to hospital births. Likewise, women who give birth in a birthing centre (see p.154) are less likely to use drugs for pain relief and less likely to have their labour speeded up artificially. They are also more likely to be satisfied with the care they receive.

Q Can I choose which hospital to give birth in or does it have to be the one nearest to me?

Although, technically, you have a right to choose any hospital in which to give birth, you should consider the practicalities of distance for attending antenatal appointments and scans at the hospital you choose, as well as thinking about how far you want to travel while in labour. A local facility is therefore probably the most sensible choice. You may have a variety of services nearby, including hospitals, GP units, or birthing centres. Discuss all your options with your midwife and doctor and try to talk to other mothers locally to see if they have recommendations.

Q My pregnancy hasn't been straightforward. Will I have to give birth in hospital?

There are several reasons why you may be advised to deliver in hospital. If this is a second baby and there were complications before, such as bleeding in pregnancy or a Caesarean, your midwife might suggest you deliver in hospital. Or if this is your first baby and there are complications, such as diabetes or high blood pressure, or it is a multiple pregnancy, you may be advised to have your baby in hospital.

Visualize your dream birth and work towards making this a reality – whether a home birth, or creating a calm environment in your hospital birthing room

ESSENTIAL INFORMATION: LABOUR AND BIRTH

Home birth
Planning a birth at home

Although only around two per cent of women in the UK choose to give birth in their own home, this number is increasing. Research has shown that mothers may have shorter and less painful labours in their own home. It is not known why this is, although it may be due to them feeling more confident and comfortable in their surroundings. You will generally have at least one midwife with you constantly once you are in established labour during a home birth. Many women hire a pool for use during labour at home, and this may progress to a water birth.

Will I be allowed a home birth? If your pregnancy has been classed as "low risk" – you are healthy and have not had any complications in this or any previous pregnancies – then a home birth is a definite option. If you desire a home birth and have experienced some complications during the pregnancy, talk to your midwife or contact a Supervisor of Midwives at your local maternity unit who will be able to advise you.

How do I plan for a home birth? If your midwife is happy for you to deliver at home, you need to talk to her about the type of home birth you wish to have, for example do you want a water birth (see p.156) or to use a birthing ball, and how do you plan to manage the pain? If you would like a water birth, you will need to hire a birthing pool in advance. You may want to set up a special area in your home to have your baby, which ideally should be near bathroom facilities. Plastic sheeting and old sheets are advisable to protect your flooring, and shower curtains make a good surface for giving birth. You will also need a supply of dustbin bags for waste.

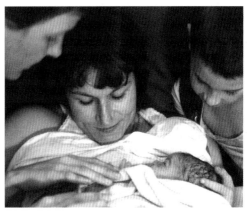

A HOME DELIVERY: Having your baby at home can be a relaxed and intimate experience, giving you control over your environment and allowing siblings to see the new baby straight after the birth.

What will happen? Most community midwives carry a homebirth pack with them, which they will bring along when you go into labour. The kit includes a blood pressure monitor; a stethoscope and/or sonicaid; a thermometer; gloves; a gas and air cylinder; pethidine; scissors; antiseptic solutions; and emergency equipment. Some midwives like you to provide towels and plastic sheets. You can use your TENS machine, and the midwife will arrange for gas and air (Entonox) to be delivered. The midwife can also ask your doctor or obstetrician to prescribe pethidine or diamorphine if you wish.

What if there is a problem? If the midwives are concerned about you or your baby's health, they will discuss this with you and it may be necessary to transfer you to hospital. This transfer is usually done by ambulance, accompanied by paramedics, your midwife, and your birth partner.

Q What additional things do I need to think about if I'm having a home birth?

It may be worth having all the items you need for the labour and birth gathered in the place you intend to deliver, and it can also be helpful to organize your items separately from the baby's items. As well as practical items, such as clothing, toiletries, and sanitary pads, you may also want to have to hand music, phone numbers, and a camera. It's a good idea to have a well-stocked fridge to ensure that you have nutritious snacks to hand during labour, as well as helping you and your partner in the first few days after the birth. Your baby will need nappies, cotton wool, vests, clothing, sheets, and blankets. If you have other children, you may need to make arrangements for them with family, friends, or neighbours, or have meals planned for them in advance and plenty of activities to occupy them.

Even though you are planning a home birth, there are occasions when things don't go quite as you wish and you need to be transferred to hospital. This can happen before, during, or after labour and so, even though you may not wish to contemplate this outcome, it's a good idea to have an emergency bag packed for such an occasion.

Hospital birthing units
Midwifery-led care

These are birthing centres run by midwives with no high-tech equipment, no input from medical staff, or use of epidurals.

Unlike "stand-alone" birthing centres, which may be some way from a hospital unit with emergency equipment, a hospital birthing unit is situated in the hospital delivery suite, or nearby, but there is still little medical intervention and doctors are not in the unit. However, if there is an emergency or you want an epidural, instead of having to await transfer to a hospital, the midwife can transfer you rapidly to the delivery suite on site.

Q Do I have a right to give birth at home?

The issue of a legal right to home birth has become a bit complicated recently because there is no right in law for women to give birth at home, and the Department of Health has issued advice to NHS Trusts saying that they should provide a home birth service "where practicable", rather than insisting that they provide one. However, the bottom line is that in law no one can be compelled to attend a hospital for treatment or care, and that includes for birth. Your local services are likely to influence your choices greatly and the organization BirthChoiceUK can help to inform your decision (see p.310).

Q What's the difference between a birthing unit and a maternity department in a big hospital?

Birthing units are run by midwives and the emphasis is on a natural birth. They can be situated next to a hospital maternity unit or on a completely separate site. Some hospitals have a birthing unit facility in the actual maternity unit, known as a hospital birthing unit (see left), where midwives provide total care in a dedicated area of the maternity unit.

As the majority of women give birth without needing medical intervention, these units provide a good alternative to a more medicalized hospital environment. The environment in a birthing unit tends to be more relaxed and flexible, which may appeal if you want a home birth atmosphere with added support. You will also have continuous support from midwives and may even be attended by the same midwife throughout your labour and birth. Furthermore, the midwives in these units are very experienced at handling a birth without medical intervention. All of these factors therefore increase your chances of having a straightforward birth.

To be eligible to give birth in such a facility, you would need to have had an uncomplicated pregnancy and be unlikely to require specialized medical care or monitoring in labour and birth. If complications do occur in labour or birth at a birthing unit, you would need to be transferred to

Getting the birth you want

Although there are no guarantees that your labour will proceed in the way you would like it to and it's probably best to approach labour with a flexible attitude, there are things you can do to make it more likely that you will end up having the type of experience you would prefer. Attending antenatal classes and being as informed as possible about labour and your choices will help you to prepare in advance. Other things women find helpful are having a supportive birth partner, making decisions with the midwife, being positive, and using a birth plan.

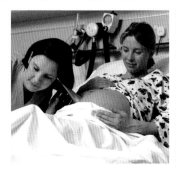

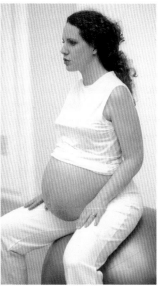

ABOVE: Communicating with your midwife helps to ensure that she is clear about your wishes and you work together. **RIGHT:** A birthing ball provides support, but also means that you can be active by rotating your hips.

the nearest maternity unit, although this is a rare occurence as most women in birthing units have been identified as being "low risk".

If you labour in a standard maternity unit, you can be subject to a range of policies and not enjoy the same degree of flexibility. However, you will have access to an epidural and, if emergency intervention is needed, doctors will be close at hand.

I'm booked for a Caesarean as my baby is breech, but I want a natural birth. Is this possible?

You need to discuss this with your midwife and obstetrician and express your preference, as your feelings are an important factor when deciding how to manage your birth. You may be able to have a procedure called external cephalic version (which is usually done around 37 weeks) to try to turn your baby to a head-first position (see p.144). However, if you have this procedure and your baby still remains in a breech position, you may be advised to have a Caesarean, although some obstetricians will support you if you wish to try for a vaginal birth (see p.183).

I don't want to be monitored in labour. Will the midwives and doctors listen to me?

Unless there is a medical or obstetric complication, such a previous Caesarean section or high blood pressure, you don't need to be strapped continually to a monitor to listen to the baby's heartbeat. Instead, a procedure called "intermittent auscultation", which means listening in regularly to the baby's heartbeat with a sonicaid, should be sufficient to monitor the baby's wellbeing. Ultimately, the choice of monitoring or listening in, if all is well, is yours. If a midwife or obstetrician wants to monitor the baby's heartbeat continuously, they should explain why.

It's a good idea to make a note of your wishes during pregnancy in a birth plan (see p.149) and discuss this with your midwife before you go into labour. If you don't have a chance to discuss this before labour, when you do go into labour, the midwife on duty will first take a medical and obstetric history and ensure that you and your baby are well, and will then ask if you have a birth plan, or you can show her the plan.

ESSENTIAL INFORMATION: LABOUR AND BIRTH

Water births
Relaxing in labour

Some cultures have used water births for centuries to provide a gentle birthing experience. Today, there is evidence to support the fact that labour may be quicker and less painful in water.

How can it help with the pain? Possibly women feel more comfortable and therefore more confident and in control in water. It is thought that water sets off a surge of oxytocin (the hormone that triggers contractions), making contractions more effective. Some women find they can move around more easily in water, which helps them find a good position in which to give birth. Some feel the benefits of immersion in warm water as soon as they get into the pool, but for others it can take 15–30 minutes before they relax. Water can

be a natural aid to relaxation as it soothes muscles and releases tension. When we feel less anxious, our bodies produce fewer "stress" hormones. This encourages the brain to produce endorphins, the body's painkillers, and promotes wellbeing. Dimmed lights and relaxing music can further aid relaxation. Some studies suggest that women have a shorter second stage of labour in water, and there may be less exertion needed to push the baby out. If contractions are too intense you can still use Entonox (gas and air).

Can the baby be monitored in water? Your baby can still be monitored by the midwife using a Pinard (ear trumpet) stethoscope or a waterproof hand-held electronic sonicaid.

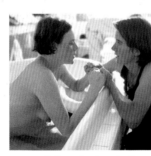

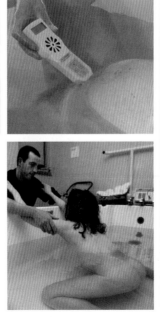

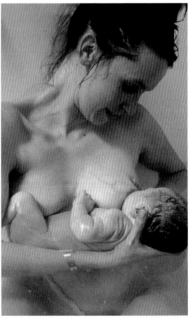

ABOVE: Labouring in warm water can help you to relax. **TOP LEFT:** Your baby can be monitored using a waterproof sonicaid. **BOTTOM LEFT:** A birthing pool enables you to move around to find the most comfortable position. **FAR RIGHT:** It's possible to deliver your baby in a pool with a trained midwife present.

Will I be allowed to have a water birth?

You can use a birthing pool providing your pregnancy is normal and there were no problems in previous pregnancies. If you want a water birth in hospital and are going to be induced (without a drip), or there are other complications with the pregnancy, you may need to negotiate this with your doctor or midwife. You can talk to a Supervisor of Midwives (who can be contacted via the maternity unit) during pregnancy to help you to make a plan to meet your wishes.

Is it possible to have a water birth in hospital?

This depends on the hospital maternity unit. Some units have their own birthing pool; some have facilities for you to hire a pool and bring it in; some units have only room enough for a pool to labour in; and others do not have the facilities for you to bring one in or the structural ability to have one in the unit as the amount of water in the pool would be too heavy for the floor to hold.

If your maternity unit does have a birthing pool, it is possible that the pool might be in use when you go into labour. To improve your chances of being able to use a pool, you may want to consider a home birth and to hire a pool (see p.153).

Can I use the birthing pool for labour and birth if I've had a previous Caesarean?

Unfortunately, it is recommended that if you have had a previous Caesarean section, your baby's heartbeat and your contractions will need to be continuously monitored throughout a subsequent labour and delivery, which cannot be done in a birthing pool. The reason for continuous monitoring in this situation is that there is a chance, although quite a small one, that your uterus may rupture. This often causes no pain and the only indication may be a change in your baby's heartbeat. If you decide you do want to labour and deliver in water after a Caesarean section, this is your choice, but you should be fully aware of the risks.

> What could be more natural to reduce stress during labour than a soak in a warm bath or even standing under a shower?

When can I get into the birthing pool?

You can get into the pool whenever you want, but some midwives suggest that you wait until you are 4–5cm (2in) dilated or in established labour. This is because some people are concerned that the water can be so relaxing that it may cause the contractions to slow down or even stop, although there is little evidence to support this. However, if this does happen, getting out of the pool and walking around for a while is likely to increase the strength of the contractions. You will need to get out of the pool if your baby passes meconium (see p.252) or if the midwife has any concerns about you or your baby.

The water temperature can be whatever you find comfortable, although 37°C (98.6°F) body temperature is usual, especially if you are giving birth in the pool, as babies can get cold quickly once they are born. Most units have guidelines on this.

Can I deliver my baby in a birthing pool, or are these just for labour?

You should ask your midwife to find out if the hospital that you have chosen to deliver at provides facilities for you to deliver in the water, or just use the pool for most of your labour. This often depends on whether the pool is big enough for the delivery. Occasionally, there may not be a midwife available who has been trained in delivering births under water, in which case you may only be able to labour in water and will have to get out for the delivery.

Q Can I bring food and drinks into the labour room?

The latest NICE guideline recommends that all women should be able to drink in labour. Water may be refreshing, but isotonic drinks may be more beneficial, as they contain energy-boosting ingredients. If established labour is progressing well and you and your baby are well, you can eat light snacks to give you energy and help labour to progress. However, if you require pethidine or diamorphine, which can make you nauseous or sick, or need an epidural, or other risk factors develop, you may be advised to drink sips of water only. You may also be offered an antacid tablet to reduce acid build-up in your stomach. This is a precaution in case you need an emergency Caesarean.

Q Who will be with me while I'm in labour?

If you have a home birth, you will be allocated a midwife who will stay with you throughout your established labour. As you near delivery, she will contact the hospital and a second midwife will be sent to support her and you through the birth. Whoever else you have at your home delivery is up to you. Things may be different in hospital, where it is generally recommended that you have just two birthing partners, simply because the space in most labour rooms is limited. Once in established labour, NICE recommendations are that you are cared for by one midwife throughout labour. In reality, although each unit will endeavour to offer one-to-one support, this may not be possible. If this is the case, the midwife will be with you as much as she can, will show you how to contact her if she is not in the room, and will be with you for the delivery. It may be wise to organize one or two people, such as your partner and a good friend, to support you during labour.

Q I've heard about hospitals being understaffed and women not getting a bed. Is this true?

There are concerns about shortages of midwives and beds. Many hospitals now employ ancillary staff and maternity support workers to support midwives. Unfortunately, there have been times when maternity units are full. If no beds are available, staff will find a bed for you at another hospital; many hospitals have "sister" units, to which they will transfer you. Most maternity units are not full for long and will organize for you to be transferred back as soon as possible.

Q I keep reading about infections like MRSA and now I'm worried about having my baby in hospital.

Although there is a great deal of media coverage of "superbugs" such as MRSA, most people have no problems at all with hospital infections. Infections are caused by germs, of which there are four major types: bacteria; viruses; fungi, moulds, and mildew; and protozoa. Hospital infections are bacterial. There are thousands of different types of bacteria. Some bacteria, known as helper germs, are friendly or good bacteria, which aid the digestion and absorption of food in the gut. Others can cause infection and illness, methicillin-resistant *Staphylococcus aureus* (MRSA) and *Clostridium difficile* (C. difficile) being two notable ones of concern in hospital.

MRSA is a bacterium that can live completely harmlessly on the skin of healthy people, but can lead to serious infection in vulnerable individuals. Good hygiene, particularly in the form of simple precautions such as hand washing, is an effective method in the prevention of MRSA infection and your chances of acquiring this in hospital are low. Even healthy relatives and friends of patients with MRSA

While in hospital, you may need to summon your assertive skills to ensure a safe environment for you and your baby carry no risk. If cutlery and plates are washed using soap and water (preferably hot) this removes MRSA, and the risk of acquiring MRSA through contact with curtains, sheets, and pillows is very low. Healthcare workers use antiseptic solutions, such as alcohol hand rubs, and more recently many hospitals have alcohol gels for hand cleaning at the end of each bed.

C. difficile is another type of bacterium mentioned frequently in the media. Hospitals prevent and control the spread of C. difficile with antibiotics, general hygiene measures such as hand washing, and by detecting cases early so that they can isolate affected patients to prevent it spreading further.

What measures can I take to prevent my baby or myself getting an infection in hospital?

Regular hand washing by yourself, staff, and visitors are likely to be adequate measures to prevent infection. Take your own soap, a flannel, and moist hand wipes with you. Always wash your hands after using the toilet and always wash your hands or clean them with a hand wipe immediately before and after eating a meal. Make sure your bed area is regularly cleaned and report any unclean toilet or bathroom facilities to staff. Breastfeeding will provide your baby with protection against infection. A new innovation, silver-lined pyjamas designed to protect against MRSA, are now on sale in the UK! Silver is thought to have particular antibacterial qualities and to be an effective agent against infection. Hopefully these measures will help you feel in control. You are unlikely to be in hospital for very long, and you and your baby should be safe.

My partner can't drive. Can an ambulance take me to hospital?

An ambulance can transport you to hospital in an emergency, for example if you are bleeding heavily. As this is an emergency vehicle driven by trained operatives, it is expensive to provide. If you call an ambulance for a non-emergency, you could be taking it away from an emergency situation and putting others' lives at risk. Could a friend or relative

MIDWIFE WISDOM

Hospital checklist
what to check before going into hospital

Part of planning for labour is finding out which facilities your local maternity unit provides and what you might need to provide yourself to help you through the labour and birth.

✳ Check if your local unit supplies equipment such as birthing balls or TENS machines or whether you need to hire these in advance.

✳ Check in advance if the hospital has a birthing pool and midwives trained to deliver babies in water.

✳ Find out if your hospital has a dedicated birthing unit (see p.154).

be on call when you go into labour? Or can you call a minicab in early labour? If you can't organize transport, discuss this antenatally with your midwife or, once in labour, call the labour ward for advice.

Can I ask for a private room in the hospital for me and the baby after the birth?

Unless you give birth in a private hospital, there are few hospitals that offer private postnatal care. Many hospitals have postnatal "amenity rooms", which are usually single rooms, with or without ensuite facilities, on the postnatal ward. These may be allocated to women who need a private room for medical reasons, in which case they are free. Otherwise, they are offered on a first come, first served basis, so state in your birth plan if you wish to have one and remind your midwife after the birth.

The cost of these rooms and their facilities can vary between units and covers the room only. The midwifery care is given by the staff on the postnatal ward and, in most units, your partner and visitors will still have to abide by the ward visiting times.

MYTHS AND MISCONCEPTIONS

Is it true that...

 Owls are bad luck?

Owl superstitions are just plain silly! If a pregnant woman hears the shriek of an owl, her child will be a girl. An owl living in the attic of a house will cause a pregnant woman to miscarry. When the time comes to give birth there should be no owls in the delivery room – if they hoot at the moment of birth the child will have a miserable life. These really are myths!

Raspberry leaf tea makes labour easier?

The evidence for this is largely anecdotal, although some studies have been conducted. Advocates of raspberry leaf tea claim it increases the muscle tone of the uterus making for more effective contractions, and therefore a shorter and easier labour. However, it's important not to use raspberry leaf tea (or extract) until the last two months of pregnancy because of the possible stimulating effect on the uterus.

Your partner weighed 10lb at birth, so your baby will be a whopper, too?

No, it's more complicated than that – it depends on the mix of chromosomes your baby inherits. So, if the father is a strapping 6ft 4in and was a huge baby, and you're a petite 5ft 2in and were a tiny baby, keep your fingers crossed that you have the more dominant genes!

My baby isn't due yet!
premature births

What is meant by premature labour?

Premature means that a baby is born several weeks earlier that the estimated "due date". While only a tiny percentage of babies will actually be born on the day that they are supposedly "due", and predicting exactly when the birth will happen is virtually impossible, most women do have their babies somewhere between 37 and 42 weeks of pregnancy. The due date (EDD, or expected date of delivery) is calculated at 40 weeks (see p.41). Technically, any baby born before the 37th completed week of pregnancy is termed premature, but the closer to your EDD your baby is delivered, the fewer problems he should have in coping with life outside the womb.

Can I do anything to reduce the risk of my going into labour early?

It is not totally understood why women go into labour, although it is thought that it is probably due to a combination of factors (see p.144). Unfortunately, most preventive measures to stop premature labour have not proved to be effective, so there may be little that an individual can do to reduce the risk of this happening. However, the most effective self-help measures towards a normal pregnancy, a positive outcome to birth, and hopefully avoidance of a premature labour, are to adopt a healthy lifestyle before and during pregnancy, including not smoking or drinking alcohol, eating a well-balanced diet, and getting some form of daily exercise. Also, good social support has been shown to help reduce stress levels and worry during pregnancy, which can have a very positive effect on your general health and wellbeing and, in turn, hopefully on your pregnancy, labour, and birth.

I'm pregnant with triplets – will my babies need to be delivered early?

A multiple pregnancy is more likely to result in a premature birth and the more babies you are carrying, the higher the risk of this happening. For triplets, the delivery that carries the least risk is an elective Caesarean section (although there is a measured risk with all medical procedures) and, if this is agreed with your midwife and doctor, a delivery date will be decided on that is in the best interests of you and your babies.

The doctors will try to seek a balance between the risks associated with premature delivery, such as the babies' development not being complete, against the increased chance of you going into your own natural labour as you get nearer to your expected date of delivery. Your consultant should discuss the timing of this with you and you should be involved in all the decisions. Every maternity unit will have their own guidelines, but the final decision will be based on not just your health, but on the health of your babies. This ensures that the babies are born at the optimum time and reduces the likelihood of problems occurring that are associated with premature deliveries.

Amazing advances in recent years in the care of premature babies has ensured the survival of some of the tiniest babies

Why are some babies born prematurely?

There are certain factors that may increase an individual's likelihood of having a premature baby. These include a previous obstetric history of prematurity of either themselves or a mother or sister; illness during pregnancy; the state of a mother's health prior to pregnancy; having a multiple pregnancy; smoking; and fetal problems, such as reduced growth, which may be due to lifestyle factors such as smoking and other fetal disorders. Most premature babies are placed in a special care baby unit (see opposite), where they will receive specialist medical care and attention until they are well enough to return home.

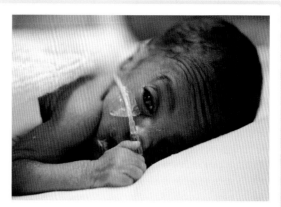

CARING FOR PREMATURE BABIES: A baby born before 37 weeks of pregnancy may need additional support with breathing and temperature control in a special care baby unit.

If I go into labour prematurely, can the doctors stop the contractions?

Usually, nothing can stop labour once it is under way, but your contractions can be temporarily slowed down with drugs called tocolytics. However, these do not always work over a long period of time and can have side effects, such as increasing your heart rate and affecting blood pressure. In general, they are not given for longer than 48 hours. If they hold off labour for this amount of time, steroids can be administered to help to mature your baby's lungs before the delivery, and this also allows you to be transferred to a hospital with an intensive neonatal unit.

Occasionally, if there is an obvious cause for labour starting early, such as an infection, then treating the infection with antibiotics may be enough to stop contractions.

My partner is in hospital as there is a risk of premature labour. How can I prepare at home?

If there is a high risk of your baby being born early, I suggest that your priority should be supporting your partner while she is staying in hospital. You will have plenty of time to prepare for your baby's arrival at home after the actual birth, as premature babies often need a prolonged stay in hospital due to a higher risk of complications.

While your partner is in hospital, she is likely to be feeling low, anxious, and possibly fairly isolated. There are plenty of things you can do to boost her morale and keep her feeling positive about her situation. You can talk to her and make a list of things that need to be bought or done at home. This will help to keep her involved and not feel so isolated in hospital, and will also help to reassure her that things will be ready for the baby. You will need the same items for your baby if he is born prematurely as you would for a baby born full term. Concentrate on the basics, such as warm clothes for your baby, a pram or buggy, and a car seat. If you haven't already done so, you could think about where your baby will sleep. This should be somewhere comfortably warm and close to you and your partner. If your partner is in hospital for a long period of time, collect shop brochures so you can make your choices together. You could also try to encourage your partner to read about breastfeeding, which will be of particular benefit to your baby if he is born early.

ESSENTIAL INFORMATION: LABOUR AND BIRTH

Special care baby unit
Caring for your premature baby

Some babies need specialist care when they are born. A special care baby unit (SCBU) is a special ward in a hospital where these babies go if they need more care. There are specially trained nurses and doctors (paediatricians) in the unit to care for your baby. If you know that your baby will need to go to SCBU while you are still pregnant, you can ask for a tour of the unit and to meet a paediatrician. If your baby is very ill, he may need to move to a neonatal intensive care unit.

Why do some babies need special care?
Sometimes a baby needs special care because he has been born early (preterm) and may need help to breathe and stay warm. Babies who are small for their dates may also require special care. Other babies may have an infection, be jaundiced, or have a congenital abnormality and therefore require special care.

What will happen in the SCBU? Your baby may be put in an incubator with monitors attached. This controls the temperature and keeps your baby warm. If your baby needs help with breathing, he will also receive oxygen through a special ventilator in the incubator. Some of the equipment looks very frightening, but the staff will be happy to explain what is going on, as they are keen for you to be involved in your baby's care; they can also help you to breastfeed. If your baby is admitted unexpectedly, you will be given a photo of him, as you may be recovering from a Caesarean, making it difficult for you to visit your baby during the first day. If this is the case, do ask the midwifery staff to take you to your baby as soon as you are able. SCBU staff love having the baby's family to visit, although they may have strict rules regarding visiting – so do ask what the policies are in your unit.

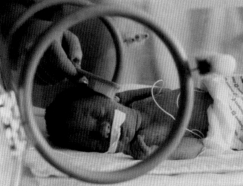

CONTACT WITH YOUR BABY: Even while your baby is in an incubator, there are plenty of ways to stimulate him and communicate. Being close to your baby will help you to cope too.

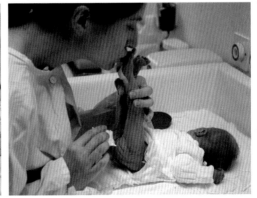

LOVING CARE: You will be encouraged to care for your baby in the special care unit, and babies needing special care have been shown to thrive from the loving touch and attention of their parents.

Why do premature babies have breathing difficulties?

Respiratory distress syndrome (RDS) is the most common complication of premature births and affects over 50 per cent of babies born before 32 weeks of pregnancy.

Lung problems occur in premature babies for several reasons. The lungs are not fully developed until the later stages of pregnancy, and an important substance known as "surfactant", which enables a baby's small lungs to mature and function effectively, does not develop until after 36 weeks of pregnancy. Also the earlier the baby is born, the more underdeveloped the lungs and muscles of the rib cage are, which results in babies becoming increasingly tired as they require more effort to breathe. Breathing problems are the commonest reason for babies being admitted to neonatal units. Premature babies are much more prone to respiratory infections than fully grown babies and may require help breathing using mechanical ventilators, which, although life-saving, can themselves cause problems for the baby's lungs.

How to cope
staying focused while your baby is in hospital

MIDWIFE WISDOM

If your baby has to spend a substantial amount of time in a special care baby unit, it can be very hard to cope emotionally. There are steps you can take to help you through this difficult time.

* Spend as much time as possible with your baby in the unit and get involved in his care whenever possible.

* If your baby's stay is prolonged, try not to feel guilty about spending time at home away from him. Instead, use this time to rest and reserve your energy for your baby.

* Keep reminding yourself that your baby is receiving the best possible care.

My premature baby has jaundice – what will be done to help him?

Jaundice is one of the most common problems in all newborn babies and premature babies are even more at risk as they have an immature liver, which normally removes bilirubin, the substance that causes the yellow tinge common to jaundice, from the body. Bilirubin is produced when the body breaks down red blood cells. It is a yellow pigment that, if not cleared by the kidneys and liver, builds up and is deposited in the skin. Babies who develop jaundice are given blood tests to measure the level of bilirubin, and the result of the blood test will determine whether they require any specialist treatment. Treatment for jaundice is given by phototherapy, which uses ultraviolet light to break down the bilirubin beneath the skin so that the baby's kidneys can safely excrete bile pigments.

Our baby, born at 24 weeks, is doing well in the baby unit, but is he likely to have brain damage?

The risk of any sort of disability in a premature baby is highest at around 23–24 weeks, becoming much lower at 30 weeks. The risk of brain damage to your baby depends on whether he is experiencing problems with his liver, kidneys, or breathing, is underweight, or has other existing medical conditions in addition to being premature. Some of the most common long-term problems in babies born very prematurely are those to do with hearing, vision, or fine coordination skills. However, overall, the majority of babies born at 24 weeks with few other medical complications do well.

If your baby is doing well after a few weeks this is a good sign. It is perfectly natural for you to continue to worry, but you may find it reassuring to talk to the doctors and nurses looking after your baby. Most specialist baby doctors and nurses working in neonatal units carry out regular brain scans on any baby they may have concerns about and you would be kept fully informed if this was the case. The doctors assess premature babies on a

Bonding with your special care baby

Having a baby in a special care baby unit can be an extremely anxious time and, apart from his physical development, you may be concerned about how you will bond with your baby. However, the staff will encourage you to be as involved as possible in your baby's care and will give you plenty of opportunity to have contact. Touching, cuddling, and talking to your baby can be a real comfort for both you and your baby. The need to touch and be touched is a primal instinct and has been shown to play a significant role in the development of your baby, as plenty of research shows that babies gain weight more quickly, cry less, breastfeed more successfully, and are discharged home earlier when continued close contact is maintained between the baby and parents.

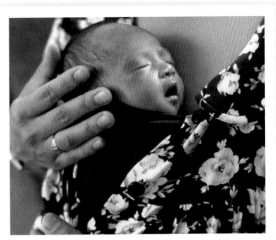

HOLDING YOUR BABY CLOSE: Once your baby is big enough to be removed from an incubator, holding him close to your body is incredibly beneficial for both of you, providing reassurance and warmth.

daily basis for any problems, especially those related to brain growth and development.

Following discharge from the neonatal unit, your baby will still be monitored very closely in outpatients. Although most serious defects can be detected from birth, it is often some time later before less obvious developmental problems can be identified, which is why this follow-up period is necessary. Although these problems can include some learning and speech difficulties, medical staff are very knowledgeable about these and a full support programme would be available.

How can we reassure our baby while he is in the special care unit?

Except in rare situations when your baby may be too ill to be touched, or if there is a high risk of infection, you and your partner will be encouraged to play a very important part in the care and wellbeing of your baby. There are many things you and your partner can do to ensure that your baby knows you are there for him and is reassured by your presence. As well

as having plenty of physical contact with your baby, touching and stroking him to help with bonding (see above), your baby will also love to hear the sound of your voice, so spend lots of time talking and singing to him. Your baby will soon come to recognize you as a comforting and loving presence.

My baby is in the special care baby unit. I'm trying to express milk every day – am I helping?

Breast milk helps to ensure that the mother's natural immunity is passed on to her baby via her milk. As premature babies are more prone to infection, expressing your breast milk is a great way to help your baby while he is in the special care unit. Breast milk is also much easier for a baby to digest, which is especially important for premature babies since their digestive tract may be less developed. This is also a great way for you to bond and develop a relationship with your baby.

This is a time of considerable stress and mothers can feel helpless. Knowing that you are doing such a great thing to help your baby will help enormously.

Q Is it dangerous for my premature baby to have formula milk?

It is perfectly fine for a premature baby to receive formula milk and is not at all dangerous if the correct formula is given. Premature babies are given formula milks that are produced specifically for their needs. These formulas are very specialized and prescribed by a doctor to meet the individual nutritional requirements of each premature baby as they grow. All artificial milks or modified infant formulas are highly processed products and have gone through rigorous health and safety checks.

Q Do all hospitals have facilities for premature babies?

Facilities vary throughout the country, and while most maternity units and hospitals have a special care baby facility, not all have a neonatal intensive care unit (NICU) where babies go if they need intensive life support. This means that babies below a certain gestation, around 24 weeks, may have to be transferred either before or after the birth to receive more specialized treatment, such as intensive assistance with breathing.

If it is thought that you are at a greater risk of having your baby prematurely, then you may well receive some or all of your care at a hospital with more specialized facilities and you will be able to view the neonatal unit before giving birth.

Q My first baby was born prematurely. How likely is this to happen again?

Fewer than seven per cent of all births in the UK are premature, and fewer than a quarter of babies born prematurely are below 32 weeks' gestation. If your first baby was premature, the chance of this happening again depends on the reason for your premature delivery last time. If it was because you went "naturally" into premature labour, with no identifiable reason, then there is a risk that it may happen again. Sometimes there may be a genetic link, which may be the case if your mother or sister

MIDWIFE WISDOM

How long will my baby stay in hospital? your baby's stay in the special care unit

How long each baby stays in the SCBU will depend on why he was there: some babies just need a few hours' observation; other babies need to stay until the time they would have been full term in the womb. Certain criteria govern when babies return home:

* When they are able to feed properly with either breast or formula milk.
* When they have gained weight and weigh a minimum of 2kg (4lb 7oz).
* When they can control their own body temperature.

had her babies prematurely. However, if it was because of a medical condition that affected you or the baby and which is unlikely to occur again, then you are less likely to have another premature labour.

Medical and obstetric conditions that can predispose women to have premature babies include multiple pregnancies (see p.128); high blood pressure (see p.87); bleeding during pregnancy, especially later in pregnancy (see p.90); premature rupture of the membranes (see p.167); increased fluid around the baby, or the presence of any disease or infection in the mother or baby, some of which may mean that your baby or babies are delivered early by elective Caesarean. Also, if you have a weakened cervix (see p.24), where the cervix shortens later in pregnancy, you are at a higher risk of premature labour. If this is known to be a problem you will be monitored during pregnancy. Some of these conditions are likely to recur in subsequent pregnancies, making it likely that you will have another premature labour, while others are less likely to reappear and you would therefore be less likely to have a subsequent premature labour.

How will I know I'm in labour?
the signs of labour

Q How will I be able to tell that I'm really in labour?

The one completely sure sign that you are in labour is that you are experiencing regular contractions that are causing your cervix (the neck of womb) to dilate or open, and this can only be determined by your midwife or doctor during an internal examination.

True labour contractions are usually painful, occur very regularly, and grow stronger and more frequent as time goes on. There are other signs that labour could be on its way, such as a mucous vaginal show or discharge (see below), but these are not true indicators that labour is actually underway.

If you are unsure about whether you are in labour, you could try timing your contractions from the beginning of one to the beginning of the next and note how often they occur. If you are in labour, then you will notice them becoming closer together and increasing in duration. If you think you are in labour, always call your midwife or your nearest delivery unit for guidance and advice.

Q What is a "show"?

During pregnancy, a plug of jelly-like mucus seals the lower end of your cervix and this prevents infection getting into your womb. This "plug" comes away towards the end of pregnancy, and although this can mean that labour is going to start soon, it can also dislodge up to six weeks before your labour actually starts. When the plug comes away, this is commonly referred to as a "show".

Q There was some blood with my show – is that OK?

Yes, it's normal for a show to contain a small amount of either fresh blood or dark old blood (like at the end of your period) as part of the clear or cloudy mucus of the plug.

Q At which point should I ring the hospital?

If you are experiencing regular contractions that are getting closer together and increasing in the amount of time that they are lasting, then labour may well have started. When your contractions are around 5–10 minutes apart, you should phone the birthing unit for further advice.

Other situations when it is recommended that you phone are if you think your waters have broken, your baby's movements have slowed and become less frequent, you experience any bleeding, or you are in pain and not due for delivery.

Never worry about phoning for advice; it is better to be well informed than to sit at home worrying about things. Always carry essential contact numbers in your bag and keep them by the phone at home, as you never know when you may need to seek advice or when your labour may begin.

Q What do people mean when they talk about your "waters breaking"?

The "waters" are the amniotic fluid contained in the membranous sack surrounding and protecting your

Even though you are facing one of life's hardest tasks, keep firmly fixed on the fact that you will soon meet your baby

baby in the womb. These membranes usually split or break towards the end of the first stage of labour. This means that the fluid continues to cushion the baby's head and prevents direct contact with the cervix at first, helping you to cope with the pain. Eventually, the pressure causes the membranes to burst, releasing the amniotic fluid, which leaks or gushes through the vagina.

What should I do once my waters have broken?

If there is quite a large gush then you will be in no doubt about what has happened. Sometimes, however, the waters break and produce a small trickle, which leaves you in some doubt as to whether they have broken. If you think your waters have broken, I suggest putting on a sanitary pad and examining it after a short while to see if there is amniotic fluid visible. If you are still unsure, then always phone your midwife or local maternity unit for individual advice. Occasionally, the membranes can break early for other reasons, for example if the mother has an infection, or they may break for no apparent reason.

Can I have a bath after my waters have broken?

If there are no complications in your pregnancy and labour then you should be able to have a bath, which you may also be using for pain relief. Indeed, using water in labour has been assessed in many trials and most show that women report a significant reduction in pain (see p.156).

Studies have found that there is no increase in the risk of infection rates in women who bathe in water following the spontaneous rupture of their membranes. If you are unsure about this, ask your midwife about your local hospital's guidelines, as most maternity units have specific policies to ensure safe practice regarding the use of water for both labour and birth.

What is a false labour?

False labour can be a number of things. It can be a series of contraction-type pains that subside after a number of hours and that do not have the length, strength, or regularity to actually dilate the cervix, or neck of the womb. Braxton Hicks contractions very close to your due date can also be

Relaxing in early labour

You will probably spend early labour at home with your partner, timing contractions and deciding when to travel to the hospital if that is where you are giving birth. As this part of labour can continue for a considerable amount of time, possibly with periods when contractions stop altogether, try to spend time relaxing in between contractions to conserve energy for later. There are simple things you can do at home to help you relax. You can have a warm bath, get your partner to massage your back, stay mobile but rest if you need to, eat nutritious snacks, and drink fluids to give your body fuel to work well later. Contact the maternity unit or your midwife if you have any questions.

THE EARLY STAGES: Staying at home until labour is established can be the most relaxing way to spend early labour. Let the unit know that labour has started and that you will come in later.

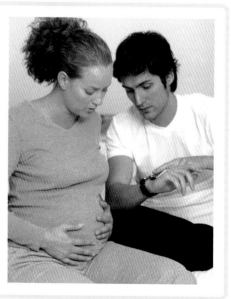

confused for labour. With these, you do experience your uterus tightening and relaxing and there is a degree of discomfort. Braxton Hicks contractions are a sign that your uterus is preparing for the contractions of labour. If this is your first pregnancy, you may be unsure how to tell the difference between these practice contractions and the real thing. Real labour contractions are more regular, powerful, and usually more painful. Some women barely notice these practice contractions, while for others they are quite uncomfortable. If this is the case, it can help to move around or have a warm bath to ease the discomfort.

Q Is it true that I will have to go to hospital if my waters break, even if contractions haven't started?

If your waters break before your contractions have started, most maternity units have a policy that you should be seen by a midwife, either at the maternity unit or at home, to determine if you and your baby are both well. The main concerns when the waters break are the position of the umbilical cord – whether it is stuck in front of the baby's head – and to rule out any chance of infection, and the answers to these two questions will determine the plan of care you will be offered.

You may be offered an examination to look at the cervix to see if there is fluid leaking and, if so, its colour, and to take a swab of the area to determine if there are any bacteria that could pose a problem for the baby. A cardiotocograph (CTG) may be performed, which monitors the baby's heartbeat over a short period to identify if there are any signs that the baby is distressed (see p.192). If all is well with you and the baby, you will be able to return, or stay at, home to await events, although a further appointment may be made to discuss further options should your contractions not start within a specified time. This timescale varies and may be as little as 24 hours or as long as 96 hours if all remains well.

Around 85 per cent of babies are born within 48 hours of the waters breaking, even if there are no contractions initially.

MIDWIFE WISDOM

Calling the midwife
is it too early to contact the midwife?

Although each woman has a different experience, here is a rough guide for when to call the midwife and when not to call the midwife.

✱ Don't worry about calling the midwife if your contractions aren't regular, occurring just once or twice an hour, as these may be Braxton Hicks (see opposite).

✱ Don't call the midwife if you have only had a show (see p.167).

✱ Do call the midwife if contractions are strong and regular, every 5–10 minutes.

✱ Do call the midwife for advice if your waters have broken.

Q How will I be able to tell the difference between real contractions and Braxton Hicks?

Labour contractions have several specific characteristics. They are very regular and over time increase in regularity and length, and they are also painful. Most start as a period-type pain or backache that again increases in intensity over time. The other difference that you may or may not be aware of is that the cervix dilates (opens up) in response to true labour contractions, but does not with Braxton Hicks. One thing that may indicate this is happening is if you experience a show (see p.167).

Q What do labour contractions feel like?

Generally speaking, women feel contractions as a painful tightening of the muscles of the uterus. Although they actually start at the top of your bump and progress to the bottom of the bump, you may experience more pain and a feeling of pressure in the lower part of your abdomen and pelvis as the baby is pushed down by the contraction.

Some women experience the pain in their tummy, while others experience labour pain as backache. Generally, contractions tend to start as something that can be compared to a severe period pain, gradually increasing in intensity; however, the degree of pain felt will be different for all women.

Q We're having a home birth – what if the midwife doesn't show up?

Arrangements for contacting the midwife when you are having a home birth will vary depending on where you live; however, certain things will be the same no matter where you are. Once you are 37 weeks pregnant, the midwives will be "on call" for your delivery. Your midwife will talk to you about the local procedure for contacting the midwife on call, which may be directly through a mobile phone or pager, or indirectly through the labour ward at your local maternity unit. If you experience labour before you are 37 weeks, you will be asked to go to hospital as this is considered "preterm" labour (see p.161).

Once you are experiencing strong, regular contractions, contact your midwife via the route you have been advised. If your labour starts in the daytime, midwives will be on duty in the area; if it's evening or nightime, it might take them a little while to reach you, so bear these differences in mind. Also, bear in mind factors like the traffic on the roads during rush hours, which may make it advisable to let the midwife know about your contractions sooner rather than later!

Playing some favourite music at home or in the delivery room can lift your spirits and encourage you to move around

Most NHS Trusts have a policy of two midwives attending your home birth; in some areas, both midwives will be there throughout the labour and birth, while in others the second midwife will be called by the first midwife nearer to the delivery so that two midwives are in attendance at the birth. In the worst case scenario, if your labour progresses rapidly and a midwife hasn't arrived, contact your local maternity unit who may be able to arrange for paramedics to attend you until the midwife arrives. Please bear in mind that it's very rare to have a home birth without your midwife being present, and that babies who do arrive quickly usually do so with very little added complication.

Q They sent my friend home from the hospital – I don't want that to happen to me.

Labours differ and are dependent on so many factors, and your friend's circumstances and your own are likely to vary enormously. Unless you have been specifically advised to go to hospital early once you think labour has started, then the best place to be in the early stages of labour is at home. In first pregnancies, the first stage of labour, when your cervix dilates to around 10cm (see p.181), averages at about 12–14 hours. So if you go to hospital very early on they may well suggest you go home until labour is a little more advanced. Although you may feel that you want to stay at the hospital "just in case", unless you have to travel a great distance to and from your local maternity unit, you are likely to be more comfortable and relaxed in your own surroundings.

Q Are there situations when you can't eat or drink in labour?

The recommendations by NICE for labour are that all women should be allowed to drink water in labour, and that isotonic, or sports water, may be slightly more beneficial because of its higher calorie value and quick absorption into the body. Eating light snacks, even in established labour, is recommended as long as you haven't had opioid painkillers, which include pethidine and diamorphine, and there are no other

MYTHS AND MISCONCEPTIONS

Is it true that...

✳ You're small-boned with small hands and feet so you'll have a Caesarean?

Research shows there's no relation between the size of a woman's feet and her pelvis. So those with dainty feet can relax. If, however, you are on the small side and your bump is growing quickly, your midwife will keep a close eye on you in the last month. If necessary, a pelvic assessment may be done by a specialist so your pelvis and the baby's head can be measured. Then – and only then – will it be determined whether or not you need a Caesarean.

✳ You'll have the same delivery as your mum had with you?

Fed up with hearing all the details of your own birth from your mum? Some say you'll have the same sort of delivery your mum had with you – early or late, speedy or forceps. However, there have been big developments in science since your mum's days so health professionals are more knowledgeable now. Also, many women are healthier and stronger these days (try telling your mum that!) so don't assume you're in for a difficult labour just because your mum had one.

✳ Your pubic hair will be shaved before you give birth?

Shaving women used to be standard procedure in labour, when it was thought it might lower the risk of infection. Nowadays pubic hair will only be shaved for medical reasons (such as for a Caesarean section) and even then it will only be shaved partially.

risk factors that would make a general anaesthetic more likely. Most women find that they want to eat in early labour, but find that they cannot face food later in the first stage although they still want to drink.

Will I be able to drive myself to hospital when labour starts?

Driving while in labour isn't advisable and could be very dangerous to yourself, your passengers, and any other road users, including pedestrians. If you are in labour, you will be having regular painful contractions and this will interfere with your ability to focus and drive a car and will also diminish your awareness of your immediate surroundings. In other words, you will be very distracted!

As the general advice about labour is to stay at home for as long as you feel comfortable, this means that by the time you are travelling to hospital you will be in very established labour and so your ability to drive would be very much diminished.

Another consideration is your insurance cover; if your driving is impaired because of pain you may well invalidate your insurance cover. The safe option is to get someone else to drive or to take a taxi.

How likely is it for a first labour to progress so quickly that you don't make it to hospital?

In first pregnancies, labour usually lasts for 12–14 hours, with contractions building in intensity and length. Most women are happy to stay at home for the early part of the first stage, and get an idea of when they want to be in hospital as their contractions get more regular. It is unusual with first babies, but not unheard of, for labour to be so quick or for you to have no sign of contractions, that you leave it too late to get to hospital. Although this also depends on your distance from the hospital, traffic delays, or other factors that may increase your journey time.

What are the signs that it is too late to go to the hospital?

Generally speaking, if you are having an uncontrollable urge to push, then that's the point

> Keep contact details close by, the car ready, and your mobile charged, so that when labour starts you will be prepared

where it may be too late to reach the hospital before your delivery. If you did find yourself in this unfortunate circumstance, contact your local maternity unit who will arrange for paramedics to attend you for the delivery of the baby. In some areas, they will also ask an on-call midwife to attend the birth. Or you can contact the emergency ambulance services yourself.

Can I check how dilated I am myself or get my husband to do this?

There is one school of thought that believes that vaginal examination of the cervix shouldn't be done routinely in a normally progressing labour by anyone, and that would include you and your partner. There are several reasons for this. One is that some women find it a very uncomfortable procedure and staff gain very little information other than that the woman's labour is progressing. Another reason is that it introduces the the risk of infection. If you are having strong, regular contractions, your cervix will be starting to dilate, and any examination should be carried out by a trained midwife or obstetrician under "sterile" conditions to limit the risk of infection. There is also the potential that whoever is doing the examination may break the bag of waters that are surrounding the baby before they would have broken naturally.

So although it might be possible to feel your own cervix depending on what stage of labour you are in, this isn't something that is generally recommended.

It's all your fault, stop the pain!
choices for pain relief

Q What is the best form of pain relief in labour?

As each woman and labour is very different, it is difficult to say which is the "best" form of pain relief. This will also depend on an individual's coping mechanisms and pain threshold. There are many different types of pain relief (see p.174) including alternative therapies such as aromatherapy, acupuncture, homeopathic kits, reflexology, and hynobirthing (using self-hypnosis to reach a state of deep relaxation); natural methods, such as water, massage, TENS, and the positions you adopt; and drugs, such as gas and air and pethidine, and epidural. Your midwife will talk to you about the different choices available and the advantages and disadvantages of each one.

Q Last time I made a real idiot of myself. I don't want to lose control again – what do you advise?

The best advice is to know your options, have an open mind, and be guided by labour and how you are feeling. Being positive and having appropriate support can not only result in a good experience, but can reduce your preception of the pain, and feeling empowered helps you to stay in control.

Q Are relaxation and childbirth classes helpful?

Relaxation and breathing techniques taught in antenatal chidbirth classes are extremely useful when used together and at the correct times in labour (see p.176). This, combined with working with your partner and the midwife, can help to make the pain more bearable and thus the birth experience more pleasurable. It is worth pointing out that people have different pain thresholds and relaxation and breathing techniques alone may not be enough to help you cope with the pain of labour, especially as labour advances. Practising breathing and relaxation techniques before labour begins increases the benefit so classes are helpful.

Q Can moving around during labour help with the pain?

Providing the labour is straightforward, it does seem to be the case that being as active as possible can help the progress of labour. Not only does this help with the pain, but it can also encourage more effective contractions so that labour is faster. As the labour advances, it may be difficult to get into a position that is comfortable, and often women move around to try to find the best one. Favoured positions are standing, kneeling, or squatting, and rocking the pelvis, either on a birthing ball with your legs astride or leaning onto the bed or into the wall.

MIDWIFE WISDOM

Being prepared
practical and mental preparation for labour

Inevitably, labour will involve a degree of pain. Although this can be a frightening prospect, accepting this and thinking in advance about how you might deal with the pain may help you to cope better when the time comes.

* Be as informed as possible about pain-relief options to help you make choices you are happy with in labour. Find out if you need to do anything in advance, such as inform staff if you want a water birth.

* Try to think about the final outcome of labour and view the pain as part of the process that brings you closer to your baby.

ESSENTIAL INFORMATION: LABOUR AND BIRTH

Pain relief choices
How to manage the pain

There are a range of pain relief options available. It's wise to think about which method you would prefer before going into labour.

Relaxation, breathing, keeping mobile, and massage: You remain in control and avoid intervention. Being upright can help the position of the baby and there are no side effects. This may not be sufficient pain relief for strong contractions.

Water: Using a birthing pool in labour and possibly for delivery can halp you to labour quicker and less painfully, with no side effects.

TENS (transcutaneous electrical nerve stimulation): Sticky pads placed on your back send small electrical impulses to trigger the release of endorphins. You control the current with a hand-held device. This may not provide sufficient relief for very strong contractions.

Gas and air: 50 per cent oxygen and 50 per cent nitrous oxygen. This is easy to use and drugs don't accumulate in your body. Some women feel sick or sleepy and find this isn't strong enough.

Pethidine or diamorphine: These can lessen the pain, but can cause sickness and affect the baby's breathing if given too close to delivery.

Epidural anaesthesia: A local injection near the spine, this is the most effective form of pain relief and doesn't enter the baby's system. It increases the chance of forceps, ventouse, and Caesarean, as you may not be able to feel when to push. You will be less mobile and will need monitoring.

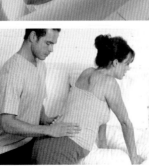
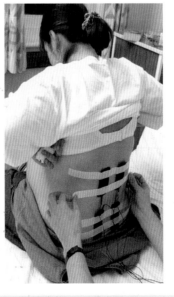

FAR LEFT: Many women find being in warm water an effective method of pain relief, whether this is having a bath at home in early labour, or labouring in a birthing pool thoughout. **BOTTOM LEFT:** A massage to the lower back is another popular way to control pain in the early stages of labour. **RIGHT:** A TENS machine gives you control over the amount of pain relief you receive and allows you to remain mobile and active during the first stage of labour.

Breathing techniques

Using relaxation and breathing techniques can help you to relax and cope with the contractions throughout your labour. Try practising techniques with your partner before labour. Learning to control your breathing has many benefits, including helping you to increase your energy reserves and let go of tension and anxiety so that you can breathe with the rhythm of the contraction. In the earlier stages of labour, you may want to practise longer, deeper breaths between contractions to help keep you calm and focused. You can also try breathing in slowly at the start of a contraction and then exhaling slowly and continuing this pattern until the contraction has passed. Later in labour as contractions become stronger, you may find taking shorter, lighter breaths helps you to ride over the contraction.

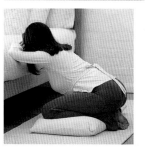

ABOVE: Deeper breaths can help to focus your mind and bring a sense of control. **LEFT:** Breathing in time with contractions helps you to bear down. Exhale to release tension after each contraction.

How can a birthing ball help during labour?

Using a birthing ball during labour has the advantage of opening up the pelvis to allow the baby to move down more easily. You can take your own birthing ball into hospital, and this may be advisable as supplies may be limited.

What is a TENS machine and how do they work?

TENS (transcutaneous electrical nerve stimulation) works by stimulating the production of endorphins, the body's natural painkillers, and also by blocking some of the pain pathways. Electrodes placed on your back or abdomen are attached to a unit that fires electrical impulses when a button is pressed, blocking pain pathways. The strength and frequency of the current can be altered according to your needs. This is a natural form of pain relief that requires no drugs and is a good way to involve your partner, who can position electrodes.

The machines will produce a tingly sensation, but this does not hurt. Some people do not like the sensation, while for others it works very well, so it's a good idea to hire a machine before labour to see if this form of pain relief suits you.

The advantages of TENS are that you are in control of your pain relief and are free to move around while you are using it. Check in advance whether the unit supplies TENS, or whether you need to hire one before going to hospital.

Will I be able to use my TENS machine at the same time as other types of pain relief?

TENS can be used with pethidine or diamorphine and gas and air, but not with water (because it is electrical) or with an epidural (because of the position of the electrodes on your back).

My midwife says that I can have my baby at home, but what pain relief will I be able to have?

There are a variety of, mainly natural, forms of pain relief that you can use in your own home. Alternative therapies, such as aromatherapy, homeopathic kits, reflexology, and acupuncture can all be used, as long as an appropriately trained person is providing them. Many women having home births opt for warm water, either in the bath or in a hired pool, as this is an effective form of pain relief. The midwife can also offer gas and air and pethidine as alternatives, if natural forms of pain relief are not working.

However, you may find that just by having your baby at home, you are less likely to need much pain relief. This is because evidence suggests that women who stay at home for as long as possible during labour, or for the whole of their labour, have a more positive experience, which includes needing less pain relief. By adopting the correct positions, using massage, and breathing and relaxation techniques, you may find that you limit the amount of medical pain relief you need.

Q Will I be able to cope through all the stages of labour using breathing techniques alone?

Relaxation and breathing techniques are extremely useful when used together and used at the correct times. It is common for women to breathe short, rapid breaths at the strongest part of the contraction. Studies show that this can cause a panic-type response in your body that can increase tension and heighten the pain. Learning to "sigh out slowly" (SOS) and keeping your shoulders down can help you in labour, if you have practised during pregnancy. At the end of labour, when it is necessary to control the head as it delivers, the midwife will ask you to pant or blow. This is two short breaths out followed by a longer breath out. Combining breathing techniques with working with your partner and the

How an epidural works

An epidural is an injection into your back that numbs your body so that you are unable to feel the contractions. For about 90 per cent of women it completely blocks the pain. Epidurals work by blocking pain nerves as they enter the spinal cord. Setting up an epidural is a medical procedure that can only be done by an anaesthetist. A local anaesthetic is injected to numb the area of the lower back before the procedure is carried out. A special needle is then carefully inserted into the space near to where the nerves enter the spinal cord. A fine tube is pushed carefully through the needle and left in place so that drugs can be run through it. The procedure usually takes around 20–30 minutes, and it takes approximately 15–20 minutes for the epidural to start working effectively.

HOW THE EPIDURAL IS INSERTED: A hollow needle is inserted into the epidural space, taking care to avoid coming into contact with either the spinal cord or its protective covering.

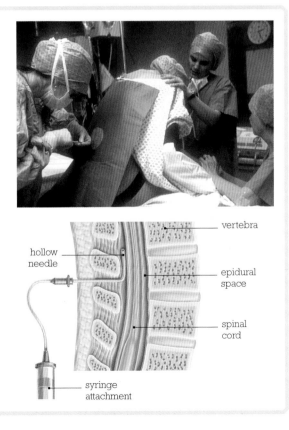

vertebra

hollow needle

epidural space

spinal cord

syringe attachment

midwife can help to make the pain more bearable and thus the birth experience more pleasurable. It is worth pointing out that people have different pain thresholds, and breathing alone may not be enough, especially as labour advances.

Can a water birth help with pain?

It is well documented that water can help with labour pains (see p.156). The heat of the water reduces muscle spasms, and the buoyancy of the water relieves pressure on the pelvis, which lessens the overall pain experienced. The water is kept around body temperature by topping up with warm water and needs to be covering your "bump" to be effective. Studies have shown that it can reduce the length of labours and the risk of tearing. Babies can be born completely under water so that they do not gasp until they hit the cold air. Most hospitals allow you to use gas and air in a pool as an additional form of pain relief.

I want to remember everything about the birth – how can I achieve this?

Probably the most effective way to remember as much as you can about your labour and the birth of your baby is to try to remain as healthy and rested as possible prior to the start of your labour, which will give you the best chance of staying strong and clear-headed during labour. Feeling strong and having plenty of energy may also help you to remain upright and active during the course of your labour, reducing the need for opioids, such as pethidine, which can create a mild state of amnesia, meaning that you may have some difficulty remembering the finer details of the birth. It's also helpful to have a partner or close friend with you throughout your labour so that they too can help fill in any blanks later, and photographs and videos are good prompts. If you do find after the birth that there are parts you can't remember, you could ask your midwife to let you see your birth notes. Or you could try to keep a birth journal between contractions!

I want an epidural but I'm afraid about having one – should I be worried?

Epidurals work by blocking pain nerves as they enter the spinal cord (see opposite). The doctor performing the procedure will be very experienced as it is a very small area they need to aim for. You need to sit very still in the position demonstrated to avoid any problems. There is a slight chance that if the needle goes in too far, it can cause a leak of fluid causing a "dural tap", which can result in a severe headache. Other fears include future backache, which may be prevented by changing your position frequently in labour. There is a very small risk (although this is highly unlikely) that damage is caused to the nerves.

I'm scared to death about going into labour – will I get an epidural?

The availability of epidurals will depend on each hospital. It is best to ask your midwife what the procedure is at the hospital you are booked at. If you think in advance that you would like an epidural, or decide in labour that you would like one, let the midwife know as soon as possible so that she can contact the anaesthetist and arrange this.

Will having an epidural slow down my labour?

As epidurals numb your feelings, this can make it hard to know when to push. As a result, it may slow the labour or increase the risk of a forceps or ventouse delivery slightly. However, if this occurs the midwife or doctor will gently lay a hand on your abdomen and will be able to feel as soon as a new contraction begins in your uterus. This will be a sign to them to encourage you to actively push, even though you do not feel the sensation of the actual contraction due to the epidural anaesthesia. Following the advice of the midwife in this way may reduce the need for an assisted delivery, as pushing with a contraction is safer and more effective in terms of easing your baby through the birth canal.

Q I'm very keen to stay active in labour – can I do this if I have an epidural?

One of the side effects of an epidural is that your legs may feel numb and unable to hold your weight, which can restrict your movements. Some maternity units do offer "mobile" epidurals. These work in the same way as a standard epidural, but you are given a lower dose of the analgesic drug. This means that you are unable to feel the pain of the contractions, but the nerves controlling your legs, abdomen, and bladder are relatively unaffected so you are still able to remain mobile. This leaves you free to move around and be upright during labour and can also mean that you do not need to have a catheter inserted to empty your bladder. A mobile epidural can also increase the likelihood of a vaginal delivery, as being able to move around will assist the progress of labour, and being less numb means that you will be able to push more instinctively during labour contractions. You may want to check in advance with your midwife whether your local maternity unit provides this facility.

Q I've heard that pethidine can make you feel sick, and the baby drowsy after birth. Is this true?

Pethidine is from the family of drugs called opiates and is the most commonly used drug during labour. It is usually given by injection and its side effects include nausea, vomiting, dizziness, or drowsiness; it can also delay the baby's breathing.

To combat the nausea and vomiting, an anti-sickness drug is usually given with pethidine. If the baby's breathing is noticeably affected, an antidote injection is sometimes given to reverse the effects of the pethidine, although this is not usually necessary and would only be given if the baby didn't respond well to other types of stimulus, such as gently rubbing the baby's back with a warm towel, or gently stimulating and rubbing the feet of a baby, which can be enough to make him inhale. Your baby's ability to breastfeed can be affected if he is drowsy, and midwives are now encouraged to

provide extra support to mothers choosing to breastfeed if they have had pethidine during labour in an attempt to overcome this side effect.

Q When is it best to start using gas and air?

Gas and air, or Entonox, is a combination of 50 per cent oxygen and 50 per cent nitrous oxide (laughing gas). It is widely available in maternity units and can be used in home births. This method of pain relief works by reducing the pain messages that the brain receives. It starts to take effect within 20 seconds, so it is advisable to time your intake of gas and air with your contractions, so that you start taking it just before or at the beginning of a contraction to get the maximum benefit, at around 45–50 seconds.

Gas and air can be used from the onset of your labour. However, some women report that they feel slightly drowsy and light-headed and therefore out of

Pethidine and diamorphine
Opiate drugs used for pain relief during labour

These drugs are useful in the early stages of labour, helping you to relax and deal with the pain, and pethidine in particular is widely used. They can only be administered in the form of an injection by a midwife or doctor, usually in the hospital or a maternity unit. As with much pain relief, these drugs have advantages and disadvantages.

✱ Pethidine has a sedative effect, relaxing the muscles of the uterus, and is especially useful if you are feeling anxious or experiencing a long labour as it helps you to rest.

✱ Both drugs can make you feel nauseous and they can enter the baby's system. If given too close to the time of delivery, they can make the baby sleepy and can even cause problems with the baby's breathing.

control while taking gas and air and therefore you may find that you want to stop taking it while you are pushing if it is distracting you too much and stopping you focusing on the contractions. Some women manage their entire labour on gas and air alone, while others find that they need another form of pain relief in the later stages of labour.

How will I use the gas and air and is it likely to make me feel sick?

Gas and air is breathed in through a mouthpiece or mask that is connected to a cylinder or pipes in the wall that lead to larger cylinders elsewhere. You administer it yourself, so are more in control of how much you take and when.

Gas and air can make your lips and mouth feel tingly and dry, and in some cases women report feeling nauseous while taking it. Using a mouthpiece rather than a mask may help to reduce feelings of nausea brought on by the smell of the gas and the sensation of having a mask over your face, and taking sips of water may help. As the effect of gas and air is short-lived, you only need to use it during contractions; taking gas and air between contractions will not help with the pain of the next contraction and is likely to increase the sensation of nausea.

I want to have a great birth but you hear such awful stories – how can I stay positive?

For every awful birth story there is an equally positive one – it does tend to be the case that you are less likely to hear about the positive birth stories as these aren't such good topics of discussion! However your labour and birth proceeds, the birth of your baby will be amazing because you will finally meet the little person who has dominated your life for the past nine months.

It is sensible to remain open minded about labour and birth, because it's impossible to foresee exactly how things will go on the day. However, there is a lot that you and your partner can do to help prepare yourselves for labour and birth so that you

Gas and air
A form of self-controlled pain relief in labour

A mixture of oxygen and nitrous oxide that is self-administered in labour.

Gas and air, also known as Entonox, is taken through a mask or a mouthpiece during labour. This dulls the pain centres in the brain and produce a sense of euphoria. This needs to be timed with your contractions as the effects are short-lasting, with the gas being breathed in just prior to and during a contraction. You will feel normal once you stop using it.

Gas and air tends to be the preferred choice for managing pain in women who want to labour as naturally as possible. The reason for this is that gas and air has several advantages, including the fact that you can remain mobile and active while using it; it can be used during a water birth; it doesn't affect the baby in any way; and it doesn't make you feel drowsy during labour, which allows you to feel more in control throughout and to remain as focused as possible on your contractions. However, although it is a widely available and a popular choice of pain relief in the UK, it doesn't tend to be used in the United States.

have the best chance of having a positive overall birth experience. For example, you can both learn as much as possible about the process of labour and birth so that you can make informed decisions in labour. You can chat with your midwife, read books, find information on the internet, and attend antenatal classes. Also, knowing how labour progresses helps to demystify the experience and therefore removes some of the fear that accompanies labour and birth. Learning basic relaxation and breathing exercises also helps (see p.173), as being able to relax as much as possible during labour helps you to feel less anxious, which in turn can help the labour to proceed as quickly and smoothly as possible.

How long will it last?
all about labour

How long will my labour last?

This is hard to determine as every woman is different and every labour is different. Also, how long your labour lasts depends on when you start timing it as the start of labour can be a gradual build-up that occurs over a fairly long period of time. Usually, labour is classed as being established when the contractions are regular and getting stronger and do not stop until the baby is born. This, coupled with the cervix opening, are indicators that labour has commenced. During the gradual build-up of contractions, labour is sometimes described as being in the "latent" phase until it becomes more established. This latent phase may last for a period of around 6–8 hours in first-time mothers.

As a general rule, if this is your first baby, you should expect to labour for around 12–24 hours in total. If you have had a baby before, your labour may be a lot quicker, providing there are no other complications, particularly if you have had a vaginal delivery in the last 2–3 years. In some cases, usually with second or subsequent babies, labours can last for only a few hours, or even minutes, and in these situations the mother may not to make it into hospital. The best advice in all cases is to speak to your midwife or hospital if you think labour has started.

I like to know what to expect. What will happen when I first arrive at the hospital?

Hospital routines vary, but generally you will be shown to a room on the labour ward, and one of the midwives on duty will come to see you. As well as asking you about your labour so far, she will probably ask to check your temperature, pulse, and blood pressure, and listen to the baby's heartbeat. She will also feel your tummy to assess the baby's position and how far the head has engaged or moved down in the pelvis (see p.148). If your contractions are regular, an internal examination may sometimes be done to reveal how far your cervix has dilated and therefore what stage your labour is at. This information will give the midwife an insight into the wellbeing of both you and your baby, and will help you both to decide on the next course of action. If your labour is in the very early stages, your midwife may suggest that you return home for a while or spend some time on an antenatal ward. If your labour is well established, a delivery room will be found for you.

How will the hospital check my progress?

An experienced midwife can tell a lot about your labour just by looking at you and observing your behaviour. For example, a woman who is chatting happily during each contraction is unlikely to be in well-established labour. A woman who is in established labour and starts to be restless and nauseous may be in the "transition" phase, approaching the second stage of labour (see p.183).

Another way in which your midwife will assess your progress is by feeling your tummy to check the strength of the contractions, and also by feeling the position of the baby's head in your pelvis.

Internal examinations also reveal a lot about how your labour is progressing. By placing two fingers gently into the vagina, the midwife or doctor can feel how far the cervix is thinning out (effacing) and opening (dilating), how the baby's head is moving downwards, and what position the baby's head is in.

What is ARM, and is it routine?

ARM stands for "Artificial Rupture of the Membranes". This means that a doctor or midwife, using a plastic "crochet hook" with a long handle,

Dilatation

In the early stages of labour, the cervix begins to soften, known as effacement, and then starts to widen, or dilate, so that the baby can pass through it and out of the vagina. The baby's head cannot pass through the cervix until it is 10cm wide and fully dilated. The time this takes varies with each labour. Some women are several centimetres dilated at the start of labour while others take several hours to reach this stage.

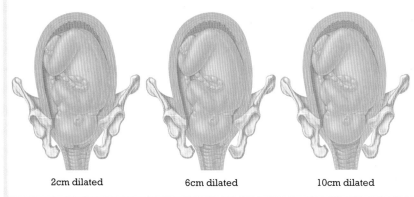

2cm dilated   6cm dilated   10cm dilated

2CM DILATED: In the early stages, the cervix starts to soften and gradually open. **6CM DILATED:** The cervix is around half way through its dilatation and now the contractions get stronger. **10CM DILATED:** At this stage, the cervix has widened sufficiently for the uterus to push the baby out.

tears a small hole in the amniotic membrane that surrounds the baby and contains the amniotic fluid and the fluid then passes out through the vagina. This procedure is also referred to as "breaking the waters" and may be uncomfortable. ARM can be used to try to induce, or speed up, labour (see p.191). The idea is that the layer of membrane between the baby's head and the cervix is removed. This enables the head to press directly on the cervix, which in turn releases the hormones that stimulate contractions and start, or help to speed up, labour.

ARM should not be performed routinely. In a spontaneous labour that is progressing normally, there is no need, and the membranes will usually rupture on their own.

Q I'm worried about being strapped to a bed and monitored. Is that essential?

If there are no complications or reasons for concern, your baby's heartbeat will usually be monitored using a hand-held device much like the one used during your antenatal appointments to listen to your baby's heartbeat. Once your labour is well under way, your midwife will listen to your baby's heartbeat for about 30 seconds to one minute every 15 minutes or so, which means that you can move around as much as you like in between.

If you have had complications in pregnancy, or problems develop during your labour, the midwife may recommend that your baby's heartbeat is monitored continuously using a "CTG", which stands for "cardiotocograph" (see p.192). This means that you will have two monitors strapped to your tummy using thick elastic belts. One measures the baby's heartbeat and the other measures the frequency of the contractions. The monitors are attached to a machine that prints out information in the form of a graph. This allows the doctors and midwives to keep a close eye on your baby's wellbeing and how she is responding to the contractions.

A CTG does make keeping active a little more difficult but by no means impossible. Leads can be moved out of the way and adjusted, and some maternity units have a wireless CTG. You can talk to your midwife about how this will be managed.

How long will the first stage of labour last?

The first stage of labour lasts until the cervix is fully open, or "dilated" (see p.181). Women tend to time their labour from the first contractions, but midwives and other healthcare professionals don't start to time a labour until it is "established", once contractions are coming regularly, roughly once every three or four minutes, and lasting for about 45 seconds to one minute, and the cervix is around 3cm dilated. Due to the difference in how labours are timed, you may hear about labours that lasted 50 hours and others that lasted two! On average, for first-time mothers labour lasts around 12–14 hours. If it continues after this time, the doctor may want to investigate why labour is not progressing.

Once labour is established, healthcare professionals usually expect the cervix to open at an average rate of half a centimetre an hour. However, there are huge variations in this average, and a labour can still be progressing normally with a slower or faster rate of dilation. Your midwife will keep you informed about how things are going during your labour, and don't be afraid to ask how things are progressing.

Is it best to stay upright in early labour?

It is thought that keeping upright and mobile can help labour to progress and make the pain easier to manage. This is because in an upright position the baby's head can press down onto the cervix and in turn stimulate it to dilate, and also gravity helps the baby to move down through the pelvis.

I'm having a trial of labour–how long will I be allowed to be in labour for?

A trial of labour is something that is done if, for example, a woman has had problems in pregnancy

Positions for the first stage of labour

In the early stages, many women prefer to walk around, and being active helps labour progress. If you get tired, sitting on a chair leaning forwards can be comfortable, as can kneeling over a birthing ball or pillows. Some women find sitting on the toilet comfy! If you want to lie down, lying on your left side is best as the pelvis isn't restricted and can open as the baby moves down, and the blood flow to the baby is not affected

LEFT: Use your partner as a support to maintain an upright position. **TOP RIGHT:** Arrange pillows or beanbags for resting in a squatting position. **BOTTOM RIGHT:** Leaning into the back of a chair can be comforting and supportive.

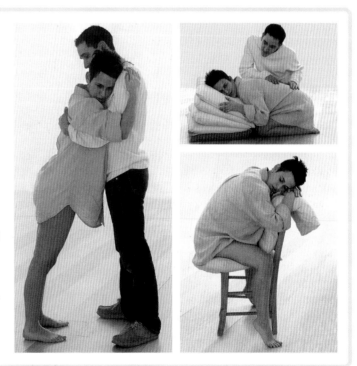

A natural breech birth

If you are having a natural vaginal delivery with a breech birth, this will be carefully handled by an obstetrician. A vaginal breech birth can be slower than a head-first, cephalic, delivery as the bottom doesn't push down as much. The obstetrician will guide the baby out. Usually, the buttocks are delivered first and then the legs will be carefully guided out. The baby may then be rotated to deliver the shoulders as smoothly as possible. Lastly, the weight of the baby helps to draw the head down for delivery.

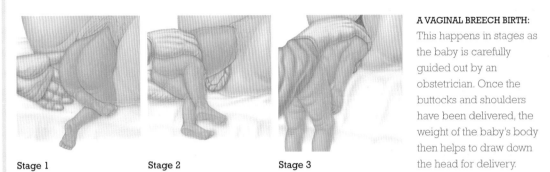

Stage 1   Stage 2   Stage 3

A VAGINAL BREECH BIRTH: This happens in stages as the baby is carefully guided out by an obstetrician. Once the buttocks and shoulders have been delivered, the weight of the baby's body then helps to draw down the head for delivery.

or has had a previous Caesarean. This allows a woman to be in labour long enough to determine if a vaginal birth may be possible. It is hard to say how long you will be allowed to labour for, as the length of time depends on how your labour is progressing and the opinion of the medical staff caring for you.

Your labour will be closely monitored, with your midwife regularly assessing its progress to check that the cervix is dilating as expected and that the baby is moving down through the pelvis. You may be offered continuous monitoring of the baby's heartbeat (see p.192) and would be close to medical assistance in the event of a Caesarean being needed.

When will I be fully dilated?

"Fully dilated" means that your cervix is fully open so that your baby can move down the vagina and be born. When your labour begins, your cervix is either closed, or only one or two centimetres open. The contractions of the uterus gradually open it further until it is completely open. Once this happens, you are in the second stage of labour, which lasts until the birth. The point at which your cervix is fully dilated can occur quite quickly after the onset of strong, regular contractions, or can take many hours.

What is meant by "transition" and why do people say it's the worst bit?

Transition describes the period of time between the end of the first stage of labour and the onset of the second, or pushing, stage. Contractions are usually at their strongest and most frequent at this point. It can last from a few minutes to over an hour, and in some cases may not happen at all. The transition period is often characterized by a woman feeling exhausted, fed up, unable to cope, shaky, or nauseous. In films and books, this is often the time when a woman swears and gets a bit mad with her partner! It is usually around this time that the first feelings that you need to push begin.

If you experience any of the unpleasant symptoms of transition, it helps to focus on the fact that your baby will soon be born. Try to keep your breathing slow and regular, and focus on your partner and midwife for additional support.

ESSENTIAL INFORMATION: LABOUR AND BIRTH

The three stages of labour
How your labour progresses

Your labour is divided into three stages. The first stage begins when you have regular contractions that widen your cervix; the second stage starts when your cervix is fully dilated and ends with the birth of your baby; and the third stage is the delivery of the placenta and membranes.

What is the first stage of labour? The first stage of labour describes the process in which your cervix dilates (progressively opens because of the womb contracting) from being tightly closed to being around 10cm – wide enough to get the baby out, or "fully dilated". During this first stage of labour, contractions generally start off gently and don't last very long – about 30–45 seconds. It is now recognized that you are in established labour only if you are 4cm dilated. Prior to this stage, the contractions you have been feeling have been

ripening (effacing) your cervix. During the early stages of labour, it is a good idea to rest and eat carbohydrates such as toast or pasta, so that you will have some energy when the contractions really kick in. This is called the latent stage of labour. Once the contractions do start coming regularly, staying active is beneficial in that it can help labour become established, as gravity will help press your baby against your cervix. Going to bed could result in labour ceasing altogether. In a first labour, the time from the start of established labour to full dilation is between 6 and 12 hours, although it is often quicker for subsequent labours.

What is "transition"? Towards the end of the first stage of labour, you may feel a great urge to push with each contraction. This period, when you are between 8–10cm dilated, is called transition. It may

The birth of your baby

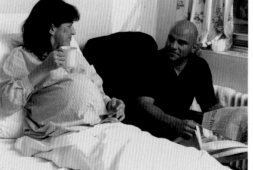

EARLY LABOUR: In the early stages of labour before contractions have become established, try to spend time relaxing to conserve your energy for the hours to come. Drinking fluids and eating a light snack is also advised in early labour.

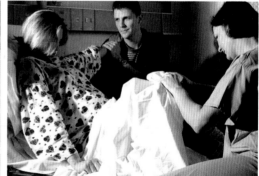

PUSHING DOWN: In the second stage of labour, once your contractions are regular and have increased in strength, you will be encouraged to actively push with each contraction to help your baby move down in the pelvis.

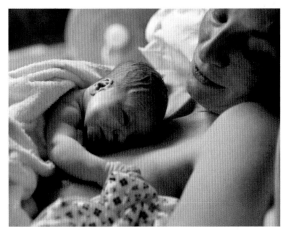

WELCOMING YOUR BABY: Letting go and enjoying close contact with your baby after the birth is a precious time.

be brief, or could last up to an hour, and is often seen as the most challenging part of labour. You will need to resist the urge to push if you are not fully dilated, and may need to use breathing techniques – such as blowing out in little puffs – to help you.

What is the second stage of labour? Once your cervix is fully opened (fully dilated), this is known as the second stage of labour. At the beginning of the second stage, you may experience a pause in contractions, but they will resume and you will be ready to push your baby out with each contraction. Your contractions will now be very close together and very strong, lasting 60–90 seconds, for which you will probably need pain relief (see p. 174). Most hospitals will limit the length of the pushing stage to less than three hours. You will soon see your baby.

What is the third stage of labour? The third stage of labour is the delivery of your placenta. This is the afterbirth that has been feeding your baby during pregnancy. You will be offered an injection of syntometrine to speed this process up and reduce the risk of heavy bleeding, or you can to wait until the placenta comes away naturally. If you choose a natural, or physiological, delivery of the placenta, this can take from 30 minutes to one hour, and you tend to bleed a bit more than if you have an injection.

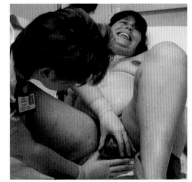

CROWNING OF THE HEAD: As the head crowns, your midwife will tell you to stop pushing and to pant instead so that the head is delivered gradually.

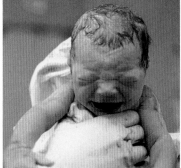

YOUR BABY IS BORN: The midwife or doctor delivers your baby, who arrives as a red and slippery bundle, covered in blood, waxy vernix, and amniotic fluid.

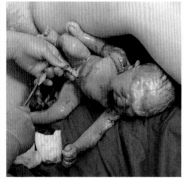

CUTTING THE CORD: The umbilical cord is clamped in two places and the midwife, or perhaps your partner, cuts the cord between the two clamps.

When can I start pushing?

Ideally, you can start pushing as soon as you feel the urge to, assuming that your cervix is fully open. The urge to push is usually stimulated by the baby moving down the birth canal, which happens at some stage once the cervix is fully open. You may experience a sensation of needing to open your bowels and may actually pass some stools or urine, as the baby is pushing on the back passage. This is a very common occurence in labour (see p.188).

If both you and the baby are well, you will be encouraged to follow the natural urge to push. Sometimes, you can feel an urge to push before the cervix is fully open. If this is the case, it is important to resist this feeling as much as possible, as pushing at this stage can cause the cervix to swell, which makes it more difficult for it to dilate. Some women find that kneeling on all fours with their head and shoulders lower than their hips is a good position for this stage of labour.

What is "crowning" and should I continue to push during this part of the labour?

This term refers to the part of birth when the widest part of the baby's head – known as the crown – eases out of the opening of your vagina. Your midwife will encourage you not to push at this stage so that the baby's head can be born in a slow and controlled way, which can help to prevent serious tears to your vagina and perineum (the muscle and tissue around the outside area of your vagina and anus). Although stopping pushing can be hard, you could try short panting breaths or slow steady breaths to help you achieve this.

Although many women are worried about the possibility of tearing during the delivery of their baby, it can be reassuring to remind yourself that midwives are very experienced and practised at guiding women and helping them to avoid tears whenever possible.

Positions for the second stage of labour

Although by this point in your labour you may be extremely tired and the contractions are lasting longer, it is best to resist any urge to lie down as this will not help the progress of the baby through the birth canal. Your partner can help support you while you hold certain positions and help you to remain upright if possible so that gravity can assist your baby. Many women find squatting or kneeling on all fours the most comfortable, or if you really need to lie down, get your partner to support one leg so that the pelvis can remain as open as possible.

TOP LEFT: Sitting upright with supporting pillows helps you to relax between contractions. **TOP RIGHT:** Your partner and midwife can support you in upright positions. **BOTTOM:** Kneeling enables gravity to push the baby down the birth canal.

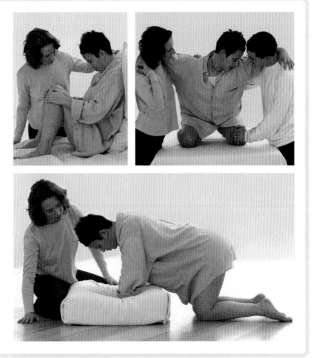

MYTHS AND MISCONCEPTIONS

Is it true that...

If you exercise a lot, your strong stomach muscles make it harder to push the baby out?

Afraid not! The fitter you are, the easier it is to give birth. For a start, you can actually support your own body so you can squat and get into good birth positions. There are other advantages, too: fit women tend to have shorter labours and get their figures back more quickly.

You'll swear at your partner and everyone else when giving birth?

Not strictly true – although no-one will blame you if you do! Giving birth can be incredibly painful, and you may feel emotional, irritable, shaky, and even nauseous. Don't worry too much about what you say and do: remember, the pain signals that labour is progressing, and your baby will be born soon.

You need a super-high pain tolerance?

Nobody likes pain, and it is often said that giving birth is almost unbearably painful. However, your body's endorphin levels will increase during labour to help you cope with the pain. So, as the intensity of the contractions build, so does your ability to handle them.

I'm scared in case I poo in labour, how will I feel?

You are not alone – lots of women are very nervous at the idea of pooing while they are in labour. It may not be what you want to hear, but in fact a large number of women do poo, usually during the second, or pushing, stage of labour. This is totally natural and happens as the baby's head comes down the vagina and pushes against the rectum, where faeces are stored. The faeces are then forced out of the anus and this is totally beyond your control. It is unlikely that you will be aware of pooing at this stage – the overwhelming sensations of birth will be more powerful! Midwives and doctors are very used to women pooing, and will simply wipe it away without a second thought. Also, sterile cloths will be placed around so it will be easily cleared away.

Will I tear when the baby comes out?

Some women do sustain some degree of tearing during the birth of their baby. Unfortunately, it is impossible to tell whether you will tear or not until the actual delivery. Some tears only involve the skin and may not require any stitches. However, others can involve the skin as well as the muscle underneath and the vaginal canal, and this will require stitches. Stitching will be performed by an experienced midwife or doctor after you have had a local anaesthetic injection. There is some evidence to suggest that regularly massaging the perineum, which is the area between the vagina and anus, during late pregnancy may help avoid tearing (see p.111). Allowing the baby's head to be born slowly can also help to prevent tears (see p.186).

What does a "skin-to-skin" birth mean?

"Skin-to-skin" is a phrase that means cuddling your naked baby against your bare skin. Many women wish to have skin-to-skin contact with their baby straight after the birth. This can help with bonding, the baby's temperature control, and the initiation of breastfeeding. As long as you and your baby are

Your newborn baby may look a bit scary – slippery and covered in blood – but embracing him in your arms is a great welcome

well, there should be no reason why this cannot be done – having your baby cleaned, weighed, and dressed can wait a moment. Most health professionals now recognize the importance of this early skin-to-skin contact, and will help you achieve this if that is what you wish. Communicate your thoughts and desires to your midwife as early as you can following admission to the labour ward, so that the midwife can plan your birth to try and meet your wishes.

What is the third stage of labour?

The third stage of labour lasts from after the birth of the baby until the placenta, or afterbirth, and membranes (the amniotic sac your baby has been growing inside) have been delivered. This stage can last for around 10–15 minutes to an hour, depending on whether you have drugs to speed it up (see below).

How does the placenta come out?

After the birth of your baby, the uterus starts to contract again and the placenta shears away from the wall of the uterus and passes out through the vagina. This will not feel the same as giving birth to the baby as the placenta is soft and squashy and much smaller! You may have had an injection to speed up this part of labour, and this is referred to as a "managed" third stage (see below). If this is the case, your midwife will apply gentle traction to the umbilical cord to guide the placenta and membranes out. If you are having a natural third stage, you won't need an injection, which may mean that this part of labour lasts a little longer, and the midwife will encourage you to deliver the placenta and membranes by pushing, and perhaps squatting over a bedpan. Your midwife will advise you as to whether a natural or managed third stage, or a choice between the two, is most suitable for you.

What happens when you have an injection for the third stage of labour?

Women are usually offered an injection of syntometrine during the baby's birth. This is a mixture of two drugs, syntocinon and ergometrine, both of which help the uterus to contract and so speed up the delivery of the placenta and membranes. This is also thought to help prevent the risk of heavy bleeding. Having this injection means that the third stage of labour lasts about 10 to 15 minutes. If you have raised blood pressure, you will be offered a slightly different injection – just the syntocinon – as ergometrine is known to stimulate a rise in blood pressure.

MIDWIFE WISDOM

What happens to the placenta?
checking the afterbirth

The placenta has sustained your baby during her nine months in the womb, and what happens to it after its delivery is a common question.

✱ The placenta will be checked to ensure it is complete and has been delivered successfully. If it looks healthy, it will be disposed of in the hospital.

✱ It may be taken away for analysis in a laboratory if there is anything untoward in its appearance.

✱ Some cultures perform ceremonies with the placenta; and in some parts of the world there is even a tradition of eating the placenta.

However, if your pregnancy, labour, and birth have been straightforward, there is no reason why you should not have a "physiological", or natural, third stage of labour.

What will happen once my baby has been delivered?

Once your baby has been born, if all is well, you will be encouraged to hold him and get to know him. The placenta and membranes will be delivered and the midwife will examine your vagina and perineum to see if you need stitches, which will be done under a local anaesthetic. When you are ready, your baby will be checked over (see p.217), labelled with your name and her date of birth, weighed, and dressed. If she hasn't fed already, the midwife will help you with the first feed. You and your partner may also be offered tea and toast, which is usually most welcome! Before going onto a postnatal ward, you will be helped to wash and go to the toilet. If you and the baby are fit and well, you may be able to go home within a few hours, sometimes straight from the labour ward, providing you have all the help you both need.

If you have a Caesarean, you will be moved to a "recovery" room near to the theatre for up to two hours to observe your breathing rate, pulse, and blood pressure. Your incision and vaginal blood loss will be checked as will your fluid levels, and the midwife will help you to breastfeed your baby. You will then be moved to a postnatal ward.

It all sounds very "busy". Will we be left alone at all once the baby is born?

Many couples look forward to having some time alone together after the baby's birth in order to start to get to know, and bond with, their baby in private. There shouldn't be a problem with this, as long as neither mum nor baby has any medical problems. The midwife will make sure you know how to call for assistance if you need it. You would usually be taken to a postnatal ward about two hours after your baby's birth, if all is well. Or an early discharge home may be an option.

I'm over my due date
do I need to be induced?

Q What is happening to my baby after 40 weeks?

In many pregnancies, there are no changes to your baby's activities after 40 weeks and his movement patterns will be the same, although your baby's head will probably move lower into your pelvis as he gets ready for labour, resulting in a lighter feeling under your ribs and a heavier feeling down in the pelvic area. In other pregnancies, mothers may notice a slowing down of movements as the pregnancy progresses. The placenta, which feeds the baby, operates on a lower efficiency after about 38 weeks, and certainly after 41 weeks. This means that your baby's growth tends to slow down the further your pregnancy goes. As it is not possible to accurately predict whether or not the placenta will continue to function well, most hospitals have an induction policy to avoid the risk of distress to the baby, which increases the longer the pregnancy continues.

Q What happens if you go over your due date?

This varies slightly from area to area, however you would normally be offered an induction of labour between 41 and 42 weeks of pregnancy, which means that your labour will be started off artificially (see opposite). Different hospitals have their own criteria for how long past your due date they will wait before suggesting an induction of labour, but this is usually between 10 and 14 days after your expected date of delivery (EDD).

If an induction is considered, your doctor or midwife should discuss all your options with you before any decision is reached. Although you are within your rights to decline induction, you should make sure that you are fully aware of the reasons why it has been suggested so that you can make an informed decision.

Q I have a long menstrual cycle. I don't think I'm as overdue as they say. Can nature take its course?

The "due date" is calculated from the first day of your last period, and assumes you have an average 28-day menstrual cycle. However, if you have, for example a 35-day cycle, your due date would be a week later. If this is the case, an ultrasound scan during the first 20 weeks of pregnancy would have measured the growth of the fetus and this would have given you a due date that reflected your menstrual cycle more accurately.

Current guidelines recommend inducing labour between 41 and 42 weeks of pregnancy if it has not begun on its own. If you choose not to be induced, you will be monitored regularly.

Q What is a "membrane sweep" and could I have this instead of being induced?

Prior to an induction of labour, at 41-plus weeks of pregnancy, it is recommended that all women are offered a membrane stretch and sweep to assess the readiness of the cervix for labour. A membrane sweep involves your midwife or doctor placing a finger just inside your cervix and making a circular, sweeping movement to separate the membranes from the cervix. The aim of this is to stimulate the release of hormones that may start labour contractions. Although this is likely to be an uncomfortable procedure, it should not cause you actual pain; you may also experience a mucus/bloodstained "show" – like a discharge – following this, which is quite normal (see p.167).

Membrane sweeps have been shown to increase the chance of labour starting naturally within the next 48 hours and therefore reduce the need for other methods of induction.

Types of induction
When your baby is overdue

Induction, when labour is started artificially, may be necessary for health reasons (your health or your baby's) or if you are over your due date. If the baby's health is at risk, your obstetrician may consider it better for your baby to be born rather than stay in your womb. For instance, a scan may show that your placenta is not working properly and your baby not growing – in this case it would be better for your baby to be born and fed orally.

How will I be induced? There are several methods that can be used to induce labour. To start with, your cervix needs to ripen (soften) and begin to dilate (see p.181). You can be given gel or pessaries of prostaglandin for this to happen. These are placed at the top of your vagina so that the drug can work on your cervix. Most units keep you in hospital after this, as the midwives will be regularly recording the baby's heartbeat on the cardiotocograph machine (CTG) to ensure that you and your baby are coping with the induction drugs. Occasionally the cervix does not ripen; if this happens, you may be given a second gel or pessary in six hours.

What happens next? If the gel still does not work, the midwife or doctor will break the bag of waters around the baby (artificial rupture of membranes, or ARM), which may cause discomfort. If you still don't have contractions, a drip will be inserted into your arm and a synthetic hormone, syntocinon, is given to start contractions. Your baby's heartbeat will be monitored while you are on the drip, as there is a risk that you may contract too much and the heartbeat be affected. Some women find this type of labour more painful and may need more analgesia, such as an epidural. If none of these works, you will be offered a Caesarean.

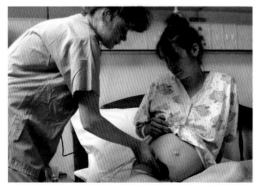

MONITORING THE BABY: The baby's heartbeat may be monitored closely on a cardiotograph (CTG) as the contractions can be strong and sudden following an induction, increasing the chance of your baby becoming distressed.

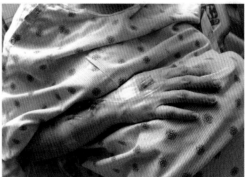

SYNTOCINON DRIP: If the pessaries and artificial rupture of the membranes fail to start contractions, you will be given the synthetic hormone syntocinon via an intravenous drip inserted into a vein in your hand or arm.

Q I don't like the sound of the amniotic hook. What exactly is this?

An amniotic hook is a long, thin piece of plastic with a hook shape at one end. This is used to make a hole in the membranes surrounding your baby to release the amniotic fluid in an attempt to kickstart labour. The procedure, known as "breaking the waters", amniotomy, or ARM (artificial rupture of the membranes), is as uncomfortable as an internal examination, and isn't usually painful, although some women do need some form of pain relief, such as gas and air, during the procedure. An amniotomy is carried out by the midwife or doctor, who will carefully guide the hooked end of the instrument into the vaginal canal with his or her fingers. He or she will then press the end against the membranes to pierce them, which can help to stimulate contractions and in turn start labour.

In some cases, contractions become established quite quickly after this procedure. If this is not the case, then you will need to remain in hospital and be induced with an oxytocin drip (see p.191).

Q Can an amniotic hook harm my baby?

An amniotic hook, which is rather like a long crochet hook used to tear a little hole in the amniotic membrane surrounding the baby and the amniotic fluid, is actually fairly blunt and shouldn't come into contact with your baby at all, so there isn't really any risk that he could be harmed.

Q Why do I need to be induced?

The main reason for induction of labour is when your pregnancy continues past your EDD, or estimated delivery date, as after this stage the efficiency of your placenta can decline, which can put the baby at risk.

Q Can I refuse an induction of labour?

You have a right to say no to any intervention and when induction is considered, your doctor or midwife should discuss all your options before any decision is reached. However, if you wish to delay induction beyond 42 weeks, then it may be

Fetal monitoring in labour

During labour in hospital, you may spend some time attached to a cardiotocograph (CTG) machine. This monitors your contractions and your baby's heartbeat to check whether your baby is showing any signs of distress in labour. Two straps are placed around your waist. One records the movement of your uterine muscle and the other measures your baby's heart rate. The machine you are attached to produces a printout of the two readings so that the midwife or doctor can review the progress of you and your baby. If your labour is straightforward and the CTG readings show no problems, then you can be unstrapped and disconnected from the machine so that you are free to move around. Your midwife may then want to monitor you and the baby again at regular intervals throughout labour.

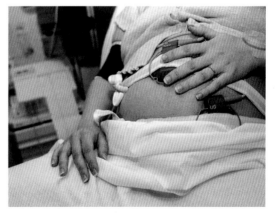

MONITORING YOU AND YOUR BABY: A CTG monitors the baby's heartbeat and your contractions, producing a printout of the readings. This monitor may be used intermittently, or more frequently if there are any concerns about you or the baby.

suggested that you attend the maternity unit for regular monitoring to check on your baby's and your own health, which may include a Doppler ultrasound to check the blood flow in the placenta. You will also be offered an ultrasound scan to check on the amount of water surrounding your baby, as this can be a good indicator of how efficiently the placenta is working and the overall wellbeing of your baby.

Q I'm scared about sudden full-on contractions after induction. Will it be more painful?

Some women do report that an induced labour is more painful than a spontaneous labour. This may be because induced labours can be longer, although this is not always the case. In a spontaneous labour, the body responds to the gradual onset of contractions with the release of natural painkillers called endorphins. In the case of induction, where the onset may be more sudden, the body has less of a chance to do this. However, some women do still get a gradual build-up of contractions after induction.

It is quite natural to be scared of pain, but you may find it a help to be prepared mentally and physically by planning which pain relief options you are going to consider and ensuring that your birthing partner knows your plans so that he or she can give you plenty of support. Many women opt for "low-tech" forms of pain relief, such as TENS, massage, being active and changing position, and aromatherapy, in early labour, and these are all options with an induced labour. If you find these are not enough, you can try gas and air, drugs such as pethidine, and even consider an epidural. If you know in advance how you are going to cope, then you will be better able to deal with the pain.

Q Will I need to be monitored continuously throughout labour if I'm induced?

If a syntocinon (hormone) drip is used to stimulate the contractions then, yes, continuous monitoring of your baby's heart rate is normally recommended. This is so the midwife and doctor can ensure that the

> Bear in mind that doctors will be considering the welfare of your baby when they recommend an induction of labour

contractions are not too close together and that your baby is coping with the contractions and not becoming distressed. During the early stages of induction you will be monitored before, during, and following induction procedures. Then intermittent monitoring of your baby's heart rate will take place. If you do need continuous monitoring, many units now have "wireless" monitors, which means that you are not physically attached to the machine and can still move around during labour.

Q Can my partner be present throughout?

Yes, your partner can be with you throughout your induction and labour, and his continued support is likely to have a positive impact on your wellbeing and help your ability to cope with the pain and stress of labour. Ensure that your partner is aware of your birth plan too (see p.149) so he can support you in any decisions you need to make. A lot of units allow up to two birthing partners, which can be a good idea if things are going to be long and drawn out.

Q What if I don't go into labour after the induction?

Very rarely, women will experience an unsuccessful induction, especially if their cervix is unfavourable, meaning that it has failed to soften and dilate. This may ultimately result in a Caesarean section being performed. As always, discuss the options with your midwife or doctor so that you are fully informed about the procedures being offered.

What can I do to help?
partners at the birth

Q **Should I be with my partner as soon as she goes into labour? I've heard that first babies take ages.**
It's true that first labours often take quite a few hours, although this is certainly not the case with everyone! When your partner notices signs that labour is beginning, such as a mucousy "show", the waters breaking, or irregular period-type pains, she may wish you to be with her. On the other hand, she may be happy to be alone, or with a friend or relative, and keep you updated by phone. Whether or not you are there really depends on how she feels, so good communication between the two of you is the key.

Once your partner is having regular, painful contractions about every five minutes, it would probably be best to be with her, if you aren't already. It is usually around this time that you should be making your way to hospital, if that is where you are planning to have the baby, or contacting the midwife if you are planning a home birth.

Q **I feel very panicky about getting my partner to hospital on time. How can I calm down?**
Your anxiety is understandable. However, not many babies are born on roadsides or in hospital car parks – that's why these stories make their way into newspapers and magazines! It is hard to advise on a definite time to go into hospital as every labour is different and follows a slightly different pattern. However, as a general rule, you should think about going in to hospital if:

＊ **Your partner has had any vaginal bleeding**.
＊ **Your partner's waters break** (see p.167). She may notice this as a gush of fluid from the vagina, or a more gradual leaking.
＊ **Your partner's contractions** (which are often described as strong period-type pains that are accompanied by a hardening of the bump) are lasting around 45 seconds each and coming regularly, at least every five minutes.

If you or your partner are unsure about how to proceed, don't hesitate to give the labour ward a call. An experienced midwife can tell a lot about how far into her labour a woman is likely to be just from talking to her about what is happening.

Q **I've heard lots of stories about blokes in the labour ward – I want to be helpful, but I am nervous.**
Many men are very anxious about being with their partners during labour and birth. This is often due to the fact that they will be watching their partner experience one of the most intense things a woman can ever do and they may be unsure of how to help.

Probably the best way to help overcome your fears is to talk to your partner about how you feel and try to discuss ways in which you could help. You will probably find that there are plenty of ways in which you can support her, such as being aware of her wishes and speaking for her if she is unable to because of the pain, repeating what midwives and doctors have said if she didn't hear or process the information, passing her a drink, rubbing her back, holding a flannel to her face, switching music on or off, and generally encouraging and reassuring her.

Attending birth preparation classes together can be very useful. You will be able to learn more about the process of labour and birth, which can be helpful, and you will learn about how to support your partner both physically and emotionally. Some classes teach birth partners massage techniques that can be an effective form of pain relief during labour. You will also be shown how you can support your partner in certain birth positions. Your partner's midwife will be able to advise you on classes available in your area.

Your role as go-between

One of the most important roles of a birth partner, whether you are the baby's father or someone else chosen to be the birth partner, is to be aware of what is happening during the labour and birth and to liaise with the medical professionals on behalf of the mother if necessary. There may be instances when you or your labouring partner don't understand why a certain course of action is being taken, and your partner may be in too much pain, or too preoccupied with labour, to be able to ask. Your job is to talk to the midwife or doctor and gather information about what is happening. This means that you will both feel fully informed about what is happening in labour and will be able to participate in any decisions that have to be made about the labour or birth.

KEEPING INFORMED: As well as providing emotional and practical support, an important aspect of your role is to pay attention to what is happening and ask questions on your partner's behalf.

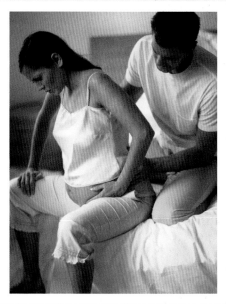

Q I really don't want to be there – how will I tell her and who should go in my place?

Honesty is the best policy, so you need to talk to your partner about your concerns well in advance of the big day. Although she may feel disappointed at first that you don't want to be there, she should appreciate your reasons if they are valid ones. Perhaps you could try to reach some sort of compromise whereby you will be with her during the earlier stages of labour, go out for the actual birth (if you are worried about this), and then come back in again straight afterwards to support your partner and meet your new baby.

It is up to your partner who else she has with her during labour. Women often choose their mum, sister, another female relative, or a close friend to be with them. However, if she can't think of anyone suitable, you may want to consider hiring a doula, who support women in labour (see p.196); there are websites that can help you with this (see p.310). Your partner may also wish to have more than one birth partner, which most hospitals are happy to accommodate.

Q What should we do when my partner goes into labour?

Although it is often hard to define when labour has started, if the signs are that your partner is in the early first stages of labour (see p.167), you can both continue with normal activities as long as she feels comfortable. Being aware of how labour progresses and how contractions build up can help you to plan your course of action. For example, if your partner's waters have broken, established labour usually follows within a few hours (although not always) and it is best to inform the hospital.

While you wait for the contractions to become stronger and more regular, try to relax as much as possible between contractions. You could make a healthy snack for you both to provide fuel for the hours ahead, practise breathing and relaxation techniques together, or run a warm bath to help your partner relax. Once the contractions are around every five minutes and last about 45 seconds, you may wish to consider going into hospital, if that is where you are planning to have your baby. Ring the labour ward first to let them know what is happening.

ESSENTIAL INFORMATION: LABOUR AND BIRTH

Birth partners
Your support during labour

The aim of a birth partner, whether this is your husband or life partner, a friend, family member, or hired doula, is to offer practical and emotional support to you throughout labour and birth.

How can birth partners help? As a birth partner's role is to support you through labour and birth, it is important that they are aware of your wishes and are prepared to liaise on your behalf or keep track of events when you are not able to. It is important that they are knowledgeable about the stages of labour and have discussed with you in advance ways in which they might help, whether through practical support such as massage or helping you with labour positions, or by offering you encouragement and reassurance.

What is a "doula"? Doula is a Greek word that means "woman servant" or "caregiver". Nowadays, this refers to someone who gives emotional and practical support to a woman before, during, and after birth. The aim is for a woman to have a positive experience of pregnancy, birth, and early motherhood. This help and support is extended to the partner and other children. Doulas can offer support in pregnancy, which gives time for the family to get to know her. In labour and birth, she can help with massage, suggesting different positions, liaising with professionals, and giving emotional support. After birth, doulas can help with feeding and baby care, as well as care of the mother. Some do housework, prepare meals, and entertain older children.

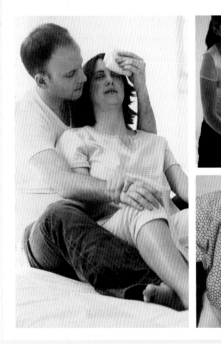

FAR LEFT: Fathers can provide invaluable emotional and practical support to their partners during labour. Being attentive to your partner's needs and comforting and encouraging her will help her to deal with the labour.

TOP RIGHT: A trusted female friend or relative is a popular choice of birth partner for many women, offering understanding and support.

BOTTOM RIGHT: Trained birth partners, known as doulas, are experienced in providing women with practical and emotional support before, during, and after the labour and birth.

Q Is massage useful, or will my partner find it irritating when she's trying to cope with the pain?

Many women find massage, particularly of the lower back, to be very helpful during labour. The sensations of warmth and pressure can be soothing and give some relief from pain during labour. Massage stimulates the body to release endorphins, which are the body's natural painkillers, and also acts as a "distraction" from pain, providing another focus. Communication is the key when it comes to massage. For example, your partner can tell you whether she wants to be massaged during contractions, or just between the contractions, or whether she wants firm or light pressure. You will probably learn simple massage techniques during birth preparation classes, or you may find some classes dedicated to massage techniques for labour. Ask the midwife what is available in your area.

It can be the case that some women find that they do not want to be touched at all during labour. If your partner feels this way, try not to take it personally – this is her way of dealing with the pain.

Q Apart from massage, are there other ways I can help my partner cope with the pain?

Every woman's experience of pain during labour is different, and they will have different ways of coping. It can be difficult to know in advance if a particular coping technique will help, but many couples find it helpful to talk before labour about how they might feel, and how the partner may be able to help. While some women find massage beneficial (see above), others will need help to focus on keeping their breathing slow and steady. It's worth practising labour positions that require the support of a partner before the actual birth (see p.182 and p.186). Having some favourite music on in the room may help your partner to relax. Above all, most women appreciate encouragement and gentle loving support from their partner, and just the fact that you are there will go a long way in helping her to cope with the pain and exhaustion of labour and birth.

(see p.182 and p.186)

MIDWIFE WISDOM

✳ Extra birth partners – can you have more than one birth partner?

Most hospitals are happy for women to have more than one birth partner, although some do set limits, depending on the amount of available space.

✱ It's common for women to have their mum, sister, or close friend with them in addition to their partner.

✱ If labour is particularly long, having more than one birth partner can mean that they can relieve each other for breaks knowing that the mother has someone with her.

✱ Some evidence suggests that having a female birth partner reduces the amount of pain relief and intervention needed.

Q My friend's husband won't be at the birth. She wants me to be her birth partner. How can I prepare?

It's a great privilege to be asked to be a birth partner for a friend and there are plenty of things you can do to prepare for the event. Obviously you will need to talk in advance about your friend's expectations for labour and familiarize yourself with her birth plan if she has prepared one (see p.149). It's important to be sensitive to your friend's wishes, for example does she want you to remain with her throughout, or would she like you to leave the room if she has an internal examination? Talk to her about how she thinks she might react under stress and in pain – is she likely to shout or perhaps become more withdrawn? – so that you can prepare yourself mentally to deal with this. It would also be wise to find out as much as possible about what birth entails – the different stages of labour and what can help or hinder them. You could suggest attending antenatal classes with your friend so that you feel fully informed. It may also help to talk to someone else who has been a birth partner and who may have

(see p.149)

some useful tips. Bear in mind that you may need to be with your friend for a fairly lengthy amount of time, so you may want to have some provisions for yourself, such as snacks and drinks. You may also need periods of relief during the labour, and there may be times when you feel your morale is flagging, in which case it can be a good idea to have someone on standby who you can phone for encouragement and support.

How will I feel when I see a male doctor examine my partner? Will I feel jealous?

If labour and birth are straightforward, it is unlikely that your partner will need to be examined by a doctor. It is only if there is some concern over the wellbeing of either your partner or the baby, or both, that a doctor's opinion is sought. Even in this situation, an internal examination is not always necessary.

If your partner did need to be examined, you would probably find that you would be too worried to be aware of any feelings of jealousy. Doctors, whether male or female, have only your partner's and baby's health in mind when they are performing any kind of examination.

I secretly want a boy – I haven't told my partner – how will I cope if it's a girl?

This is certainly not an unusual feeling to have and I think that many prospective parents have a preference, secret or otherwise, for a baby of a particular sex. While it may take you a little while to become accustomed to having a baby of your "less preferred" gender, you may well find that you have no problems at all bonding with the baby if it is a girl. Seeing your own newborn baby for the first time is something that no-one can prepare for, and many parents feel a strong rush of emotion straight away. Others take a little longer to fall in love with their baby, and this is fine too.

Whichever sex your baby is, it takes time to get to know him or her. You will probably find that you relish watching every little movement and expression,

touching and stroking his or her little body, and will enjoy learning about all the different aspects of baby care. By being involved with your baby from the beginning, you will quickly experience the joy of parenting your son or daughter.

I can be quite panicky in stressful situations. What if I pass out?

The image of the father-to-be fainting onto the floor of the delivery room is often portrayed in cartoons and on birth congratulation cards, but it is far from funny if it actually does happen! Fortunately, it is probably much less common than you may think.

It is understandable for any birth partner to feel anxious and tense – you are watching someone you care about in pain, and you are in unfamiliar surroundings experiencing probably the most significant moments of your life! Focusing on your partner and attending to her needs may help to keep you occupied and distracted and less likely to dwell on your own anxieties. Also, developing a trusting relationship with your partner's caregivers

MIDWIFE WISDOM

Remaining calm
– keeping your cool under pressure!

Even though the birth of your baby is one of the most memorable and exciting events of your life, it can also be hard to witness your partner's pain and to stay calm under pressure.

✽ Being mentally prepared to see your partner experience considerable pain can mean that you are more likely to respond in a reassuring, rather than anxious, way.

✽ Breathing and relaxation techniques can help you to stay calm and focused too.

✽ If you do start to feel flustered, it may be wise to leave the room briefly, if there is an opportune moment, to refocus.

will help you feel able to express any worries you are having, and hopefully you will be given the reassurance and information you need.

If you do find yourself feeling even the slightest bit woozy, try and leave the room as the midwife will be focused on caring for the mother and baby. If you do not have time to leave the room to seek help, and you feel faint, dizzy, or light-headed, try to sit down immediately, with your head lower than your hips, or lie down with your feet raised. Try to stop yourself "panic breathing" (breathing quickly and lightly), and take slow, deep breaths. You should find that the feeling passes quite quickly. The midwife will probably ring the buzzer for assistance. A good tip is to ensure that you are not too hot – take shorts and a T-shirt with you as delivery rooms can be quite stuffy – and make sure you eat and drink regularly to prevent your feeling faint due to low blood sugar.

Q Our little boy suffered a lack of oxygen at his birth. He is fine, but I'm anxious about this delivery.

Unborn babies are designed to cope with a moderate lack of oxygen during the birth, which is quite normal. Some babies do suffer a greater lack of oxygen, and midwives are often alerted to this by observing the baby's heart-rate pattern. If there is any cause for concern, the baby can be delivered quickly, either by forceps or ventouse, or by a Caesarean section. In most cases, the baby is born in a healthy condition, or responds quickly to resuscitation after the birth.

Every labour is different and there is no reason why your next baby should react to labour in the same way as your first, but your baby's heart rate will, of course, be monitored very closely, so you should feel reassured by this.

Q Will I be able to help the midwife cut the cord after the birth?

It is popular for the baby's father, or another birth partner, to cut the umbilical cord after the birth. Midwives and doctors are usually happy for this to

Having a trusted birth partner – whether your husband, best friend, or mum – can help you labour more effectively

happen, as long as there are no problems with the mother or baby that would necessitate the cord being cut very quickly.

The cord is tougher than most people think, but the midwife will guide you and show you how to cut it safely. Be warned that it usually takes quite a few attempts to sever it completely!

Q Will I be able to video or photograph the birth and do I need to agree this in advance?

Most hospitals are happy for you to film or photograph the birth of your baby, if that is what you both want. However, before you embark on this, you should first check that the midwives or doctors who will be conducting the actual delivery have no objection, as some professionals do not wish to be filmed for legal reasons.

While some couples treasure having a visual record of probably the most special and momentous time of their lives, other couples prefer to start filming or photographing their baby after the actual birth. It is important to consider the impact that being filmed or photographed at such an intimate and vulnerable time could have on your partner, and she should not feel in any way pressured to be filmed. Also, it might be worth thinking about how filming the event may affect your actual participation in the birth. If you are concentrating on filming or taking photographs, you may not be as involved in the birth as you could be and may not be providing your partner with all the support that she needs.

When planning how to record the birth of your baby, bear in mind that clear communication between you and your partner before the labour, and with the midwife and doctor once labour has started, is important to ensure that everyone's wishes in this matter are respected.

Q Can we take food into the delivery room?

Most hospitals are happy for you to bring your own food and drink into the delivery room, although most are able to provide your partner with light refreshments should she want something. It used to be the case that women in labour weren't allowed to eat or drink, but nowadays this is not the case. Research on the subject has concluded that it is perfectly safe for women to control their own food and drink intake during labour.

However, hospitals don't tend to provide food for birth partners, so it would be wise to pack plenty of snacks. There is usually a canteen on the hospital campus somewhere but getting supplies from there may mean you are away from your partner for a time. Alternatively, vending machines may be available.

What and how much your partner eats should be guided by her appetite. She should try, however, to stick to light, easy-to-digest foods that will give her plenty of energy, such as fruit juices, bread and honey, dried fruit, digestive biscuits, or bananas. Once labour is well established, it is likely that she won't feel much like eating as her body needs to focus on delivering the baby.

Good communication and getting information from carers is key – we are less stressed when we feel involved in decisions

Q I've heard that natural or water births are best for the baby. Should I ask my wife to have one?

Most childbirth experts would agree that a straightforward vaginal birth is the safest form of birth for both mother and baby. It is also generally considered safe to use water as a method of relieving the pain in uncomplicated labours (see p.156). However, it is sometimes not possible to achieve a straightforward vaginal delivery due to certain situations that can arise during pregnancy, labour, and/or the actual birth. If a problem with either the mother or baby occurs, the medical team will advise on the safest way of delivering the baby.

It is important that your partner thinks herself about the type of birth she would prefer and does not try something she is uncomfortable with. So it is not really your job to make decisions on behalf of your partner, and it's also wise to be prepared to be flexible and to see how labour unfolds.

Q My wife doesn't remember much about the birth. How much should I tell her?

It's best to be honest about your memories of the labour and birth, even if this was a daunting experience for you both. You are likely to be the best person to explain to your partner about how she coped, and sharing your memories may help her to feel comfortable about expressing her own emotions about the birth, particularly if it was fairly traumatic. In this case, an important part of your partner's (and your) acceptance of what happened during the birth is to recall the sequence of events and to try to understand why things went the way they did. This is especially important if you feel that your partner's care didn't go according to the birth plan. If this is the case, you may even want to talk to the midwife who cared for your partner during labour and birth about what happened. You can ask her to go through your partner's notes with you both and explain exactly what happened. You can also ask for a postnatal "briefing" to discuss the birth by contacting the head of midwifery at your local unit.

MYTHS AND MISCONCEPTIONS

Is it true that...

✳ You have to pant while giving birth?

Some natural childbirth practitioners advocate "patterned breathing" or panting during childbirth, while others recommend natural deep breathing, and techniques that rely on positioning and relaxation. Patterned breathing or panting can be useful if it helps you manage contractions, but it's best to just do what feels right for you.

✳ Each labour gets easier?

This may or may not be true for you. Generally speaking, second labours are shorter in duration, but that is not always the case. Shorter does not always mean easier: your second baby could be bigger than your first, or positioned differently; there are many factors that affect your experience of giving birth.

✳ You will feel the urge to push?

Feeling the urge to push is instinctive, natural, and overwhelming, right? Well, believe it or not, this is not always true. Many women do feel an urge to push, but sometimes pushing is painful and women will avoid pushing at all costs. Other times medications, such as an epidural, will interfere with the sensation of needing to push. Your midwife will help you understand what's happening and guide you as to when it's safe to push.

Why isn't the baby out yet?
assisting the birth

Q What is an assisted delivery?

An assisted delivery is one that uses either forceps or a ventouse, or suction cup (see p.204), to help extract the baby from the birth canal if the baby is not making good progress during labour or there are complications during the second stage of labour in a vaginal delivery. You will still be helping to deliver your baby with your contractions, but the instrument used will be helping to guide the baby out of the birth canal.

Q How is an assisted delivery carried out?

Assisted deliveries are carried out using either forceps or ventouse (vacuum extraction) by a doctor (or specially trained midwife). Forceps are metal instruments specially shaped to fit around the baby's head, whereas in the ventouse method, a vacuum is created by attaching a cup-like fitting to the head and using a mechanism to create suction to help draw your baby out.

Q How do they decide whether to use ventouse or forceps? Will it be my choice?

Both forceps- and ventouse-assisted births are relatively safe procedures and, although each has pros and cons, it's best to be guided by the doctor, as the choice of instrument usually depends on the position of the baby and the doctor's preference or experience, although your opinion will be taken into consideration. Although forceps used to be the most widely used instrument, ventouse has increased significantly in popularity. Many consider ventouse easier to use and less likely to cause damage and tearing to the mother. However, this method is also more likely to cause swelling to the baby's head where the cup was placed.

Q What is a "prolonged second stage" and does this mean that the delivery will be assisted?

It is difficult to define a "prolonged second stage" as it depends on certain factors, for example if it is your first baby, the position and size of the baby, if you have an epidural, if the contractions are effective and how often they are coming, how well you are pushing, and if the pelvis is an adequate size. There is some evidence to suggest that if the baby has progressed further into the pelvis, and there is no sign of distress, then there is no need to put a time limit on labour. However, it does tend to be the case that hospitals have guidelines as to how long they will allow a woman to push for before deciding that intervention may be necessary. Usually, after about one and a half hours, doctors may decide to assist the delivery to reduce the risk of fetal distress and of the mother becoming exhausted.

Q I had a forceps delivery as in the end I was too tired to push. Is this likely to happen again?

An assisted delivery is more common during a first birth than in subsequent ones. The first pregnancy and birth causes the pelvic ligaments to stretch,

The decision to assist a vaginal delivery may prevent the need to perform an emergency Caesarean section which can make subsequent births easier, and the uterus is often more efficient in contracting the second and subsequent times around, which also means that labour is usually shorter. Often, even if the baby's head is not in the best position for birth, for example if the baby is in a posterior position, where the back of the head is towards the mother's spine and lower back, it may be delivered without assistance during a second delivery. Therefore, it is likely, but by no means certain, that you will have a normal vaginal delivery next time.

Q Can I refuse to have forceps or vacuum extraction and what are the alternatives?

No-one can go against your wishes if you do not want to have a particular procedure. However, it's usually best to have a flexible approach to labour. Although you may wish for certain things not to take place, the doctor or midwife is likely to have a good reason for wanting to carry out a procedure and has your and your baby's best interests at heart. If an assisted delivery is suggested, asking the midwife or doctor to explain and support this decision can help you to come to terms with it. Usually the only other alternative to an assisted delivery would be a Caesarean section; however, this may be difficult if the baby has gone too far into the pelvis.

Q Will I have an anaesthetic before they use the forceps?

Suitable pain relief, such as a local anaesthetic injection, or an epidural, will be given before the procedure. The doctor will then help to pull the baby out while the mother pushes. The forceps and ventouse cup are removed after the head has been delivered, and the body is delivered normally.

Q What can go wrong at an assisted birth?

Forceps and ventouse can cause bruising, swelling, and marks on the baby's head or face, although these usually resolve without any problems within a few days. In rare cases, cuts and severe bruising on

Assisted delivery
When is this necessary?

An assisted delivery, using forceps or a ventouse vacuum extraction, may be carried out for one or more of the following reasons:

✻ The mother is exhausted from a long labour and has insufficient energy to push.

✻ The baby is showing signs of distress during the second stage of labour.

✻ The baby's head is in a slightly wrong position – if you are in the second stage of labour, forceps or ventouse can often be used to turn the head around and deliver the baby.

✻ Forceps are sometimes used to protect the delicate head of a premature baby during birth.

✻ Forceps are sometimes used to deliver the head of a breech baby.

✻ If the baby is particularly large – this can be the case when the mother has had gestational diabetes (see p.87).

the baby can occur. The paediatrician, a doctor who specializes in babies and children, may prescribe a paracetamol-based medicine to ease any discomfort that the baby may feel. There is also an increased risk of the baby developing jaundice, where the baby looks yellow due to the presence of the waste product bilirubin (see p.164), particularly in cases of severe bruising. The levels of bilirubin in the baby will be checked if the doctor is concerned and the condition can be treated, if necessary.

For the mother, the two main concerns are that there is an increased risk of tearing or being cut during the procedure – and hence an increased risk of more bleeding (which can be dealt with straight away) – and, rarely, damage may occur to the tubes that lead from the bladder.

If the situation warrants an assisted delivery, the benefits of delivering babies by these methods far outweigh the risks. If the procedure is not successful, an emergency Caesarean may be necessary.

ESSENTIAL INFORMATION: LABOUR AND BIRTH

Helping your baby's birth
All about assisted deliveries

A delivery may be assisted using either vacuum extraction (or ventouse), which involves a small suction cap (metal or plastic) being placed on the back of your baby's head and very gently pulled, or forceps, metal tongs that guide the baby out.

Why might this be necessary? There are several reasons why the obstetrician, and in some units the midwife, will advise this type of birth. Generally an assisted delivery is carried out because the mother is too tired to carry on pushing after a prolonged second stage of labour, and the ventouse suction cap or forceps can help accelerate the baby's progress through the birth canal. An assisted delivery may also be necessary if your blood pressure has risen suddenly, or if there are signs of fetal distress. You will be given either an epidural or local anaesthetic before the procedure is carried out.

Is it safe? This is a safe way for your baby to be born, although there is a very small chance that your baby may bleed under his scalp and may need to go to the neonatal unit to be cared for and monitored after the birth. After vacuum extraction, most babies will have a little bump (a "chignon") where the soft cup has been attached to the head, and the baby's head may look slightly elongated. Babies delivered by forceps may have marks on the sides of the head where the tongs were. However, any swelling or marks should disappear within a few days.

Will I need an episiotomy? An episiotomy – a cut made between your vagina and back passage to make more space for your baby to be born in order to prevent tearing – is sometimes carried out if you have an assisted delivery, and is more likely with a forceps delivery (see opposite).

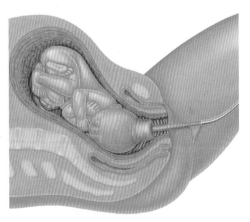

VACUUM EXTRACTION: A suction cup is attached to the baby's head. This creates a vacuum, which is then used to help draw the baby down the birth canal.

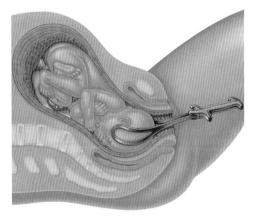

FORCEPS DELIVERY: The curved metal tongs are placed gently on either side of the baby's head and then, in time with the contractions, they help to guide the baby down.

Episiotomy

An episiotomy is an incision, or cut, made with scissors into the area called the perineum, which is the piece of tissue between the vagina and the anus. This area stretches and thins during the birth to allow for the baby's head to be born with ease. An episiotomy is performed only in an emergency situation. An example of this is if the baby needs to be born quickly, or sometimes during an assisted delivery, for example with forceps (see opposite), to prevent uncontrolled tearing. Before the procedure is performed, a local anaesthetic is gently injected into the muscle to reduce the discomfort or pain during the procedure. An episiotomy will need stitching afterwards, and this is usually done by the midwife who has been involved in your delivery or by the obstetrician involved in the birth. Although episiotomies used to be routine around 10 to 15 years ago, they are now performed only when really necessary. You should be informed why one is being recommended and give your verbal consent before the procedure is carried out.

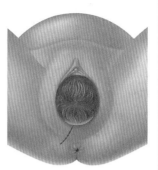

MEDIO-LATERAL CUT: The incision may be done at an angle, moving away from the vagina and into the surrounding muscle.

What is an episiotomy and why might this be done?

An episiotomy is a cut along the muscle between the vagina and anus, known as the perineum, to widen the area where the baby will be delivered (see above). This is done only when absolutely necessary and will not be performed without your consent. There are several reasons why an episiotomy may be recommended, including if the baby is in distress, to speed up the delivery of the head; in cases of forceps or ventouse deliveries; if the baby's head is too large to pass through the vagina; if the perineum has not stretched sufficiently by the end of the second stage of labour to allow the smooth passage of the baby's head through the vagina; if there is a complication in the vaginal delviery of a breech baby; or if the mother is finding it difficult to control her pushing while the baby's head is crowning (see p.186), which means she is more likely to tear significantly during the delivery.

Usually, local anaesthetic is injected into the muscular area first and the procedure is performed at the strongest part of the contraction, as this distracts you from what is being done and assists with a quick delivery.

The thought of having a cut down there is terrifying. What can I do to prevent this?

Some studies have shown that massaging the perineum regularly in pregnancy, using an unscented vegetable oil, can reduce the risk of tearing (see p.111) as this helps to make the area more flexible and may consequently help to stretch the area as the head is being born. Wash your hands thoroughly before massaging the perineum. Although an episiotomy may be a worrying prospect, if you are advised to have one, this may prevent uncontrolled tearing.

Why might they do an emergency Caesarean section?

Emergency Caesareans are carried out for several reasons. The baby may be showing signs of being very tired, picked up by the fetal heart monitor or a blood test carried out during labour, and this could lead to the baby being distressed, known as fetal distress, in which case a Caesarean may be recommended. Rarely, the umbilical cord comes down before the baby, a condition known as cord prolapse, and this is an emergency that requires immediate delivery by Caesarean.

They said I need a Caesarean
all about Caesarean births

Q What's the difference between an emergency and elective Caesarean?

Caesareans are classified as elective or emergency. An elective Caesarean indicates that a pre-planned decision was made during pregnancy to deliver the baby by Caesarean before the onset of labour. An emergency Caesarean is when a situation arises, usually in labour, that means the safest route for delivery is by Caesarean section.

Q Is it fair to say that most doctors prefer Caesarean deliveries these days?

Although the Caesarean rate has risen over the years, it would be unfair to say that this is due to doctors' personal preferences; it is more likely to be due to over-caution on the part of the medical staff. NICE guidelines on Caesareans are quite specific on the reasons why a Caesarean should be considered and offered as an alternative to a vaginal delivery. However, they also recommend that as currently one in five women will have a Caesarean section, all women should be offered some information about the procedure in antenatal classes. If a Caesarean section is considered to be the most appropriate mode of delivery for you, then you should also be made aware of the benefits and the risks to you and your baby and of the possible implications on future pregnancies before you give your consent.

Q Are there any factors that might reduce the likelihood of having a Caesarean?

Research shows there are certain factors that decrease the likelihood of having a Caesarean section and these include:

✱ **Having one-to-one support** from another woman during labour; whether a midwife, a doula, or a supportive friend or relative. This is thought to reduce your chances of having a Caesarean.

✱ **Waiting until after 41 weeks** to have an induction of labour, if your pregnancy has been uncomplicated.

✱ **Having a home birth** reduces the likelihood of a Caesarean if you have had an uncomplicated pregnancy.

✱ **Having appropriate tests during labour**, such as a fetal blood sample and fetal electronic monitoring, will confirm any indications that your baby is distressed before going ahead with a Caesarean.

Q I've got a small pelvis; I'm not too posh to push, but they said I may need a Caesarean. Is this right?

Cephalopelvic disproportion (CPD) is the term used to describe a labour that is not progressing due to the size or shape of the mother's pelvis in relation to the size and position of the baby entering it. Problems may occur if a baby is unusually large or a mother unusually small. True CPD is rare and even if it is a concern in pregnancy, it is often thought best to give labour a try, although you may be cautioned that a Caesarean is a possibility. Certain signs signify CPD in labour; for example if the baby does not descend through the pelvis, or the cervix does not dilate; in these situations, a Caesarean would be necessary.

Q The midwife wrote LSCS in my notes – what does that mean?

The most common type of Caesarean section is a lower segment one (LSCS). This refers to the 12–15cm (5–6in) cut made along the bikini line. The other type of incision is a "classical" or vertical cut, although this is extremely rare nowadays and would only be used if, for example, there was a vertical scar from a previous Caesarean, or in an emergency situation, such as a haemorrhage, although even then it is rare.

Q I want to be asleep during the Caesarean section. Will I have that option?

It is preferable that you are awake in the operation as most surgeons and anaesthetists agree that it is safer for mothers and babies to have an epidural or spinal anaesthetic. Also, you will be able to have your partner with you, and will see and hold your baby straight away. In addition, some women even manage to breastfeed while the operation continues or straight after the operation in the recovery room. There are also greater post-operative risks for the mother and baby with general anaesthesia, including respiratory problems. If you are afraid of the operation, talk to your midwife or doctor. You may be able to visit an operating theatre and discuss the procedures.

Q I haven't had problems, but I just don't want to go through birth. Can I opt for a Caesarean?

If there are no medical grounds for a Caesarean and this is purely down to your fear of labour pains, then to opt to have a Caesarean is a drastic decision. A Caesarean is major abdominal surgery, and although it is sometimes preferable, it is not a favoured method for many reasons, such as the risk of post-operative problems occurring as a result of surgery; a higher risk of secondary fertility problems, or the second baby being born by Caesarean; and an increased risk of postnatal depression. It would be better to talk to your midwife about the pain-relief options available and ensure you receive the most effective type for

A Caesarean doesn't mean you have failed – you have probably done what is in the best interests of you and your baby

you. Having somebody you know and trust with you in labour can reduce your anxiety levels greatly. If you still feel that you cannot go through with labour, you may need to talk to your consultant obstetrician as the final decision will probably be his or hers.

Q I've had two Caesareans and now have been advised to have an elective one. Is this necessary?

It is common practice to advise women who have had more than one Caesarean section or operation involving cutting the womb to have an elective Caesarean. This is because the risk of the womb rupturing during labour is slightly higher with each of these procedures. Usually, women who have had one previous Caesarean can have a "trial of labour" (see p.182), but this will depend on the reason for the last Caesarean and how your current pregnancy is going. If you do have a trial of labour, this will be carefully monitored and any indications that may suggest a rupture beginning would result in a Caesarean without question. It is usual to prepare the mother for a Caesarean in case an urgent one is required by having an epidural anaesthetic in place, as this will reduce the time delay if intervention is needed. Ultimately, whether you opt for an elective Caesarean or for a trial of labour is your decision and the consultant will be able to advise on the risks and benefits of each method.

Q I heard that Caesarean babies are brighter because they don't have a traumatic birth. Is this true?

No, this is not the case at all. Full term, healthy babies are designed to cope with the stresses of a natural labour and birth and should not be affected in any way by this experience. The type of birth on its own does not affect a baby's abilities, although if a baby becomes "distressed" during the delivery, on rare occasions this can cause problems that persist into later life (although usually the baby is born fit and well). It is the case that you can help your baby by staying healthy in pregnancy, for example by eating well and not smoking or binge drinking.

ESSENTIAL INFORMATION: LABOUR AND BIRTH

Caesarean births
How the procedure is carried out

A Caesarean birth is when your baby is born during an operation in which the surgeon lifts out your baby through a short incision made through your abdomen (generally below the bikini line) and through the wall of your womb. This operation is carried out under anaesthetic, which could be spinal anaesthesia, epidural, or occasionally by general anaesthetic. There are many different reasons why a Caesarean birth happens. Sometimes the decision can be made during the pregnancy, which is called an elective Caesarean, and sometimes the decision is made during labour, which is known as an emergency Caesarean.

Today the Caesarean birth rate is 25 per cent in the UK and rising. Look at the statistics from your local hospitals to see what their Caesarean rates are to help you decide where to have your baby. If you are considering an elective Caesarean, you should bear in mind that this is not without risks to you or your baby, or even to your next pregnancy. The decision to have a Caesarean section should be made by weighing up all the risks and then making a decision that is right for you.

Can I avoid a Caesarean? There are a few things you can do to help prevent a Caesarean section, for instance having someone with you throughout your labour, especially a midwife; having a homebirth (if you have no risk factors like high blood pressure); having an external cephalic version (turning your baby while you are about 37 weeks pregnant) if your baby is in a breech position (their bottom coming first); having a senior obstetrician involved in the decision not to have a Caesarean; and, if it is thought your baby is distressed, taking a fetal blood sample before deciding to carry out an emergency Caesarean.

What type of anaesthesia will I have? There are different types of anaesthesia for Caesareans, all of which prevent you from feeling the operation. General anaesthetics (which make you go to sleep) are only used if your baby needs to be born quickly or you have a rare blood disorder with low levels of platelets (these help your blood to clot). More often, an injection is put into your back, which is either a spinal block, when the drug is injected into the spinal fluid, an epidural, or a combined spinal epidural; you are awake to experience your baby being born and there are fewer complications this way.

You will have an intravenous drip in your arm and a urinary catheter (a tube draining urine from your bladder) put in just before you have your

The procedure

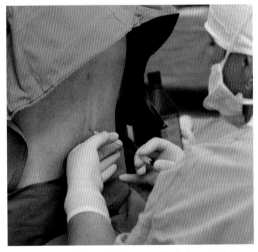

PREPARATION: A fine, hollow needle is inserted into your back and you will be given either an epidural or a spinal block. The operation will start once the anaesthetic is working, in around 20 minutes.

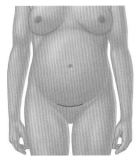

BIKINI LINE CUT: A horizontal incision is made just above the top of your pubic area, along your bikini line. Once the wound has healed, the scar is barely visible.

How much can I do after a Caesarean? Once you get home, take it easy and let the pain guide you as to how much you do. You can start gently exercising as soon as you want and most hospitals give you information as to which exercises you can do safely. Using your vacuum cleaner, driving, and strenuous exercise are definitely not recommended. You can drive again after six weeks, depending on your insurance company.

Caesarean, and these will stay in place for about 24 hours. If you wish to breastfeed, you can feed as soon as the baby is born, while the operation is still happening. It is important that you are pain-free after your Caesarean, so ask the midwives for more pain relief if you need it, ideally before the pain builds up. To prevent blood clots forming in your legs, you will be given an injection and after 24 hours, or preferably sooner, you will be encouraged to get up and walk around.

Will I have to have a Caesarean next time? The reason you had a Caesarean this time will determine the advice from your doctor as to whether you have a VBAC (vaginal birth after Caesarean) or have further Caesareans for subsequent babies. If you feel negative about the birth of your baby, you should try talking to your doctor or hospital and get expert help, as it is common to feel unhappy if you had an emergency Caesarean when you were expecting a vaginal birth.

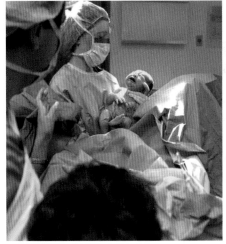

THE BIRTH: Once your baby has been lifted out of the uterus, she is likely to give her first cry. The umbilical cord will then be clamped and cut.

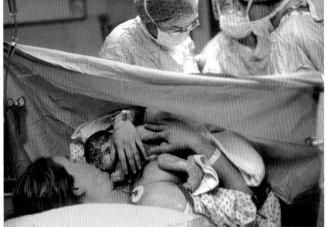

YOUR FIRST HOLD: While the surgeon is completing the operation, delivering the placenta and stitching together the uterus and the various layers of tissue, the baby is handed to the mother or father to enjoy a first hold and cuddle.

Q What type of pain relief will I be given before the operation?

There are two main types of anaesthesia, or pain relief, prior to a Caesarean section: general and regional. A general anaesthetic is the procedure whereby the mother is put to sleep before the Caesarean. Although this is a relatively quick and safe method for the mother and baby, it is not common practice as it is thought preferable for the mother to be awake during the operation so that she is able to expereince the birth of her baby, rather than having to wait until she recovers from the anaesthetic and is possibly too groggy to respond to her baby. There is also a slight risk of the mother inhaling vomit during the operation, and the possibility that the anaesthetic will affect the baby's responses after the birth (see p.207).

A regional anaesthetic is given either as an epidural (see p.176), a spinal block, where the anaesthetic drug is injected into the fluid surrounding the spinal cord, or a combined spinal epidural. In both cases, a needle is inserted into the back and medication is given through a narrow tube to numb the abdomen downwards. Although this takes longer to perform than a general anaesthetic, the anaesthetist will be very skilled at inserting the needle. He or she will use a cold spray to ensure that you are totally numbed and the procedure will not start until the anaesthetist is completely happy that this is the case. On very rare occasions when the procedure can be felt, a general anaesthetic will be given straight away. The regional option is safer and

Don't fret about your Caesarean scar. This will fade with time until it is a barely noticeable thin white line

the birth experience is not missed. The choice will ultimately be yours, unless certain conditions dictate the safest option.

Q Who will be in the operating theatre?

Although it may seem like a crowd, all of the people in the operating theatre have a role. An anaesthetist will be present to make sure you do not feel the procedure and he or she will be helped by an operating department assistant. The main surgeon and his or her assistant will be performing the Caesarean section. A midwife and sometimes a paediatrician will receive the baby. A scrub nurse will pass the instruments to the surgeon and a "runner" will be there to fetch things and count the instruments with the nurse. Your permission must be gained for students to be present. You may wish to have your husband, partner, friend, or a family member present with you, which is usually agreed with the team leader in advance (although it is very common for your partner to be there).

Q How will I be stitched and how long will my scar be?

If you have the most common type of Caesarean, a "lower segment Caesarean section", a 12–15cm cut is made along the bikini line. The other, less common, type is a "classical" or vertical incision. During a Caesarean, the surgeon needs to cut through several layers of fat and tissues before making an incision in the uterus. These internal layers will then be restitched after the operation using soluble stitches and then the layer of skin will be stitched or clipped at the end. Clips, or staples, are usually removed about three days after the operation, whereas stitches are left in for about five days. The removal of clips or stitches is usually a fairly painless procedure.

Q Can my partner still cut the cord?

It is important during a Caesarean section that the procedure is carried out under sterile conditions. This means that all of the staff around the operating table, and the instruments, will be sterile (the highest level of cleanliness). The staff have to undergo a specialized washing technique called "scrubbing" and then use a gown that has been washed and packed to certain standards. This is to reduce the risk of infection to the mother and baby. If your partner was allowed to cut the cord, this would mean that the same principles would apply. It would therefore not be practical or possible to ensure that every partner was trained in this technique. However, it may be possible for your partner to "trim" the cord away from the table as an alternative. This is sometimes necessary when the midwife has cut the cord and applied the cord clamp, but there is still too much cord length, and it is often a good opportunity to involve dads.

Q Will I be able to watch my Caesarean section operation if I want to?

Usually the mother is fully awake for her Caesarean section, with the exception of some emergency situations when it might take too long for the anaesthetist to insert the spinal anaesthetic, in which case a general anaesthetic will be given. However, whether the mother would literally be able to watch the Caesarean section is a different matter. During a Caesarean when the mother is awake, it is usual for a screen to be erected to stop her and her partner from seeing anything. To see the operation, the screen would have to be taken down. You would also need to have your head raised, which would present difficulties for the surgeon, as the operation requires that the mother lies fairly flat so that the surgeon can get to the baby and the abdomen. Although the operation itself may sound thrilling, you may not be thinking this when it is actually happening to you. On occasion, even a planned Caesarean section can run into difficulties, and in the worst case scenario, the mother will have to be given a general anaesthetic.

Many obstetricians, however, do drop the screen, if you wish, at the point of your baby being delivered from the abdomen, and the parents are shown the baby so that they can see what the baby looks like

MIDWIFE WISDOM

Your partner's role
how partners can help during a Caesarean

You may think that there is little a partner can do during a Caesarean, but this is not the case as your birth partner still has the important job of supporting you during the operation.

✱ If the Caesarean is an emergency procedure, partners can make sure that the reasons why this is necessary are clear.

✱ If you are awake for the procedure, your partner can remain in the theatre, sitting by your head and offering you reassurance throughout the operation.

✱ Once your baby is born, you and your partner can welcome her together.

and its gender. Then the screen is put back up to deliver the placenta and stitch up the incision. If you do wish to watch more of the operation, you should discuss this with the surgeon and the anaesthetist prior to the operation. Likewise, if you don't want the screen to be lowered at all, make this clear to the operating team beforehand.

Q What are the reasons for Caesarean sections?

There are various reasons why a Caesarean section might be carried out. You may be advised to have a Caesarean if the baby cannot enter the pelvis due to the baby's size or position or the shape and size of the pelvis; if you have a low-lying placenta; for a multiple pregnancy or breech baby; if your labour is not progressing; if you had a previous Caesarean section or traumatic birth; if you have severe pre-eclampsia; if the baby's growth is severely reduced; if you have had heavy bleeding in pregnancy; and for certain other medical conditions. The doctor will advise you of the reasons why a Caesarean section may be the safest option.

Q Is a baby born by Caesarean section any different to a baby born vaginally?

The condition of a baby following a Caesarean section depends greatly on the reason for the operation. If the Caesarean section is being performed as an emergency situation because the baby's wellbeing is in question, there will be differences between this baby and one born by a planned Caesarean section or vaginal birth. For example if the baby is distressed, its skin colour, activity levels, and breathing rate may all be affected. Each baby is assessed, initially by the midwife and/or a paediatrician, and is then given a score out of 10, known as the Apgar score (see p.217). This looks at the baby's colour, heart rate, stimulation response, how the baby is breathing, and the muscle tone, and the midwife will perform a detailed examination of the baby a little later to examine the baby's skin, fontanelles, ears, eyes, mouth, nose, body, genitals, spine, anus, and heart and breathing. A baby born by a planned Caesarean will have a nice rounded head as it hasn't been pushed through the birth canal, and

is likely to have a good Apgar score. However, a baby who hasn't been through the birth canal has less chance to clear her airways and may swallow amniotic fluid. This can mean that a baby is mucousy for a few days, which may interfere with feeding.

A baby who has been born vaginally and has not been compromised in the labour and delivery may have a slightly misshapen head, as the head moulds to assist its passage through the birth canal, although this soon resolves. A vaginal baby's Apgar score will depend on the stress the baby has been through during the delivery. All being well, both babies will be fit, well, and of a similar condition within 24 hours.

Q What pain relief will I be given after the Caesarean?

As long as you are not asthmatic, do not have pre-eclampsia, and have not bled a lot during the operation, you will be offered a painkilling suppository straight after the Caesarean operation. If you do have any of these conditions, you will be offered an alternative, such as codeine and paracetamol. If you have your Caesarean under a spinal anaesthetic, this will continue to work for an hour or two after the operation. If you are coming round from a general anaesthetic, the pain is likely to be worse and the surgeon may therefore inject a local anaesthetic into the wound to reduce the pain. After the operation, you will be offered regular pain relief, which is likely to be paracetamol four times a day and diclofenac three times a day. If you are breastfeeding, many doctors are now more reluctant to offer regular codeine or codeine-based medication as this may pass through to the breast milk. Instead, codeine may be offered just for the "breakthrough" pain, when the initial anaesthetic wears off, although many doctors offer a liquid morphine-based analgesic or injections of morphine instead, which are unlikely to be addictive as they are given irregularly and in small quantities.

The best way to manage pain relief following a Caesarean section is to inform your midwife as soon as you feel any pain, as the sooner your pain is controlled, the quicker you will be able to move

MIDWIFE WISDOM

*

Taking things slowly
getting back on your feet

Moving around in the first couple of days after a Caesarean is quite uncomfortable, but the sooner you become mobile, the faster your recovery will be. However, it's important to exercise caution and move with care.

* When getting out of bed, move on to your side and use your elbow to lever yourself up, then slowly lower your legs onto the floor.

* When standing, or if you cough or sneeze, place your hands over the site of your wound to avoid discomfort.

* At first, walk short distances only and avoid steps. If you feel dizzy, sit down and rest, then try to walk again in a little while.

Recovering from a Caesarean

Although you should remain mobile after a Caesarean operation, it is also important that you get plenty of rest. A Caesarean is major surgery so you will need to avoid lifting and carrying heavy loads for the first few weeks. As this may be difficult if you have other small children or are at home alone, you should try and recruit as much help as possible after the operation. You should avoid doing any shopping, which usually involves lifting, or driving for a few weeks. Check with your insurance company when they are happy for you to drive again and make sure that you feel comfortable wearing a seatbelt and doing manoeuvres, including emergency stops. It is generally thought to take up to six weeks to fully recover.

TAKING IT EASY: It's important to accept that you have just undergone major surgery and that you need to allow yourself as much rest as possible to aid your recovery.

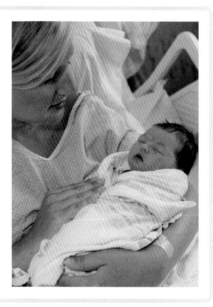

about and this will, in itself, speed up recovery and reduce the risks resulting from immobility, such as deep vein thrombosis.

Will I still be able to hold my baby straight after the birth?

In most units, the midwife or paediatrician will show you your baby quickly before reviewing your baby's condition (see p.217). Once the paediatrician and the midwife caring for you are happy that your baby is well, she will be well wrapped and placed across your chest while you are on the operating table. Although it might be hard for you to hold your baby at this point due to your position, this will be the first opportunity for you to feel and see your baby.

Once you have been transferred to the recovery area after the operation, the midwife will first make sure that you are well by checking your pulse, breathing, and blood pressure, and by looking for any signs of heavy bleeding. She will then attempt to get you into a comfortable position, probably lying on your side, to enable you to enjoy some skin-to-skin contact with your baby and to breastfeed your baby should you so wish.

How soon will I be able to go home after a Caesarean section?

Only a relatively few years ago, women who had had a Caesarean were kept in hospital for around five to seven days, and a few years before that, 10 to 14 days was the average amount of time spent in hospital. Nowadays, mainly due to the recognition that women do recover much better in the comfort of their own homes – where they are likely to get more sleep and rest as they are not being disturbed by other babies – and also sometimes due to economics, lack of space, and reduced maternity staffing levels, women are usually discharged from hospital at around two or three days after their Caesarean operation.

There are individual circumstances when this might not be the case, for example if the mother is not coping well after the birth, if she is on her own at home, or if she is having problems breastfeeding her baby, then her discharge home may be delayed. If a baby has been admitted to the special care unit in the hospital, many maternity units will allow the mother to stay for up to 10 days.

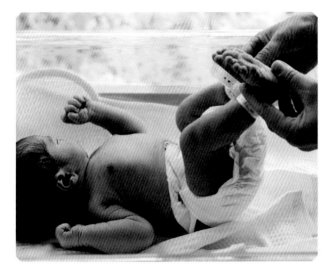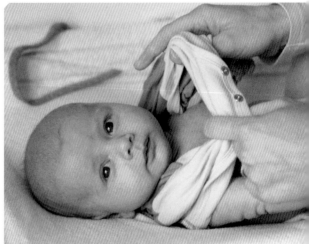
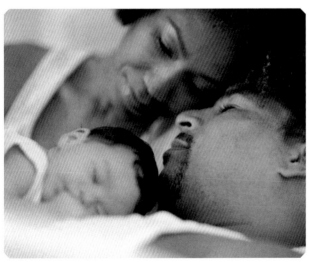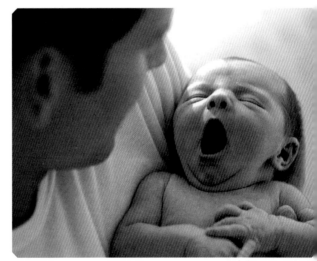
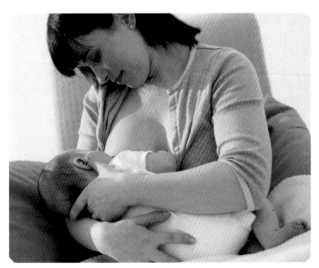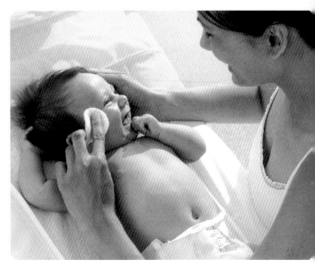

New parents

 He looks like a pixie
is my baby OK?

 Breastfeeding your baby
why breast is best

 I don't want to breastfeed
bottlefeeding your baby

 I just want to go home
the first days with your baby

 I'm scared of dropping him
caring for your newborn baby

 Losing a baby
coping with a devastating loss

He looks like a pixie
is my baby ok?

Q What will happen once my baby is out?

The midwife will first check your baby's breathing and that the airway is clear of mucus or amniotic fluid. A few babies need some help with breathing and are given oxygen after being born. This may be done on the bed, although usually it is done close by on a piece of equipment called a resuscitaire. If this does happen, it is usually only a matter of minutes before the baby is breathing normally and will probably be handed back to you. Other initial checks will be carried out, known as the Apgar score (see opposite), either straight after the birth, or shortly after you and your partner have spent some moments holding the baby.

While your baby is being checked, the midwife will see if you need stitches; if you do you will be given a local anaesthetic to numb the area. The stitches may be done while your baby is feeding, or your partner can enjoy skin-to-skin contact with your baby while you are being stitched. You should have had an earlier discussion with the midwife about your preferences for the delivery of the placenta: the two options are a physiological third stage, when you deliver the placenta naturally, or a managed third stage, when drugs help your uterus to contract and the midwife helps to ease the placenta out (see p.188).

Q What is the Apgar score?

Apgar is an assessment tool used just after the birth to assess the health of a newborn baby and whether they need any medical care (see opposite). Although it was developed in the 1950s, it's still used as a simple and quick, but effective, assessment.

Q What if there is a problem with my baby's breathing?

If there are signs that your baby is having problems breathing, the midwife will give immediate treatment and also ask a paediatrician to check your baby. Sometimes just gently rubbing a baby's skin can improve breathing or a baby may need a little more oxygen. If you had pethidine as pain relief in labour, this can have an effect on the baby's breathing and your baby may have to be given an injection of a drug called Naloxone to reverse the effects. If there are continued concerns about a baby's breathing, then the baby will be transferred to the special care baby unit for a short time for observation (see p.163).

Q Will I be able to have skin-to-skin contact with my baby after the birth?

This shouldn't be a problem, especially if you have had a natural delivery. It is thought that skin-to-skin

---

MIDWIFE WISDOM

** **The bonding process**
getting to know your newborn baby*

You may fall in love with your baby the moment you set eyes on him, or find that your emotions are initially mixed. Whichever your response, there are ways to help you and your baby "bond".

* Some quiet time with your partner and baby after the birth is precious as it helps you relax and get to know your new arrival.

* Try not to feel perturbed if you don't experience an instant rush of love for your baby. Bonding can be a slower process, which doesn't mean that your relationship will be less special. Nurturing and caring for your baby daily is equally important.

Apgar score

These tests are carried out at about 1 minute, 5 minutes, and 10 minutes after the birth. Your baby's skin colour, heart rate, responses, muscle tone, and breathing are assessed. In black and Asian babies, the colour of the mouth, palms of the hands, and soles of the feet are checked. Each is given a score of 0, 1, or 2; a total of 7 or more at 1 minute is normal. Below 7 means that some medical help may be needed.

Apgar score	2	1	0
Skin colour	Pink all over	Body pink, extremities blue	Pale/blue all over
Breathing	Regular, strong cry	Irregular, weak cry	Absent
Pulse/heart rate	Greater than 100 bpm	Less than 100 bpm	Absent
Movements/muscle tone	Active	Moderate activity	Limp
Response after certain stimuli	Crying or grimacing strongly	Moderate reaction or grimace	No response

contact shortly after the birth has many beneficial effects for both the mother and baby. As well as assisting the bonding process, it helps to regulate a baby's temperature, breathing, and heart rate. Skin-to-skin contact also helps to establish breastfeeding, as this is a time when most babies show their natural instincts and root around looking for food, latching on for their first breastfeed. The National Institute of Clinical Excellence (NICE) recommends that skin-to-skin contact continue for at least an hour after the birth, unless you wish it to stop sooner.

Will they clean up my baby first?

This is something to discuss with your midwife before the birth. She will ask your preferences for whether to deliver your baby straight on to your tummy or, as some women prefer, on to the bed to be cleaned and dried before being handed to you.

When will my baby be weighed?

Your baby will have a head-to-toe check, be weighed, and have his head circumference and body length measured. This may be done very quickly after the birth, but more usually it is done once you have had the opportunity to cuddle your baby.

What is vernix?

Most babies born before 40 weeks have some vernix, a white waxy substance, on their skin that protects them while they are in the amniotic fluid. After 40 weeks this begins to disappear. If it is present after birth, it doesn't need to be wiped off as it will gradually be absorbed into the skin.

How will the cord be cut?

Once your baby is born, the usual practice is to place a plastic cord clamp on the cord about 1cm (⅓ in) away from the baby's tummy, and then to clamp another about 3cm (1in) away from the first cord clamp using artery forceps; the cord in between the clamps is then cut using cord scissors. Recently there has been some debate about the best timing for clamping and cutting the cord. The most recent research suggests that delaying the clamping of the cord for 2–3 minutes is most beneficial for the baby. This is because the cord continues to pulsate for several minutes after the birth and so delaying cutting it allows more blood to pass from the placenta to the baby. This boosts the baby's oxygen supply and blood volume, which in turn raises iron levels and reduces the risk of anaemia developing.

Although some maternity units are changing their policies in line with this research, most are continuing with the practice of clamping and cutting immediately. If you have a preference as to the timing of clamping and cutting the cord, you can include this in your birth plan. If your birth partner would like to be involved in cutting the cord with the midwife, discuss this prior to the birth; this should be possible, providing all is well at the delivery.

Do all newborn babies look the same?

Babies vary in appearance at birth and a variety of factors play a part. Sometimes parents are surprised that instead of a soft-skinned baby they are faced with a red-faced, wet, screaming individual. Some aspects of your baby's appearance may be temporary and related to the birth or your baby adapting to life in the outside world, such as the shape of his head, which may have been affected by the birth, or the colour of his skin (see p.219). If your baby is born late, at around 42 weeks, he may have drier, flakier skin than babies born around 40 weeks; if he is born prematurely, he may still be covered in the fine downy hair called lanugo, which will gradually disappear. Also, the type of delivery can affect the way your baby looks after birth. If you have a Caesarean, your baby is less likely to have a distorted or "squashed" appearance to his head as he has not had to squeeze through the birth canal.

I've heard that sometimes the genitals are quite swollen. Why is this?

The hormones produced by your body in pregnancy, namely oestrogen and progesterone, cross the placenta and so are present in the baby during pregnancy and immediately after the birth. One of the side effects of these hormones can be swollen genitals in both newborn boys and girls. In girls, the swelling can be accompanied by a reddening of the skin and some baby girls may have a vaginal discharge. As the hormone levels drop, the discharge may include a small amount of blood, all of which is normal. Hormone levels can also cause swelling of the breasts in both boys and girls. After the birth, any swelling and discharge settles quite quickly as the baby does not produce hormones and levels drop to zero in the first week.

Will he be wrinkly?

A newborn baby's appearance changes over the first hours and days of life. Immediately after birth, babies tend to have a wrinkly appearance because they have been in a bag of fluid for the last nine months, much the same as we get if we stay in the bath for too long. As their skin adapts to being in the outside world, the wrinkles disappear. If a baby is very overdue, the skin can appear quite dry and in most cases will flake off. In this situation, it will also appear wrinkly due to a lack of moisture. Once a newborn baby's skin starts to flake, there is nothing that can be done to stop it, and you should not use any moisturizing products to try to prevent it. Rest assured that the layer of skin underneath will be fine.

My baby's face is covered in spots. Will they go?

Newborn babies have very sensitive skin. They have been protected in a safe environment in pregnancy and following the birth their skin needs to adjust to the outside world. That is why rashes and spots may occur. The most common rash in newborns is called *erythema toxicum neonatorum*, which occurs in around 50 per cent of newborn babies and is usually noticeable around 1–5 days after the birth. This consists of small red spots that appear and disappear all over the skin apart from on the palms

Don't worry if you grimace when you see your baby – it's normal to see a wrinkly face covered in blood, but this is a fleeting moment

Your newborn's appearance

Your baby's appearance straight after the birth may not be what you expected. Straight after the birth, the skin can look dark red or purple, but quickly changes to a lighter colour as he begins to breathe air through his lungs for the first time. His hands and feet may look a little blue for the first 24–48 hours; this is normal, but blue-tinged skin elsewhere at this time isn't normal and should be assessed. A baby's head shape sometimes concerns parents; as the baby passes through the birth canal, the bones of the skull are designed to overlap, which means that after the birth the head can looked quite pointed. However, this resolves within 24 hours. Sometimes there is bruising on the scalp due to the baby's position in labour that tends to disappear in the first week.

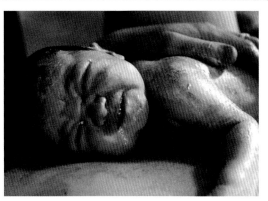

HOW YOUR BABY LOOKS: A newborn's appearance immediately after the birth is quite different to how he will look in a day or two. Your baby may be covered in the thick, waxy substance called vernix and may have marks and bruises sustained during the birth process, which usually disappear within a few days.

of the hands and soles of the feet. It isn't harmful and it doesn't indicate an infection. It can't be passed on to others and it usually disappears within two weeks without any treatment. Milia is another noticeable skin change occurring in about 40 per cent of newborn babies. These are pin-head-sized white spots, which usually appear over the nose and cheeks, but can also occur on other parts of the face. These are blocked-off pores containing some sebum (an oily substance produced by the skin) and, again, they disappear without treatment.

My baby has a big red strawberry mark on his head. Will it be there for ever?

Birth marks are fairly common and most disappear in the first few years of life. Strawberry birth marks start as a red dot and tend to grow in size for about a year, but usually disappear by five years. Other marks include pink patches of skin, called stork patches, and Mongolian blue spots, which are patches of skin with a bluish tinge that occur on babies of Afro-Caribbean or Asian descent. They usually occur at the bottom of the back but may extend over the bottom and are due to the concentration of pigment cells in the skin; they often disappear by three to four years of age. Port-wine stains are larger red marks that tend to occur on the face and neck. These birth marks are permanent, so you may want to talk to a skin specialist about whether there are treatments to reduce them.

Should I be careful about using products on my baby's skin?

Yes, you do need to exercise caution. As a baby's skin is very sensitive, it can react to any chemicals that it comes into contact with, including some baby bath products. The very best option is to use nothing other than plain water on a baby's skin until he is at least a month old, and to continue to take care over which products you use in the following months.

You can use oils to massage your baby. Pure vegetable oil or olive oil is best; avoid aromatherapy or mineral oils, which may be harmful to a baby's skin, and nut-based oils, as there is a possible link between these and the development of nut allergies.

ESSENTIAL INFORMATION: NEW PARENTS

Newborn tests and checks
Top-to-toe examinations

Between 6 and 72 hours after the birth, your baby will receive a detailed examination from a doctor or midwife. The aim of this is to detect any abnormalities in a baby that may not have been picked up by the antenatal scans during pregnancy. If you need to see a specialist as a result of these tests, an appointment will be made at a later date. Other tests are carried out in the couple of weeks following the birth, usually in your home by the midwife or health visitor.

The first examination During this initial examination, your baby will be weighed and measured and his heart and lungs will be listened to using a stethoscope. The roof of his mouth will be checked to make sure that there is no cleft, or split, in his palate and his eyes will also be examined. His limbs will be checked to ensure that they match in

length, and that his feet are properly aligned with no sign of clubfoot. Your baby's tummy will be felt to check that the internal organs are the right size and in the right place, and the pulses in the groin will also be checked. The genitals will be examined, and the spine will be checked to make sure that all of the vertebrae are in place. His hip joints will also be looked at to ensure that these are not dislocated and not "clicky", which could lead to instability later on. Your baby's reflexes will also be checked (see p.223).

The newborn blood spot test This is most commonly referred to as the Guthrie or heel-prick test. It is usually the next check that your baby will have, and it takes place between days 5 and 7 after the birth. This newborn blood spot screening test is carried out to identify babies who may have

How your baby is checked

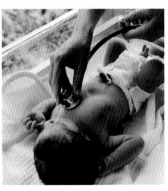

HEART AND LUNGS: A stethoscope will be used to listen to your baby's heart beat and his lungs and check that both of these sound normal.

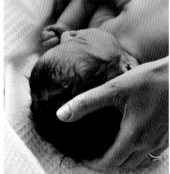

HEAD EXAMINATION: The shape of your baby's head will be checked and the soft spots on the skull, known as the fontanelles, will be examined.

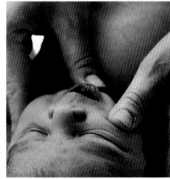

MOUTH AND PALATE: The midwife or doctor will check that there is no split in the roof of your baby's mouth that could indicate a cleft, or split, palate.

rare, but potentially serious, conditions and may consequently need treatment at some stage.

Conditions that are identified Blood spot tests screen babies for phenylketonuria (PKU), a rare metabolic condition; congenital hypothyroidism; cystic fibrosis; sickle cell disorders, which can lead to severe anaemia and other serious health problems.

PKU is an inherited condition in which babies are unable to process a substance in their food called phenylalanine. Early treatment involves a special diet, which can prevent severe disability. If screening has shown that your baby suffers from congenital hypothyroidism, early treatment will involve thyroxine tablets, which can prevent permanent physical and mental disability. In some areas of the UK, babies are also screened for cystic fibrosis.

How the blood test is done The blood test involves the side of your baby's heel being pricked and four drops of blood being carefully placed on a special card. The test is often done while your baby is feeding, as this makes it less painful or alarming for your baby. You can

get the results from your doctor, although you will be contacted if anything is detected. Sometimes further testing is needed. Most babies screened will not have any of these conditions, but, for those who do, early treatment can be vital to ensure long-term health.

Your baby's hearing test A hearing test will be carried out when your baby is around 2–3 days old. Around 1 or 2 babies in every 1,000 will have some degree of hearing loss, and 90 per cent of these are born to parents without hearing problems themselves. The hearing test involves one of two checks. For the first, the specialist will put a small earpiece with a microphone next to your baby's ears, and, for the second test, headphones are placed over your baby's head. Clicking sounds are then made and the brain's responses are recorded and a read-out is given on a computer screen. A very small number of babies will need further testing (around 3 per cent). It is important that any hearing loss is picked up within the first six months of life so that special support can be given to the parents to ensure normal language development later on.

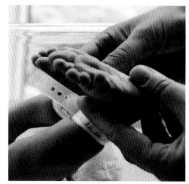

FEET AND HANDS: Each hand and foot is checked and the number of digits counted, and the feet are looked at to check that they align properly.

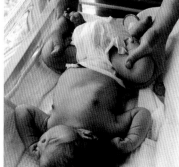

HIPS: The legs are bent gently upwards and then the hips are rotated to check that there is no sign that the hips are dislocated, or "clicky".

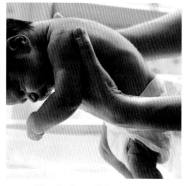

SPINE: Your baby will be turned over and his spine will be examined to check that it is straight and that there are no other abnormalities present.

Q Will my baby have any blood tests before we leave the hospital?

Apart from the newborn blood spot tests (see p.220), other occasions when a blood test may be required include:

✳ **If a baby is ill** and his general health needs to be assessed, which is most commonly done by checking blood sugars.

✳ **If a baby shows significant signs of jaundice,** to check the bilirubin levels and rule out a more serious underlying condition in the baby, such as anaemia or an infection.

✳ **If the mother is Rhesus negative** (see p.79), although blood is usually taken from the umbilical cord at birth to determine the baby's blood group and Rhesus factor.

If the hospital does suggest taking blood from your baby, then a midwife, doctor, or other health professional should clearly explain to you the reasons why they recommend this course of action and ask for your consent prior to blood being taken from your baby.

Q I've heard that they check babies' hips. Why is this?

All babies have two hip checks (see p.221) as part of the recommended child health screening programme. The checks are done in the first couple of days when the baby has a physical assessment, and at 6–8 weeks of age when the physical assessment is repeated.

The two conditions that are being screened for are congenital dislocated hip and developmental dysplasia of the hip, also known as "clicky hips". The screening may be carried out by a doctor or a midwife, or later by a health visitor. If a problem is found, a splint may be recommended to align the hip correctly and ensure the socket develops normally.

Q Why do they measure the baby's head?

Measuring a baby's head is done to assess wellbeing, development, and brain growth. Many babies have their head measured straight after the birth, but this probably isn't the most accurate measurement as the head may have changed shape as it passed through the birth canal. It is not until a few days later that it settles into its normal shape. Your health visitor usually takes a measurement at one of her visits in the first few weeks after the birth and this is generally used as the baseline measurement on your baby's growth chart. Measurements taken throughout the first year are plotted on this in a personal child health record that you will be given by your health visitor.

Q Why do some newborns have jaundice?

Just over half of all newborns suffer from jaundice. Usually it isn't noticeable until 2–3 days after the birth and clears by 14 days. The most common cause is high levels of haemoglobin (the oxygen-carrying part of the blood) before birth. Once babies are born and breathe for themselves, their haemoglobin count doesn't need to be so high; these blood cells die off and are processed as waste by the liver. In small babies, the liver is immature and takes a while to cope with the workload. The result is that instead of this waste product, known as bilirubin, being passed in the urine and

---

MIDWIFE WISDOM

✳ ## Vitamin K
an essential vitamin for your baby

After the birth, you will be asked if you would like your baby to receive a vitamin K supplement. This is an essential vitamin for helping the blood to clot, and as babies receive very little of it from their milk diet there is a small risk that they could suffer internal bleeding. There are two ways to give babies this supplement:

✳ By an injection. Only one dose is needed to prevent vitamin-K deficiency.

✳ By mouth. Two doses are given in the first week and breastfed babies may have a further dose after a month.

Newborn reflexes

Babies have several reflexes that are present from the moment of birth and are part of their survival skills.

* **Startle, or moro, reflex.** If a baby's head is not supported, this produces a falling sensation and she will fling out her limbs. It's important that you always support your baby's head.
* **Rooting reflex.** If you touch your baby's cheek, she will turn her head in search of food.
* **Grasp reflex.** If you put a finger in your baby's palm, she will grip it tightly with her fingers.
* **Stepping reflex.** If you hold your baby upright on a surface, she will make stepping actions.

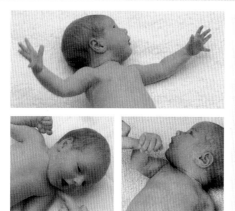
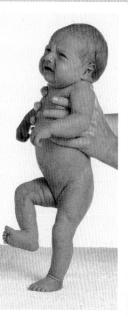

TOP: If your baby feels unsupported she will fling out her arms and legs. **BELOW LEFT:** Your baby instinctively "roots" for food when you touch her face. **BELOW RIGHT:** A baby's grip is surprisingly tight. **RIGHT:** Your baby steps up and down automatically on a surface.

stools, it stays in the body for a while and gives the skin a yellow/orange colour. In a healthy full-term baby who is feeding well, jaundice will resolve on its own without any treatment. Sometimes, if there has been bruising, the baby is slow to feed, or is premature, the bilirubin levels continue to increase, and in these cases phototherapy (ultraviolet light treatment) is needed to reduce the bilirubin levels in the baby.

Any jaundice that occurs within 24 hours of birth and any that continues after 14 days is investigated to rule out and treat any medical problems.

How much will he cry, or will he be asleep all the time?

Many factors influence your baby's sleep pattern, such as the type of delivery you had; the gestation of your baby; his health at birth; and the method of feeding your baby, with bottlefed babies tending to sleep for longer stretches. However, all babies need a lot of sleep, approximately 16 hours each day, which consists of short intervals of sleep intermingled with shorter periods of wakefulness through the day.

My baby's foot is turned in and we've been told he may need a splint. What is wrong with him?

This is known as talipes and affects 1 in 1,000 babies. It's more common in boys and affects one or both feet. Talipes may be positional or structural. Positional talipes is caused by pressure compressing the foot while it's developing, as a result of its position in the womb. This may be resolved with exercises to help the foot regain its natural position. Structural talipes is more complex and is caused by several factors, including a genetic predisposition. This needs prompt treatment while the tissues are soft to manipulate the foot. Splints, strapping, or casts may be used to hold the foot in place. In some cases, if this is not effective, an operation to straighten the foot may be suggested. Both surgical and manipulation methods have a good success rate. Your child will have regular reviews in childhood and adolescence, particularly during growth spurts, and more surgery may be needed in adolescence. There are organizations to contact for support and advice (see p.310).

ESSENTIAL INFORMATION: NEW PARENTS

The first 12 hours, step by step
What to expect after the birth

It's hard to imagine how you will feel at the start of your life with a new baby. What is more certain is that you will most likely be shattered after the birth, and will probably experience a whole range of emotions, from euphoria at meeting your new baby and relief that the labour and birth are behind you, to tearfulness brought on by sheer exhaustion and anxiety at the prospect of caring for this tiny human being. You may feel incredibly protective towards your baby and overwhelmed by the immense responsibility of looking after him. All of these feelings are normal and part of the huge adjustment you make after having a baby. Here is what to expect in the first 12 hours.

1–3 hours Once your baby has been delivered and providing you both are well, you should be able to hold him straight away and enjoy your first cuddle. The cord will be cut by the midwife, or possibly by your partner. After the birth, you will need to push again to deliver the placenta (see p.188). If you had an episiotomy or tore during the birth, you will be given an anaesthetic before being stitched. Minutes after the birth, your baby's condition will be assessed using the Apgar score (see p.217). Within the first hour, he will be weighed, measured, cleaned, and wrapped in a blanket.

If you are planning to breastfeed, you should be able to put your baby to the breast as soon as possible; he may root for your nipple straight away, or may simply enjoy being held close to you and having skin-to-skin contact. If you had a Caesarean, you will be moved to a recovery room once the operation is completed; once in the recovery room, the midwife will help to position you comfortably for the first breastfeed. Also, in the first few hours after the birth, you and your

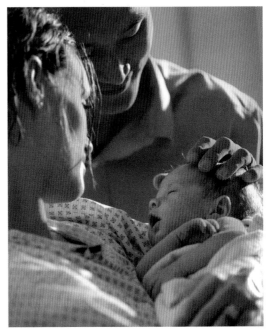

THE FIRST CUDDLE: Holding your baby after the birth is an incredibly precious moment, whether you are feeling exhausted, relieved, or tearful.

partner will be offered some tea and toast, which is usually extremely welcome.

4–5 hours By this stage, you may be recovering on the postnatal ward. If you haven't already done so, you may want to shower and freshen up after the birth. You may need to have someone with you at first in case you are feeling unsteady. If you had a Caesarean, you won't be able to shower yet, but the midwife will be able to give you a bed bath. During this time, you are likely to have your blood pressure, temperature, and pulse rate checked by the midwives, and any stitches you have will be checked intermittently to ensure that they are not bleeding excessively or loose, and there are no signs of infection. You will also be offered medication to help you cope with any pain. Although you may be sore after the birth, it's a good idea to start moving around as soon as possible as this will help your recovery by building up your strength and helping your circulation. Movement will also encourage your bladder and bowel to start working sooner. Passing urine after having stitches can sting, so you may want to try pouring a jug of warm water over your genitals when you go to the loo. If you had a Caesarean birth, moving around will be more difficult, but it is still important to start to be active to avoid the risk of blood clots developing.

6–12 hours Your abdomen will be palpated to check that the uterus is returning to its normal pre-pregnancy size and your bleeding, known as lochia (see p.264), will be checked to ensure that it is not excessive and there are no signs of clotting. Your baby may want to

feed and you can practise positioning him at the breast so that he latches on correctly (see p.228). The midwives or maternity support staff will help you to get started with breastfeeding. You may find you experience fairly strong afterpains while feeding as your uterus contracts down (see p.264). You should also receive practical advice on how to change your baby's nappy and top and tail him (see pp.250–1). Don't worry if you feel apprehensive about the practical care of your baby and try not to feel intimidated if there are more experienced mums on the ward; you will find that your confidence grows quickly as you become practised at handling your baby. The midwives have a supportive role to play on the postnatal ward, so don't be afraid to ask for help.

Often, a sense of camaraderie builds up on the ward, and your stay in hospital can be a good opportunity to talk to other mums and share information and experiences. You may feel well enough to start receiving visitors and, if all is well with you and your baby and you feel ready, you may be able to return home!

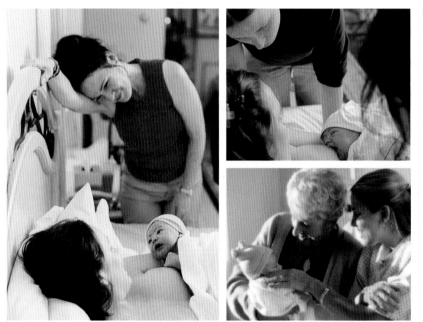

FAR LEFT: Following a home birth, you will be able to take things at your own pace and rest and receive visitors as and when you wish. **TOP LEFT:** Hospital staff will assist you with breastfeeding, helping you position your baby at the breast so that he can latch on correctly. **BOTTOM LEFT:** Once you're settled on the postnatal ward, you will be able to receive visitors. Close family, particularly new grandparents, are usually keen to see the new arrival.

Breastfeeding your baby
why breast is best

Q Can I get breastfeeding advice before the birth and will I get help in hospital?

If you are planning to breastfeed, ask about specific breastfeeding support or sessions available in your area prior to the birth (see opposite), as having additional information beforehand is extremely useful and will help you in the first few weeks when you are trying to get breastfeeding established.

You should get breastfeeding support while in hospital, both in the delivery suite and on the wards; this may come from a variety of sources, not just from the midwife. Many maternity units have maternity support workers who offer support with breastfeeding. Other units encourage local voluntary breastfeeding support workers to come into hospital to offer women guidance while they are staying in hospital and then afterwards at home. Some babies will breastfeed well without problems, while others take a little while to learn, so ask for help and assistance as and when you need it. There are a few tips to remember to help you make a good start:

✱ **Skin-to-skin contact at birth** is recommended to encourage milk production.

✱ **Good positioning and attachment at the breast** is very important. Hold your baby close to you and facing your breast, with her head, shoulders, and body in a straight line (see p.228–229), and make sure that her nose or her top lip is opposite your nipple, so she is able to latch on easily.

✱ **Ensure your baby can reach the breast easily**, without having to stretch or twist.

✱ **Always move your baby towards the breast** rather than your breast towards the baby.

✱ **Feed your baby on demand,** allowing her to feed as often as needed for as long as she wishes.

✱ **Avoid supplements of water or formula milk** unless there is a medical reason for this that has been fully explained to you.

✱ **Avoid giving your baby bottles or dummies** while you are establishing feeding as this can create "nipple confusion" as nipples and teats require different sucking techniques.

✱ **Try to relax** and enjoy your baby's feeds.

Q Should I put my baby to the breast as soon as she is handed to me after the birth?

Holding your baby close to you as soon as possible after the birth is recommended, partly to encourage breastfeeding, and skin-to-skin contact is advised so

Benefits of breastfeeding
Giving your baby the healthiest start in life

There are several unique advantages to breastfeeding, the main one being that breast milk arrives on demand as the perfect food for your baby. Other benefits of breast milk include the following:

✱ Breast milk protects babies from infection.

✱ It reduces the risk of some diseases.

✱ Breastfeeding is thought to increase a child's IQ later in life.

✱ It can reduce the risk of allergies. It has also been reported that babies who are formula-fed are more likely to have breathing problems such as asthma, and gastric problems such as colic. Constipation is also more common among formula-fed babies, and hence there are more hospital admissions from bottlefed babies.

✱ There are greater benefits for the mother if she breastfeeds, such as increased weight loss.

MIDWIFE WISDOM

Thinking ahead
being practically and emotionally prepared

It's wise to think about how to prepare for breastfeeding before the birth.

* Address your perceptions about breastfeeding and those of your partner and family, and deal with negative stories. This is because some of the problems associated with breastfeeding include embarrassment and a lack of confidence in your ability to produce enough milk.

* Purchase nursing bras and try to attend your antenatal classes, where breastfeeding will be discussed. The National Childbirth Trust (NCT) and La Leche League (LLL) also run classes on breastfeeding (see p.310).

that your baby is close to the breast. Your baby may root for the nipple and some babies will latch on instinctively, while others may just sniff and lick the nipple. Don't be worried if your baby does not latch on straight away as babies are born with enough nutrients to last several hours before getting hungry.

What is colostrum?

Colostrum, commonly called the first milk or premilk, is a watery, white/yellow substance produced by the breasts for the first few days. Most women do not notice it until after the birth, although it starts being produced from as early as 20 weeks in pregnancy and may leak during pregnancy. Although colostrum is not abundant, it has a high concentration of nutrients. It is high in protein and vitamin K and it also contains antibodies and white blood cells to protect your baby against infection. Colostrum helps your baby to excrete waste products and lines the stomach with a protective layer that helps fight against foreign substances, such as bacteria, in the body. It is also thought that colostrum helps to prevent allergies.

Help! My breasts are like huge beach balls. Will they stay like this if I carry on breastfeeding?

Between three and six days after birth, your breasts prepare to increase their milk production and may be tender, throbbing, lumpy, and uncomfortably full. This is due to the blood and lymphatic flow to the breasts increasing and a larger volume of milk being produced. This is normal, but if milk isn't effectively removed at each feed, breasts can become swollen, or engorged. This should be a temporary condition, as long as your baby latches on well and feeds on demand for as long as she needs. Some mothers find it helpful to massage the breast during feeds to encourage milk flow. Wearing a supportive feeding bra and alternating hot and cold flannels can relieve the discomfort.

When will my milk come in?

After the birth, your body produces the hormone prolactin, which tells your brain to produce milk, and most women start to produce breast milk between days three and six. Which day your milk comes in may also depend on the type of birth you had, as some studies suggest that milk production is delayed if you have a Caesarean. A delay can also occur if a woman is on medication, such as insulin, to control blood sugar levels. Also, although this is a natural process, certain factors can affect when, and how much, milk is produced, such as a woman's thoughts on breastfeeding and how relaxed she feels, and if a mother is undergoing any stress or anxiety.

There are so many different formula feeds around nowadays – is breast really still the best?

It's true that there are many types of formula milk, with each one striving to be as close to breast milk as possible. However, there are some nutrients and bacteria-fighting cells present in breast milk that cannot be artificially produced. Breast milk contains everything a baby needs for at least the first three months. As well as promoting the benefits of their own brand, all formula brands also acknowledge that breastfeeding is the best option.

ESSENTIAL INFORMATION: NEW PARENTS

Getting started
Establishing breastfeeding

Each mother has a different experience when starting to breastfeed. Both you and your baby will be learning and practising together, which can seem quite strange for something that is supposed to be so natural. Some babies will simply attach themselves onto the nipple ("latch on") straight away, while others will take longer and may need help from a midwife. Sometimes, the type of labour and birth that you experienced can affect how quickly you establish breastfeeding.

How should I start the first feed? Many babies begin to breastfeed if left "skin-to-skin", lying directly on you near your breasts, for about 45 minutes. Your baby can smell your milk and will naturally start to make mouthing movements and turn her head to your nipple. At first, your baby will need only a small amount of food because she has

a store of water and fat in her body to provide nourishment until milk is available. She will, however, have a strong urge to suckle.

How should I position myself for feeds? For subsequent feeds, it is worth taking the time to check that you are in a comfortable position (see below, right). It might help if someone holds your baby while you make yourself comfortable – perhaps with cushions behind your back, or a cushion to lie your baby on.

How should I position my baby? The key to successful breastfeeding is ensuring that your baby is in the right position and has a good "latch". Move your baby so that her nose is opposite your nipple and "tummy to mummy" (your baby's tummy is lying across your tummy) in a straight line and held

Latching on

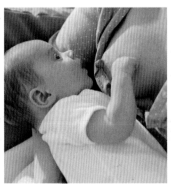

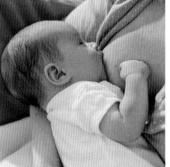

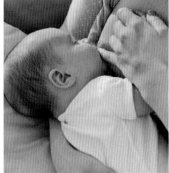

PUTTING YOUR BABY ON THE BREAST: Hold your baby so that her head and body face you and she is level with your breast, with the nipple pointing to her nose.

LATCHING ON: Make sure your baby has the whole of the nipple and most of the areola in her mouth and that her bottom lip is curled back.

REMOVING HER FROM THE BREAST: Gently slide your little finger into the corner of your baby's mouth to break the seal and remove her without pulling your nipple.

close to you (see below). Wait until she opens her mouth really wide (this ensures that her tongue is in the right position) and then move her mouth onto the breast.

How do I know if my baby has latched on properly? It is important to make sure that the whole of the nipple and areola are in your baby's mouth. This enables your baby to get a good sucking action and prevents your nipples from getting sore or cracked. The baby's bottom lip should be curled back, and sucking will be long and deep (rather than little chomping movements). You may also notice that her ears move as she sucks. When your baby has latched on correctly, you shouldn't feel any pain (or, possibly, only a slight pain when she first starts to suck). If it still hurts after she has begun sucking, she is not latched on correctly and you should ease her off the breast and start again after adjusting her position.

How do I take my baby off the breast? Do this by sliding your finger gently inside your baby's mouth – this will break the seal it forms around your breast.

Structure of breasts

Before pregnancy **During pregnancy**

muscle, milk-producing gland, fatty tissue, milk duct

HOW MILK IS PRODUCED: While pregnant, you have high levels of progesterone and oestrogen. After the birth, these levels decrease, allowing the levels of the hormone prolactin to rise, which stimulates the body to produce milk. The milk is produced in special cells called alveoli in the breasts and is transported to the nipple along the breast ducts.

Comfortable feeding positions

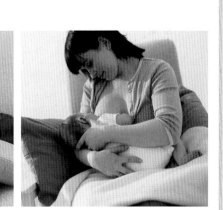

LYING DOWN: Some mothers find that breastfeeding lying down is the best position for them, particularly if they have had a Caesarean delivery. Keep your baby's body tucked in close to you and her head level with your breast so that she doesn't have to pull on your nipple.

TUMMY-TO-TUMMY: Sitting comfortably with your back and arms well supported by cushions, hold your baby so that you are tummy-to-tummy, supporting her with one arm.

Q I'm expecting twins – can I still breastfeed?

Lots of women successfully breastfeed with twins, although it may take extra planning, as life is easier if both babies adopt the same routine and are fed together. Most women think that they won't produce enough milk to satisfy twins; however, milk production works on on a supply and demand basis, so the more your babies suckle, the more milk you produce. You can either fully breastfeed with both babies latching on, or express milk (see p.234–235) and alternate when each baby latches on. Expressed milk may be cup-fed to minimize the risk of a baby taking to a teat and possibly preferring this to the nipple. The Twins and Multiple Births Association has plenty of advice on caring for twins (see p.310).

Q I've heard that it's harder to breastfeed straight after a Caesarean – is this true?

Women who undergo a Caesarean are likely to be in more pain than those who have had a vaginal birth, and studies have also shown that postoperative pain can affect breastfeeding. Also, following major surgery, it's not easy to move around for a day or so. These factors make feeding more challenging initially. However, most hospitals provide good post-delivery pain relief, which helps women to breastfeed. Adopting feeding positions that don't put pressure on your stitches also helps (see below). Even if breastfeeding does not happen in the first 24 hours, it is important to allow skin-to-skin contact between you and your baby as soon as possible.

Q Will I need a special bra?

It is important that your breast is free during feeding. With a normal bra, you would have to remove a garment, so yes, it is advisable to purchase at least two nursing bras. Nowadays there are lots of attractive bras available. The bra should have a zip or drop-cup fastening to allow one cup at a time to be undone. Ask a trained assistant to measure you, as a poorly fitted bra can contribute to problems such as mastitis (see p.233). It's best to wait until 36 weeks before choosing a bra as your breasts continue to grow. The average increase is around two cup sizes.

Breastfeeding after a Caesarean

Breastfeeding after a Caesarean section can be more challenging than following a vaginal birth as your baby may be sleepy from the effects of the drugs and you will be feeling uncomfortable from the stitches. If your baby is asleep most of the time, do encourage her to wake for a feed every couple of hours. Finding a comfortable position to feed is important for the let-down reflex. You may find lying on your side facing your baby easier and this is a recommended position after a Caesarean. In the days following the operation, when you are more mobile, you can try feeding sitting up with your baby lying on a pillow to alleviate pressure on your wound.

SIDE BY SIDE: Holding your baby so that she is lying alongside you, tucked under your arm with your hand supporting her head, can be a comfortable position after a Caesarean as there is no pressure on your abdomen.

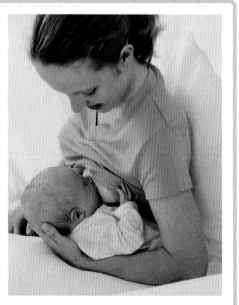

MYTHS AND MISCONCEPTIONS

Is it true that...

✳ I've got inverted nipples so I can't breastfeed?

Babies breastfeed not "nipple-feed" and if your baby latches on well, this shouldn't cause difficulties. About 10 per cent of women have flat or inverted nipples. The best way to find out whether you can breastfeed is simply to try. There are various techniques that may help – do ask for help from your midwife if you're having problems.

✳ My milk can "dry up" just like that?

This is unlikely. Aside from daily variations, milk production doesn't change suddenly. There are things which may make it seem as if your milk has decreased, such as an increase in your baby's appetite (so-called growth spurt) or certain medications (for example, contraceptive pills). Ask for help if you need it, but don't worry too much – your milk supply is triggered by sucking stimulation, and should be just right for your baby's nutritional needs.

✳ I've had a boob job so I can't breastfeed?

This isn't true: many women can breastfeed after implants, but not all. In most cases the implant is separated from the breast by a layer of muscle, but there may be some trauma to the tissue in the placement process. This may decrease the likelihood of successful breastfeeding. If the milk comes in successfully, most women with implants can breastfeed safely. If you're thinking about getting implants but want to breastfeed, it's safest to wait until after you've given birth and fed your last baby.

Breastfeeding is such a struggle. What are we doing wrong?

Although breastfeeding is supposed to be a natural process, for some mothers and babies it can be a challenge. There are a few basic guidelines to help you relax your baby and get her to latch on properly (see p.228). First, try not to force the nipple into your baby's mouth. Instead, wait for your baby to lean towards the nipple. For this to happen, your baby must be turned towards you with her head, shoulders, and body in a straight line (see p.229). Your baby's lower lip should be below your nipple. To soothe your baby, you can try stroking her lip with your nipple, or squeeze a few drops of milk onto her lips. If your baby wants to feed, she will open her mouth to receive the nipple. If so, draw her closer so that she can latch on across the nipple and around the areola (the darker skin around the nipple). Once she is in the right position, you shouldn't be able to see any of your nipple, just a small area of the areola. It should also feel comfortable. Although you shouldn't force the nipple on your baby, you can move her towards the breast so that her mouth touches the nipple and is encouraged to open wide. Avoid bending forwards, as this can give you backache and may encourage a poor feeding technique.

There are key signs that your baby is properly latched on. These are that the bottom lip is curled back, the chin touches the breast, the mouth is wide open, your areola shows more above her top lip than under her bottom lip, and the sucking pattern changes to long deep sucks.

How often should I breastfeed my baby?

This is commonly asked by mothers as they feel that the baby should have a routine or pattern. However, it is best not to schedule feeding times and force your baby into a pattern of, say, every 3–4 hours. All babies, but particularly breastfed ones, should be fed on demand. All babies are different and you will soon become familiar with your baby's signs of hunger. For example, your baby may "root", or search, for the nipple, may not settle, and may make crying or

Troubleshooting
How to alleviate discomfort and pain

Sore, cracked nipples are a common complaint among breastfeeding women and a source of great distress, often leading women to abandon breastfeeding altogether. Knowing what steps you can take to prevent this happening, or how to alleviate any discomfort, will help to make breastfeeding a more relaxing experience.

* Make sure your baby latches on properly and is removed from the breast gently (see p.228). If your breasts are engorged, expressing some milk first helps your baby to latch on more easily.
* Keep your nipples dry between feeds. Let the air get to your nipples and use breast pads to soak up leaks of breast milk.
* Relieve sore nipples with a chilled cabbage leaf. You can use a nipple cream if necessary, although most midwives suggest avoiding these if possible.

whimpering sounds. A baby can only hold about 1–2 ounces of milk in their stomach, so some babies may be hungry after an hour, while others may hold out a bit longer. If your baby dirties a nappy just after a feed, it is likely that she will become hungry again sooner, usually within an hour of the feed. It is also important to allow your baby to feed for as long as possible on each breast before changing side, to ensure that she gets the full benefits of the milk.

What can I do to help my baby get enough milk?

There are steps you can take to ensure successful breastfeeding and that your baby gets enough milk.
* **Hold your baby close to you** as soon as possible after the birth. She will start to "root" for your nipple when she is ready to feed.
* **Feed your baby as often as she demands** in the first few hours and days after the birth. This will enable your body to synchronize with your baby's

needs. Feeding on demand in this way also helps your milk to come in around days 3–5.

✳ **Check that your baby is latched on** correctly (see p.228). When your baby is in the correct position, you will both feel comfortable and relaxed. If the baby is not latched on correctly, it may become painful for you, and you are more likely to stop breastfeeding earlier.

✳ **Allow your baby to feed on one side** as long as possible. This is because the consistency of breast milk changes during the feed. The first part, or foremilk, is lower in fat compared to the hindmilk. The longer she feeds, the more milk you will produce.

✳ **Avoid giving your baby a bottle** and/or a dummy until feeding is established as this may lead to nipple confusion. In some cases, a baby may find it hard to latch on, or reject the nipple in favour of a teat. If this continues, your milk production will fall significantly.

✳ **Some women believe** they should not exercise as it may affect milk production, but this is not the case. Studies have revealed that even high-intensity exercise does not affect breast milk production.

Q How will I be able to tell that my baby has had enough milk?

Although you can't measure the exact amount of milk your baby gets, the breasts work on a supply and demand basis, so your body responds to your baby's sucks and the amount of milk she takes and produces more according to her needs. Usually, babies feed for at least 10 minutes each feed in the first few days after the birth and you may need to offer both breasts before she is satisfied. You can tell that your baby is feeding well as her lower jaw will move steadily while she is on the breast. When she is full, she will fall asleep or release the nipple and be contentedly awake. You should not break the feed, even to change breasts. Your breasts may feel softer and less tense after a feed. Another sign that your baby has enough milk is the amount of wet and dirty nappies she produces. (Breastfed babies tend to have runnier poo than bottlefed ones, see p.242.) If you think that your baby is not satisfied, ask your midwife or health visitor for advice and support before using formula milk.

Q I get wet patches on my clothes and find breastfeeding so messy. Do you have any advice?

Your breasts leak when they are full and overflow, or when the let-down reflex kicks in, for instance when another baby in the room cries or when you feed from the other breast. To avoid this, try expressing to stop your breasts becoming too full. Breast pads can help: there are disposable and washable ones available. If one breast leaks when your baby feeds on the other, put a plastic, washable breast shell inside your bra before you start to feed. If the shell is sterilized, you can save the milk that it collects and freeze it. This can be given to your baby at a later date or donated to a milk bank at your local hospital, if you have one. When you're out, carry a change of clothes, bra, and breast pads. If you feel a let-down, cross your arms and hug yourself, pressing gently against your breasts, which may stop the flow. You will probably leak most in the first few weeks of breastfeeding, while you are establishing the right supply for your baby. Many women find that the problem disappears after the first six weeks.

MIDWIFE WISDOM

✳ Avoiding mastitis
an infection of the milk and surrounding tissue

Mastitis is a painful infection of breast tissue that occurs when the breasts are engorged (hard and swollen) and a milk duct blocked. Dealing with engorgement helps prevent mastitis.

✳ Don't stop breastfeeding as you need to release your milk.

✳ Express little and often to relieve some pressure (which also makes it easier for your baby to latch on), and feed little and often to drain your breasts.

✳ Place a warm flannel on a sore breast.

✳ Begin each feed from the sore side as your baby's sucking is strongest at the start.

ESSENTIAL INFORMATION: NEW PARENTS

Expressing breast milk
Providing additional milk supplies

You can express breast milk as soon as you feel ready after the birth, although some women prefer to wait until breastfeeding is established, at around four weeks. Expressing milk means your partner can start to help with feeds and you may be able to get out for periods.

How is it done? Most women use a pump to express their milk. There are many different types available, ranging from manual to electric ones. The other way to express your milk is manually. To do this, support your breast with one hand, making a c-shape towards the back of your breast and gently squeeze in a downward motion, moving towards the nipple; stop, and then repeat until you have enough milk. You will soon learn where the best place is to put your finger and thumb. Sometimes it is difficult to get a "let-down reflex" when you are expressing – try thinking of your baby and you should soon be making lots of milk.

How should breast milk be stored? It is important that you put the expressed breast milk into a sterile bottle liner or a sterile bottle. This can then be stored in the fridge for 24 hours, or in the freezer for up to three months. Label each bottle or container with your name (if your baby will be with others at a nursery), and the date and time you expressed it. To defrost the milk, warm it gently in a bowl of hot water – don't use your microwave. Do not keep milk in the fridge door, as the temperature fluctuates.

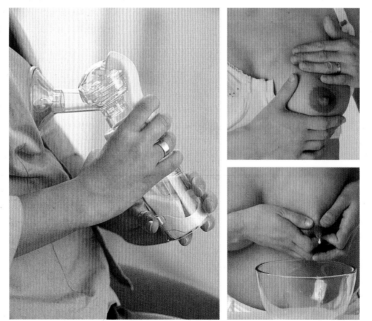

FAR LEFT: Before using a breast pump, try to stimulate the let-down reflex by using a warm flannel, having a warm shower, or looking at your baby. **TOP AND BOTTOM LEFT:** When expressing by hand, use the techniques, above to stimulate your flow of milk. Hold your breast in one hand while you gently massage it with your other hand. Then, with your fingers positioned underneath the nipple and your thumbs on top, gently start to squeeze around the nipple to release the milk.

Q Do I have to watch what I eat and drink if I'm breastfeeding?

Yes. Generally, it is important to remember that your baby receives all the nutrition she needs through your breast milk, so having a well-balanced diet is really important (see p.50). However, there are certain foods and drinks that will affect your baby's digestion. For example, if you eat lots of fruits, such as grapes and oranges, it can cause loose stools or diarrhoea in your baby. You are advised to avoid high amounts of salt as this can cause your baby to become dehydrated. It is also advisable to avoid alcohol. Not only can it make your baby quite sleepy, but there have been studies linking this to cot death.

Q Can all women breastfeed? My mum says she wasn't able to.

The majority of women are able to breastfeed. You may find that the system of maternity care hindered your mother's breastfeeding, as there was a time when mothers were told to feed only every four hours. Learning as much as you can about breastfeeding in advance makes you more likely to succeed. A common myth is that breast size affects the ability to feed, but this is not the case. Breast surgery may affect breastfeeding, but even after the most invasive surgery, it is possible that a portion of the original glands and ducts remain intact. Hopefully you will feel confident enough to give breastfeeding a try.

Q I want to go back to work six weeks after the birth. Is it worth starting to breastfeed?

Yes, most certainly. Even if you only breastfed for the first week, your baby would benefit from the colostrum. So continuing breastfeeding up to six weeks is good. It is estimated that around 40 per cent of women stop breastfeeding at around six weeks, which may also coincide with the fact that they are no longer receiving visits from a midwife or health visitor and therefore have a lack of support. Once back at work, you can express your milk, either at work, depending on the facilities, or in the mornings and evenings at home.

> For many, breastfeeding is a natural extension of pregnancy and birth. The benefits you give your baby are beyond measure

Q What are the benefits of expressing milk?

Expressing breast milk (squeezing milk out of your breasts, see left) enables your baby to receive all the benefits of breastfeeding if you are unable to be with your baby for every feed. Mothers express their milk for many reasons. Some like to give their baby breast milk from a bottle if they are going out when a feed would normally take place, while others who are going back to work express several feeds' worth so they can continue to breastfeed their baby. Mothers of premature babies being cared for in a special care baby unit might express all their baby's feeds.

Q When can I start expressing?

You can start expressing as soon as is practical after your baby is born. Also, studies have shown that expressing as soon as possible can greatly increase long-term milk production. For mothers who breastfeed and are returning to work, expressing should start at least a week before so that the baby can get used to receiving the milk from a bottle or cup. Once you start expressing, if possible, you should express around every three hours, including once in the night when prolactin levels are highest, aiming to express 6–8 times in a 24-hour period. As breast milk is made on a supply and demand basis, the better your baby feeds, or the more often you express, the more milk you will make for your baby. An Australian study found that women who express milk are more likely to continue breastfeeding for up to six months.

I don't want to breastfeed
bottlefeeding your baby

Q I don't want to breastfeed – can you tell me what to do?

If you do not want to breastfeed, you can either bottlefeed your baby expressed breast milk or formula milk. There are many women who do not breastfeed because they receive a lack of support and find that the advice available is insufficient. However, having a go at breastfeeding, even if this is just for one week, will benefit your baby.

If you have chosen to bottlefeed you will need to decide on a few things. First, you need to work out which type of formula you want to use. Take some time to look at the many brands on the market and opt for one that you feel will be right for your baby. Ask your midwife or health visitor for advice if you are not sure. You will also need to purchase bottles, teats, and a sterilizing unit. This can be confusing as there are lots to choose from, so you will need to take some time to find out about the available options and which unit will work best for you (see p.239).

Q Bottlefeeding sounds so complicated. Are there "dos" and "don'ts" to remember?

Yes, it is important to bottlefeed safely. The NHS provides guidelines for safe bottlefeeding.

* **Always make sure you use a sterilized bottle,** cap, and teat for each feed.
* **Ideally, make up one feed at a time** and discard any leftover milk at the end of a feed.
* **Use boiled tepid water** that has been left to cool for up to half an hour before making up a feed.
* **Put the water into the bottle** before the formula.
* **Don't pack the formula into the scoop;** instead, level it off gently with a knife.
* **Warm the feed** – not in a microwave, but in a bowl of hot water – and test the temperature before giving it to your baby.

* **Avoid swapping scoops** from different makes of infant formula milk as different scoops may be different measurements.

Q I feel guilty for not breastfeeding – should I?

No! The main thing is to ensure that your baby receives the best possible care in life that you are able to provide. If it is not possible for you to breastfeed, then formal milk feeds are a safe option. However, you need to feel comfortable with your decision and not be swayed by others. You may want to look at the advantages and disadvantages of both breast- and bottlefeeding. That way you'll be sure you've made the right decision for you and your baby without feeling guilty. Once you have made an informed decision, communicate this confidently to family, friends, and your healthcare provider.

Q Is formula milk as good as breast milk?

Breast milk is universally considered the ideal nutrition for your baby, and the World Health Organization (WHO) recommends exclusive breastfeeding for the first six months of life as it provides all the nutrients a baby needs. However,

Once you decide how to feed your baby don't look back. Be confident in your ability to choose what is right for you both

Bottles and teats
Getting ready to bottlefeed your baby

There are a variety of bottles and teats available in different styles.

You will need between four and six bottles and teats. As well as larger bottles measuring 250ml (8fl oz), you may also want a couple of smaller bottles of 125 ml (4fl oz). Teats come with different sized holes to make the flow of milk faster or slower to suit your baby's needs. Some teats are therefore recommended for newborns and some for hungrier older babies.

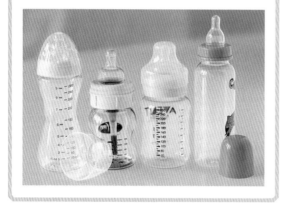

there are a variety of high-quality, nutritional baby formula milks available that scientists and medical experts have spent years developing. Most infant formula milks are derived from cow's milk, but are modified to resemble breast milk as closely as possible. If you feel confused, discuss the different brands with your midwife or health visitor.

What exactly is in formula milk and how similar is this to breast milk?

If you read the labels on different brands of formula, there are not many variances. The Infant and Dietetic Association website (see p.310) provides a table comparing the contents of the five main brands

available in the UK. Baby milk must provide energy, fat, protein, carbohydrate, vitamins, minerals, and trace elements, and the quantity of each nutrient is specified by law. The proportions of energy supplied by protein, fat, and carbohydrate in infant formulas are similar to those in mature breast milk.

✱ **The fat content.** In infant formulas this is based on blends of dairy or vegetable fats that are chosen partly depending on their levels of unsaturated fat. Omega 3 fats may be added as these are vital nutrients for growing brains and bodies. Formula milk does not have the fat-digesting enzyme, lipase, which accounts for the unpleasant-smelling stools of formula-fed babies.

✱ **The protein source.** In formula milk, this is either cow's milk, in the form of casein or whey, or soya (see p.240). The amino acid content of formula is equivalent to that of breast milk to meet the needs of the rapidly growing baby.

✱ **Lactose.** This may be included in formula; mature breast milk contains about 7 per cent carbohydrate in the form of lactose, which is thought to be important for brain development.

✱ **Vitamins, minerals, and trace elements.** These are added to formulas to meet the nutritional needs of the baby and to comply with legal requirements.

✱ **Iron.** This is vital to your baby's wellbeing, being essential for healthy blood, growth, and development, and this is added to formula brands.

✱ **Other components.** Infant formula may contain other components that are found naturally in breast milk, such as long-chain polyunsaturated fatty acids (for brain and membrane development), oligosaccharides (to aid digestion and immunity), or nucleotides (to promote healthy growth and development and to help the immune system).

There are some components of breast milk that cannot be replicated in formulas. For example, breast milk contains important antibodies that help protect babies against infection and illness and these are not present in formula milk. However, prebiotics, which are nutrients found in breast milk that strengthen a baby's natural immune system, may be added to some brands of formula.

ESSENTIAL INFORMATION: NEW PARENTS

How to bottlefeed
Preparing and giving feeds

Bottlefeeding, using formula or expressed breast milk, can seem daunting at first, but becomes easier once you get into a routine.

How do I start? You will need at least 4–6 bottles and teats, with at least one or two sterilized and ready. You can sterilize by steaming, microwaving, boiling, or using a sterilizing liquid. Your choice will depend on the cost and what you find easiest. Before sterilizing, rinse a bottle first with warm soapy water using a bottle brush, taking care to clean the top of the bottle and inside the teat.

How do I make up a feed? Wash your hands and make up a feed according to the instructions. Put the correct amount of tepid boiled tap water into the sterilized bottle first and then add the right number of level scoops of powder. Never add extra powder as this could make your baby ill. Don't put a half-finished feed back in the fridge – throw it away and use a fresh bottle next time.

How do I give the feed? Test that the milk is not too hot by putting some on the inside of your wrist (never use a microwave to warm up milk). Find a comfortable position and always hold your baby's head slightly higher than his body. Put the teat gently into his mouth and slowly tip the bottle so that only milk, not air, gets into the teat. You can wind your baby – gently pat or rub your baby's back – halfway through the feed, or wait until the end. Throw away any milk that is left over.

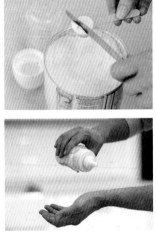

PREPARING A BOTTLE: Measure the powder using a knife to level the top. Add to the water then warm the bottle and test the temperature on your wrist.

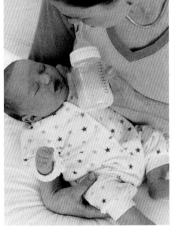

GIVING A BOTTLE: Stroke your baby's cheek to stimulate the sucking reflex and gently insert the teat into his mouth, being careful not to push it too far in.

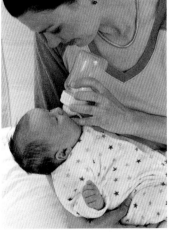

FINISHING THE FEED: Towards the end of the feed, tilt the bottle so that its neck is completely filled with milk. Slide your finger into his mouth to break the seal.

Sterilizing equipment

Before using new bottles and teats, and each time you use them, wash and sterilize them. Wash them in warm, soapy water with a bottle brush, and rinse thoroughly. Sterilizing methods include:

✱ Electric steam sterilizing, which takes about 10 minutes, plus the time it takes for equipment to cool.

✱ Microwave steamers, which take around 5 minutes. The equipment remains sterile for up to 3 hours if the lid is left on.

✱ Equipment can be sterilized by boiling, which takes around 10 minutes. The pan must not be used for another purpose and you may find that teats wear out more quickly.

✱ Cold water sterilizing tablets can be used either in a special sterilizer, or in a suitable clean container with a lid. This takes around 30 minutes and the equipment can be left in the solution for up to 24 hours; the solution needs to be changed each day.

✱ Dishwashers need to be set on a high temperature and some parents prefer to wait until after a year before using these.

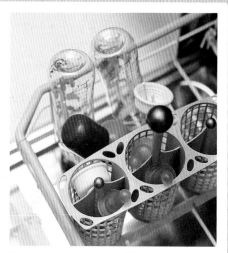

KEEPING BOTTLES CLEAN: Whichever method you choose, it is important to sterilize bottles and teats to keep them germ-free.

Q Is it OK to combine breast- and bottlefeeding?

Yes, it is possible to combine breastfeeding with bottles of expressed breast milk or formula, and many women choose to do this rather than stop breastfeeding altogether. You may also decide to do this if you are returning to work.

Feeding from a bottle uses a different technique to feeding from the breast, and your baby may take a little time to get used to it, which can make it quite a struggle to introduce bottles. It may help to warm the teat and to get someone else to offer the bottle the first time, as your baby may be able to smell your milk if you hold him and will be likely to want to be breastfed instead. Holding him in a different position, such as propped up against your front and facing away from you, may also help.

Before deciding to introduce the bottle, it's worth considering that breastfeeding does get easier and that there is a lot of extra work involved with bottlefeeding in terms of preparing feeds. Also, as your breast milk is produced on a supply and demand basis, introducing bottles for some feeds will affect your milk production. If you do want to combine the two, talk to your health visitor or a breastfeeding counsellor about how to manage this so that you can maintain breastfeeding.

Q Will people treat me like a failure if I can't breastfeed and have to use formula?

Many mothers do feel pressure from friends and family to breastfeed their newborns. It is unlikely that you will be treated as a failure, as Western society is very accepting of bottlefeeding and, on the contrary, it is a continual effort to try to promote breastfeeding in our society. In November 2007, the Department of Health actually banned baby milk manufacturers from advertising infant formula for children under six months old on television and in parenting magazines.

Guidelines aside, although breastfeeding is a wonderful experience, it can sometimes be very hard work to establish. If you find that you are struggling to establish breastfeeding, it's worth seeking help from your midwife, health visitor, or breastfeeding counsellor before giving up completely. However, if you find you simply cannot breastfeed, or you choose not to, you should try not to feel guilty as formula-fed babies grow and develop perfectly well. This is your baby and you will have your baby's best interests foremost whatever action you decide to take.

Q Which formula milk should I buy?

There are a number of brands that have a very similar nutritional content and you may need to chat to your local midwife or health visitor, or even family and friends with little ones, when trying to decide which one to use. Sometimes, babies are born prematurely and may need a special formula, or occasionally may react to a particular brand. If your baby was born full-term and is healthy, it is usually down to personal preference.

Manufacturers modify cow's milk to make formula for human babies by adjusting carbohydrate, protein, and fat levels, and adding vitamins and minerals. There are two main types of formula milk, which have different ratios of the two proteins in milk: whey and casein. Those that are suitable for babies from birth contain more whey than casein. The ratio of whey to casein in these milks is similar to that of breast milk, so it is thought to be easier for new babies to digest. Milks that are marketed for the "hungrier" baby (known as "follow-on" milk) are casein-dominant and take longer to digest.

Q Why do some people use soya-based formula and is it safe?

Soya-based formula is made from soya beans, which are modified for use in formula with vitamins, minerals, and nutrients. Some parents consider giving a soya-based formula if their baby has an intolerance or sensitivity to cow's milk formula. Soya infant formulas are nutritionally similar to cow's milk-based formulas. The protein used in soya formulas is an extract of the soya bean, which has a high protein content. However, the UK government recommends that you should always seek the advice of a health professional before giving soya-based formula to

your baby. The current Department of Health advice is that soya formula milk should not be given automatically to babies with a sensitivity to cow's milk, as there are other types of formula that are suitable for most babies with an allergy or intolerance that may be more favourable than soya. So if you are considering soya milk, make sure you seek medical advice first.

The carbohydrates used in soya milk contain glucose syrup, which may damage your baby's teeth over a period of time, so if you are using soya formula, make sure you take your baby to the dentist once his teeth come through and tell the dentist that your baby has a soya formula. The Food Standards Agency also highlights concerns that soya-based formula could affect reproductive health. This is because soya contains phytoestrogens, substances found naturally in some plants, which may mimic or block the action of the hormone oestrogen. As this is a potentially sensitive time in a baby's development, it is not clear whether soya-based infant formula could affect a baby's reproductive development.

Q How should I hold my baby when I'm giving him the bottle?

Bottlefeeding can be a wonderful time for bonding with your baby by holding him close. Find a position that both you and your baby like – think about whether you are right- or left-handed and the age and size of your baby. You can cradle your baby, or simply sit your baby on your lap. You will help reduce wind by giving your baby his bottle in as upright a

Your baby's nutritional needs constantly change. No sooner are you sure of their requirements than they grow and change position as possible. Also take care to tilt the bottle so that the teat and neck are always filled with formula and never leave your baby to feed unattended by propping the bottle up. Ask your midwife or health visitor for further advice.

How long do you need to sterilize bottles for?

The recommendation is that you sterilize bottles and teats for at least the first year of your baby's life. It is during this time that they are most vulnerable to germs and viruses, which if contracted could cause illness and possibly dehydration.

Can I make up feeds in advance?

Ideally, you should make up each feed fresh. The Department of Health and Food Standards Agency's recommendations on the preparation and storage of formula milk advise that the risks associated with using powdered infant formula milk are reduced if each feed is made up fresh, as the longer the formula is stored, the greater the risk of bacterial growth. They do acknowledge that there are times when this is not practical, for example if you are going to leave the house for an extended period, or if you are dropping off a baby at a childminder's or nursery. In this case, you should prepare the feeds in separate bottles as instructed and then store them in the fridge (see below). This is a departure from previous information so can seem unusual to mothers who have previously bottlefed. Discuss this with your midwife and health visitor.

How long can pre-made feeds stay in the fridge?

Although it is not recommended that you make up bottles of infant formula milk in advance to store in the fridge because of the risk of bacteria developing, if you need to do this, store them in the back of the fridge, not the door, to ensure they are below 5°C (41°F) and never store feeds for longer than 24 hours (although this is considered too long for young babies). Formula milk is not suitable for freezing.

MIDWIFE WISDOM

Taking a break
sharing bottlefeeding with your partner

One of the major plus points of bottlefeeding is that anyone can feed your baby, allowing you to have some time off and rest.

✱ Getting your partner involved in feeding is a great way to help him bond with and feel close to your baby.

✱ Sharing feeds gives you a break and you can take it in turns to do night feeds.

✱ If you are switching from breast- to bottlefeeding, it may be easier to get someone else to give your baby the bottle, as your baby may reject the bottle from you, wanting to be breastfed instead.

Is it safe to warm a bottle and take it out to use later on?

Carrying warm formula milk in an insulated carrier is not safe, as warm milk is a good breeding ground for bacteria. The safer option is to make a feed up fresh for your baby just before it is required. If you are out, you can carry boiled water in an insulated container ready to mix with formula powder when you need it. Ready made-up milk feeds that come in little cartons are a more expensive option, but are handy for instantly decanting into a sterilized feeding bottle. If your baby is reluctant to take milk at room temperature, you could use a travel bottle-warmer, which can also be used to heat up containers and jars of baby food.

What precautions should I take making feeds with bottled water when I'm travelling?

When using bottled water to make up a feed, make sure the seal is still intact. Use still, not sparkling, water, and avoid water with high concentrations of the minerals sodium, nitrate, or flourine. Boil the water in a kettle in exactly the way you would boil tap water at home and wash and sterilize your feeding equipment as usual. Large bottles of mineral water should be stored in a fridge after opening. For convenience, you may prefer to use smaller bottles of mineral water if you are travelling from place to place. For extra convenience, ready-to-feed milks are available in cartons so you do not have to carry bulky tins of powdered milk with you. Although more expensive, these cut down on the amount of work you have to do and mean that you can be sure of good hygiene in the absence of adequate facilities.

Q I've heard that bottlefed babies have smellier poo – is this true?

This does seem to be the case. Bottlefed babies may have one bowel movement a day or only have a bowel movement once every three or four days. Both are normal. A bottlefed baby's stools are pale brown, smelly, and more formed than those of a breastfed baby. Some baby formula milks give a greenish tinge to the stool. It is thought that unabsorbed fat causes the unpleasant-smelling stools in formula-fed babies. Breast milk is better absorbed, which means the stools usually have less odour.

Q Will my baby get more wind if he is bottlefed?

Wind refers to the air in your baby's tummy. It is swallowed along with milk during feeds, but also when he cries. It will fill his tummy before he has drunk enough milk and be uncomfortable. Also, the faster flow of milk from a bottle can make babies take in more gulps of air. Some babies suffer with wind and need burping after every feed. Breastfed babies tend to get fewer problems with wind than bottlefed ones as they control the flow of milk at the breast and so suck at a slower pace, swallowing less air with the milk. They also have smaller and more frequent feeds and may be fed in an upright position, both of which can reduce wind.

Some babies have trouble bringing up wind and their discomfort is obvious. You can reduce wind by feeding your baby in an upright position and tilting the bottle so that the teat is full of milk and not air. If your baby doesn't burp after a couple of minutes, he probably doesn't need to. Wind your baby by gently rubbing his back or placing him over your shoulder. Some babies only seem to be able to get rid of wind through hiccuping. If the wind is severe, your health visitor or doctor may suggest medication.

Q Is it OK to give my baby water as well as milk?

Formula milk does tend to be less thirst-quenching than breast milk as the strength of formula doesn't vary, whereas breast milk varies in consistency, with the beginning of a feed tending to be more watery. If your bottlefed baby still seems hungry after a feed, it could therefore be that he is thirsty and some cooled boiled water may help to placate him. In hot weather he may need regular top-ups of water.

Avoiding tummy upsets
The importance of hygiene while bottlefeeding

Small babies are more susceptible to gastro-intestinal infections so it's important to observe strict hygiene while bottlefeeding.

One of the most important aspects while bottlefeeding is to ensure that all the equipment involved in the bottlefeeding process is sterilized properly and spotlessly clean with no trace of old milk. This means sterilizing the bottles, teats, and lids (see p.239). If your baby doesn't complete a feed, don't be tempted to give it to him later to finish as germs that are present in the baby's mouth may have transferred to the bottle and can then breed in the milk. When you are travelling or out for the day, you need to take care transporting feeds. Ready-made formula is probably the safest way to feed your baby while on the move, or adding formula to the water when you need it. Changes in water in different regions sometimes cause tummy upsets in bottlefed babies.

I just want to go home
the first days with your baby

Q I hate the thought of being in hospital for long – how soon can I go home with my baby?

In most maternity units, there is a degree of flexibility as to how long you remain in hospital after the birth. If you wish to stay for as brief a period as possible, talk to your midwife about this. In the past, postnatal stays tended to be longer – in 1997–98, the average stay in England was 2.2 days, and was 5.5 days in 1981. Nowadays, the minimum length of time in hospital is about six hours and many mothers just stay overnight to rest and gain some confidence. In some areas, you can move to a doctor's unit or birthing centre. To help make the transition home as smooth as possible, plan your return, making sure you have plenty of support in place.

How long you stay in hospital will largely depend on your type of delivery. If you have a vaginal delivery, you should be able to return home fairly soon, but a Caesarean may mean you need to stay in for about three days. Also, if your baby is born early, or is unwell, or struggling to feed or maintain his temperature, then you will be advised to stay in hospital until your baby is ready. When babies are premature, mothers may have to leave them in the special care unit and visit regularly.

Q Will I have any privacy in hospital? I don't want to be on a ward.

There is usually an attempt to make maternity wards as cheerful as possible, although the reality is they are often busy and lacking privacy. Your delivery room is likely to be a single room and may have ensuite facilities. Postnatal ward facilities vary tremendously in different locations; there may be single rooms, small rooms, or traditional Nightingale wards with a corridor of beds. Each bed will have curtains to pull around it for extra privacy, and bathroom facilities can vary.

Q Where will my baby sleep when we're in the hospital?

Mothers and babies usually remain together for 24 hours a day. You should only be separated from your baby if there is a medical reason for this, for example your baby needs special care, and you should be fully informed before agreeing to this. Your baby will usually sleep in a cot attached to the bed or next to it. This is recommended by the World Health Organization (WHO) and UNICEF who run a programme called The Baby Friendly Initiative. This works with healthcare systems to ensure a high standard of care for mothers and babies, and many maternity units are guided by their advice.

Q My friend's baby slept almost continuously for the first day or so. Is this normal?

The birth process is tiring for the baby as well as the mother and so it is not unusual for the first 24 hours to be fairly quiet, as your baby rests after the birth. Babies are often very alert and ready for a feed immediately after the birth, but then have a long

Take the chance to ask the midwife any questions you have so that you will feel confident caring for your baby once you are home sleep. Also, if you had drugs, such as pethidine or diamorphine, during labour, these can linger in the baby's system and contribute to the drowsiness. If your baby does sleep a lot at first, make the most of the opportunity to rest while still offering regular feeds – your midwife will advise you. After the first 24 hours, you may still find that your baby is feeding erratically, maybe every hour for five hours, and then having a four-hour sleep. Rest assured there is no set pattern in the early days; your baby should feed when she wants to and you shouldn't expect any routine to emerge at this stage.

Will the hospital help me with the everyday care of my baby if I'm having problems?

While you are in hospital there will be midwives and maternity support workers to help you. They have plenty of advice and information to offer so don't be afraid to ask about anything that is worrying you, such as specific questions about your baby, or any aspects of baby care (see below). However, do bear in mind that maternity units tend to be extremely busy and this, coupled with the fact that presently there is a shortage of midwives nationwide, means you may have to be patient and prepared to wait a while at times before someone is free to help you. Before you go home you will also be given contact numbers in case you need help or advice in between your postnatal checks.

Once you are home, your community midwife and your health visitor will be available to offer advice and support. They will also be able to give you details of local mother and baby groups, and postnatal drop-in clinics, all of which offer support and information for new mums and their families and give you the chance to meet other mums.

Do we need a car seat straight away or can I hold my baby in the car?

If you intend to take your baby home in the car, it is a legal requirement for them to travel in a car seat appropriate for their age. Indeed, it is illegal for children to travel in a car without a correctly fitting and fitted car or booster seat until they are over

Getting advice in hospital

Although the arrival of your baby is a time of incredible excitement, it can also seem overwhelming and you may feel daunted by the enormous task of looking after and meeting the needs of this tiny new baby. One of the benefits of your stay in hospital, as well as recovering from the birth, is to help you feel confident in the care of your baby. There are several aspects of baby care and feeding that the hospital midwives can help with.

✱ Staff can help you to establish breastfeeding by guiding you on technique. Some hospitals have a dedicated breastfeeding counsellor on site.

✱ The midwives can help you with everyday care by demonstrating topping and tailing, bathing techniques, changing a nappy, and dressing and undressing.

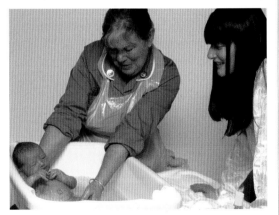

BATHING HELP: Take advantage of your time in hospital to ask the staff on the postnatal unit advice on baby care and breastfeeding techniques. They will be able to advise you on many aspects of your baby's care, which will help to increase your confidence.

Leaving hospital
the procedure for returning home

Each hospital varies, but generally, before being discharged from the hospital, several checks take place.

* You will be examined by a midwife or doctor to check that your uterus is starting to return to its pre-pregnancy size.

* If you had stitches, these will be checked to see if they are healing properly.

* Your baby will undergo various newborn checks (see p.220) and will need to be signed off by a paediatrician.

* If you need to take any medication home, this will be dispensed and you will be told how to arrange your postnatal check.

1.35 metres in height. Small babies and children need the protection that baby seats and child seats are designed to provide. So, yes, you do need to get your car seat ready before the birth to take your baby home from the hospital.

I'm going to be on my own when I go home and I'm worried I won't manage.

It's only natural to feel anxious about your new responsibilities when you arrive home with your baby. Being a single parent is increasingly common so don't be afraid to ask for help. Your midwife and health visitor will visit you to help with any baby-care problems and you will be given contact telephone numbers before your discharge from hospital in case you experience problems or need advice in between postnatal visits and checks.

When you are on your own, it's a good idea to arrange for a group of reliable friends or family members who are willing to assist you with babysitting, morale boosting, and provide general all-round back-up in the early days. Over time you can establish a network of other single parents in your area with whom you can share your problems and solutions. Also, ask your midwife or health visitor for contact details of local postnatal groups and organizations that support single parents.

My mum is coming to stay with me but I don't want her to take over. How should I approach this?

Overbearing mothers and mothers-in-law can be a problem, however well-intentioned they are. You will find it's not just mothers who insist on issuing lots of advice and information, but friends and other relatives can be just as vocal. Although this advice is often useful, some of it may be old-fashioned or simply conflict with your own ideas on how to care for your baby.

Even though you may be feeling vulnerable after the birth, practise being clear and assertive about the way in which you want to do things and make sure that people understand and respect your views and that your partner supports you in this too. It may help to pass on leaflets or books that you have read so your mother can see how things have changed since she brought up her children, and what advice you are following. You could suggest other ways in which she could help, such as shopping, cooking, and cleaning, so that you are left with the care of your baby. Most mums just want to help in some way, so it's up to you to channel her enthusiasm.

Will I get any sleep at all in the early days?

You will get sleep but whether it is of the same quantity and quality that you are used to is questionable. Although young babies need a lot more sleep than adults, approximately 16 hours each day, they do not take all of this sleep in one long stretch as they need to wake up for frequent small feeds. Up to the age of three months, babies have "sleep–wake" cycles throughout the day with longer spells of sleep at night.

The length of these cycles varies from baby to baby, but on average your baby will sleep about two hours at a time in the day, and four to six hours at night. All babies wake up a number of times throughout the night. The length of time your baby sleeps for during the night may also be affected by how she is fed. Several studies suggest that breastfed babies take longer than formula-fed babies to develop a pattern of sleeping through the night. This is because breast milk is easier to digest than formula milk, so babies get hungry more quickly and wake more often in the night. Most babies are physically capable of sleeping through the night from the age of six months.

Q Should my baby be in her own room or in with us and, if so, for how long?

In the early days, when your baby is fed frequently, often every two to three hours, you may find it more convenient to have her closer to you. UNICEF recommends that babies share their mother's room for the first six months of life as this helps to sustain breastfeeding and is also thought to help protect babies against cot death (see p.276).

As your baby grows and develops, her needs and sleeping patterns will change. One of the main changes is that your baby will start to sleep longer between feeds at night and often this is the stage that many parents decide is a good time to move their baby into their own room. You may also find that, if your baby is a light sleeper, she may sleep better in her own room as she is less likely to be disturbed by you and your partner.

There are plenty of people to turn to for breastfeeding advice. Keep numbers for your midwife and helplines close to hand

Q I'm a really deep sleeper and I'm worried that I won't hear my baby crying. Is this likely?

This is a common worry for many new parents, but you should rest assured that it is highly unlikely you will sleep through your baby crying. Many new parents find that they do not sleep as deeply following the birth of their baby, which may be partly an unconscious worry about sleeping too deeply and not attending to their baby's needs. Having your baby sleep in the same room as you to begin with and using a baby monitor later if your baby moves into her own room will help you to feel confident about hearing your baby at night. It's a good idea to try to catch up on some sleep during the daytime and take a nap while your baby is sleeping, as this will mean that you are not totally exhausted when you go to bed at night. You should also learn to trust the greatest prompt of all, your natural inbuilt maternal instincts!

Q Who can I turn to if I have problems with breastfeeding?

Although breastfeeding comes naturally to some mums, for many others it can prove surprisingly difficult. Initially you will have midwives and maternity care assistants on hand in the hospital to assist you with breastfeeding. Once you return home, your community midwife and health visitor can continue to advise you, but obviously they will not be available 24 hours a day. If you continue to have problems with breastfeeding, there are many helplines and local support groups available for which your hospital, doctor's surgery, and health centre should have contact details. Also, there are plenty of Internet sites that have forums, which are useful for discussing problems and comparing experiences. Some midwives and health visitors run local drop-in breastfeeding sessions, and some breastfeeding groups meet informally in cafés, so enquire whether there are any of these groups locally. The National Childbirth Trust (NCT) (see p.310) also has a national network of trained breastfeeding counsellors and a helpline for you to call.

First days at home

Regardless of whether or not this is your first baby, on your return home you are likely to be both physically and mentally exhausted. If this is your first baby, although the transition to motherhood is exciting, it can be daunting and, once home, you may be surprised at how big an adjustment this is. While some families want to share their joy with family and friends as soon as possible, others decide to have some quiet time together at first to get to know the new arrival and get used to their new roles. Try to put worries about housework and clearing up to the back of your mind – these will keep. Hormonal changes may mean that you feel quite low and weepy about three days after the birth, known as the "baby blues" (see p.281). Getting as much rest as possible will help you to recuperate and begin to feel normal once more.

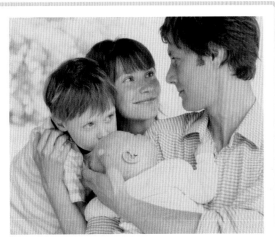

BEING TOGETHER: The first days as a new family are a unique and special time. Give yourselves plenty of quiet time alone to relax and get used to your new relationships and family unit.

Q I don't want to go home too soon – can I stay in hospital if I want to?

When you leave hospital is something that you will agree with the hospital midwives and doctors, and it will be dependent on your particular needs and circumstances. Although you obviously can't remain in hospital indefinitely, generally you won't be transferred home until you feel ready to return. The midwife will ensure that you are confident feeding your baby, whether this be breastfeeding or bottlefeeding, and that you are confident providing everyday care for your baby, which is good preparation for returning home.

When you go home, your care will be transferred back to the community midwife, so you will continue to receive support, information, and advice as necessary. Also, planning in advance support for when you return home may help you to feel more confident about leaving the hospital. As well as support from your partner, try to enlist the help of family, friends, and close neighbours to help you cope in the first few weeks after the birth.

Q We had so many visitors in hospital last time it was exhausting. Can I stop this?

Many people seem to believe that if you are in hospital then they can visit whenever they want to, whereas most people, even close family, wouldn't just turn up on your doorstep unannounced if you were at home with your baby. If you know in advance how you will feel then you really need to be assertive this time and let people know your wishes. It is possible to do this in a diplomatic way without offending people by simply telling friends and maybe family too that you would prefer to have some quiet time with your partner and children during the first few days to recuperate and get to know your new baby. Most people will understand this sentiment and will be more than happy to wait for a few days until you are feeling ready to see them.

If you are discharged fairly early from hospital, it may be easier to control the flow of visitors as you will be able to dictate visiting on your own terms. You can then take the time that you need to settle down to a new family life.

I'm scared of dropping him
caring for your newborn baby

Q Even though we have a toddler, I'm still scared I'll drop the baby. Do other dads feel like this?

This is a normal and natural feeling and affects the majority of all new dads (and many mums!). Babies seem to be such fragile little creatures, especially because of their size compared to you. However, they are in fact quite resilient to inept handling and are a lot stronger than they look. Remember the tough journey they have just undergone to be born! If you have so far avoided handling your baby much, try to overcome your fears by watching your partner or midwife change your baby or bathe him, then offer to help so that you can give your partner a rest. Once you have changed a few nappies, or done some winding sessions, you will find that your confidence in handling your baby begins to grow quickly. The more contact you have with your baby, the more confident over time you will become, and your partner will also benefit from the added support and help you are providing and from knowing that she can feel confident leaving you in charge of the baby sometimes.

Q Our baby screams whenever he goes near water. How can we make bathing him less stressful?

There is no right or wrong way to bathe a baby, but with a little care and organization it can actually become quite a playful and fun experience (see p.250–251). This may seem hard to believe at the moment, and it is certainly the case that many newborn babies initially scream throughout their bathtime. However, the main reason why babies do this is because they don't like to feel cold. To keep your baby comfortable during a bathing session, make sure that the room you bathe him in is sufficiently warm and draught-free, which will

help him to relax and feel less distressed. Also, always gather everything you need ready before the bathing session so that you don't have to go and fetch items mid-way through a session, leaving your baby lying on a towel and letting him get cold.

If you are feeling stressed during your baby's bathtime, he may be sensing this, which could be adding to his upset. The biggest fear that mums and dads have is of dropping their baby while bathing him, so you could initially try bathing at ground level to help you to build your confidence. Also, remember to communicate with your baby all the time while you are bathing him – talking to him constantly in a soothing tone, or singing to him, will help to distract and reassure him and in turn you are likely to feel far more relaxed, which will have a positive effect on your baby.

If you are still concerned about handling your baby, then seek help from your partner, if he or she is more confident, or talk to your community midwife who will be more than happy to offer you additional advice and support.

Q Our newborn sleeps so much – it's wonderful, but should I be waking him for a feed?

While many newborn babies sleep for what seems to be a very short amount of time, some do sleep for quite long periods. One factor that may influence how long your baby sleeps is how he is fed. The makeup of formula milk is very different to that of breast milk and sits in a baby's stomach for longer. So formula-fed babies tend to sleep for longer periods and are, in fact, encouraged to do so to prevent overfeeding and constipation. However, a bottlefed baby shouldn't be left without a feed for more than six hours and it is recommended that bottlefed babies should have no fewer than six feeds a day. So if your baby sleeps well at night, daytime feeds will need to be closer together and you may need to wake him to give him feeds.

Breastfed babies are very different feeders. Many feed 10–12 times a day, or even more, and there are times when they "cluster feed" and the feeds blend into one very long feed. However, there are some breastfed babies who do not feed regularly and appear sleepy. These babies may be tired, sedated by maternal medication during labour, or just very sore as a result of the birth.

Straight after the birth, babies have fat and fluid stores that can sustain them for a day or two. However, if your baby is very sleepy for the first 24–48 hours, you should still try to stimulate him every few hours and wake him for feeds. There

are several things you can do to encourage a sleepy baby to feed, such as lying your baby naked on your chest so that you get skin-to-skin contact, which can encourage him to root for the nipple and feed; massaging him; dripping expressed milk onto his lips; and changing his nappy to encourage him to wake. However, do not force him to feed by, for example, pushing him towards the breast, as this could put him off breastfeeding.

You can also start to express milk every two to three hours to stimulate your breasts to produce milk. The midwife will examine your baby to make sure that he is not becoming dry or passing dark urine; that his bowel movements are changing colour to yellow; and that he is not jaundiced, as being a little drowsy is one of the signs of mild jaundice.

Holding your newborn

New parents, particularly first-timers, sometimes worry about picking their baby up or carrying them properly. However, newborn babies are not as fragile as you think. Although, of course, you still need to take care when handling your baby, it's best to trust in your ability. The more you practise, the easier it will become and you will find that your confidence will soon grow with experience. The main point to remember is that babies need to be supported at the head and lower body as their muscle tone is not developed enough to support themselves. The same principle applies if you are cradling your baby, holding your baby upright over your shoulder, or sitting him on your lap. Once you have been shown the technique by your midwife, you might like to practise without being watched.

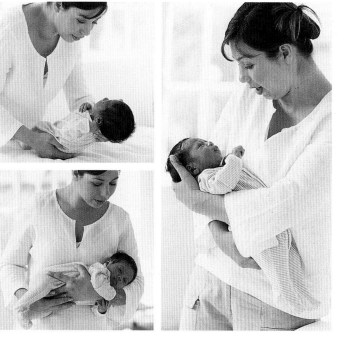

TOP: Support the back of the head when lifting. **ABOVE:** Holding him face down is comfortable for your baby.

ABOVE: Cradling your baby in your arms allows you to keep his head supported and enables you both to make eye contact.

ESSENTIAL INFORMATION: NEW PARENTS

Bathing and washing
How to clean your baby

There are differing views on how to bathe and wash a baby, but the general opinion seems to be that less is more. Some say it is unnecessary to bathe your baby for the first month, others say if you want to, just use water and, if you wish, pH-neutral balanced products. Always read the label and avoid anything with sulphur in it. Your baby's newborn skin is so delicate and thin that if you use harsh or highly perfumed products the skin's protective barriers can be damaged; skin may then become dry and more vulnerable to infection. A baby's skin also absorbs certain chemicals that may contribute to conditions like eczema and asthma later in life.

When should I bathe my baby? The vernix, the waxy-like substance that covers your baby at birth, should be left to absorb into his skin as it is the most amazing moisturizer. If your baby's hair needs a wash, just use water and a baby comb to remove any debris. You can "top and tail" your baby in the first few days of life, using cotton wool (organic if possible) and water, gently washing his face (being careful around the delicate area of the eyes) and nappy area. This allows your baby's skin to adjust to the outside world. Later, when you bathe your baby, hold him gently in water two or three times a week.

What should I use to clean my baby? Use water and cotton wool in the first month. If your baby's eyes become sticky, use cotton wool dipped in cooled boiled water to clean them – gently wipe the eyes with an in-to-out movement, using a new piece of cotton wool for each wipe. Use cotton wool to wipe around the outside of the ears and nose.

Topping and tailing

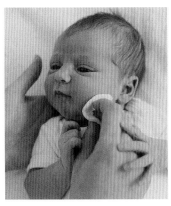

FACE AND NECK: With damp cotton wool, clean the face and in the neck creases. Wipe eyes from the inner to outer corners, using a new piece of cotton wool for each eye.

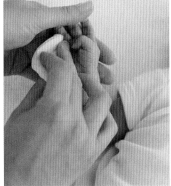

CLEANING THE HANDS: Uncurl the fingers and with a new piece of cotton wool, wipe the backs and fronts of the hands and in between the fingers. Pat dry with a towel.

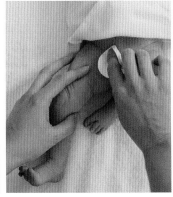

LEGS AND FEET: Wipe the legs and feet with a fresh piece of cotton wool, cleaning in between the creases in the skin. Gently dry the skin with a towel.

Bathing your baby

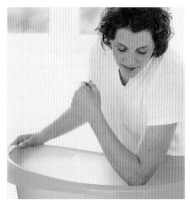

TESTING WATER: Test the water temperature with your elbow or the inside of your wrist. The water shouldn't feel too hot or too cold. If you want to check the water with a thermometer, the temperature should be 29°C (85°F).

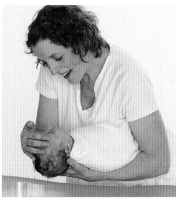

HAIR WASHING: Wrap your baby securely in a towel with his head exposed, then tuck him, feet first, under your arm – whichever feels most comfortable. Support his head with your hand and gently wet his hair with your free hand.

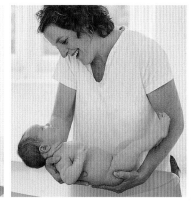

PUTTING HIM IN THE BATH: Dry your baby's hair and unwrap the towel, then lower him into the water. Keep his head well supported by putting an arm under his shoulders and gently grasping his upper arm furthest away from you.

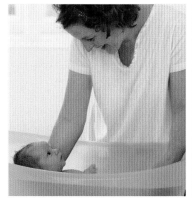

BATHING YOUR BABY: Once in the water, your baby's head should rest naturally on your wrist and then you can use your free hand to gently wash him.

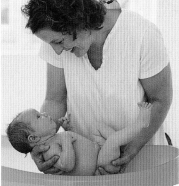

LIFTING OUT: When you have finished bathing your baby, gently lift him out of the bath, making sure you are supporting him firmly across the shoulders and bottom.

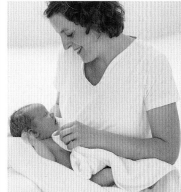

DRYING YOUR BABY: Wrap your baby in a towel and gently dry him; make sure he is dry in between the skin creases and don't use powder on the nappy area as this could irritate.

I'm scared to touch my baby's cord stump – should I clean it?

The cord stump is the end of the umbilicus that housed the arteries and veins that fed your baby and removed his waste products in pregnancy. It is common for parents to not want to touch the stump. However, the stump can become infected as its base can become moist, and harmful bacteria that live naturally on our skin may grow in this moist area before it falls off, usually by the tenth day. If the cord stump is clean, there is no need to touch it, but if it becomes soiled, it should be cleaned with damp cotton wool. Once the stump has fallen off, the "wound" needs cleaning until it heals, as the navel and surrounding area can also become inflamed. If the stumps smells offensive or is sticky, contact your midwife or doctor.

What is meconium?

Meconium is a waste product from your baby's bowels. It is dark brown/green in colour and its texture is quite sticky and globular. Meconium is formed from as early as 12 weeks gestation and contains dead skin cells and debris from the amniotic fluid that the baby swallows and digests throughout pregnancy. It is usually expelled after birth in the first few stools, but it can be passed in pregnancy or labour when it may be a sign that the baby is distressed. If meconium is seen before the birth, the baby will be monitored carefully during the labour and birth.

How often should I change my baby's nappy?

Your baby's own toilet habits will dictate how often to change his nappies. However, you should check his nappy fairly regularly, as wetness and the ammonia contained in urine and the digestive enzymes in stools can quickly irritate a baby's sensitive skin. Some babies need changing around 6–8 times a day, while others require a nappy change as often as 10–12 times a day, for example, breastfed babies who poo much more frequently than bottlefed babies. As your baby gets older, he will need changing less frequently.

Is there anything I should look out for when changing his nappy?

A baby's urine is pale after birth and then darkens within the next few days. There may be a pinky-orange stain in your baby's nappy, which is concentrated urine from when he was in the uterus and is quite normal. As long as your baby passes urine at least four times a day and there is no blood present, there is nothing for you to worry about. The black-green meconium passed after the birth (see left) gradually changes to a yellow colour as normal digestion begins.

Breastfed babies tend to pass stools that are runny and mustard-yellow, which can look similar to diarrhoea, while a formula-fed baby's stools will be much firmer and a seedy pale yellow. Some babies have a bowel movement with every feed, as feeding stimulates peristalsis, or muscular contractions, in the gut; others, particularly bottledfed babies, may only pass a stool once a week. If your baby's stool is hard and dry, or there is any mucus or blood in the stool, talk to your doctor.

How should we deal with nappy rash?

Nappy rash is sore for the baby, but also distressing for parents, who may feel that they should have been able to prevent it. There are several reasons for nappy rash, including if the baby's urine or stools are concentrated, causing them to be more of an irritant; if a barrier cream has not been used; or if the baby has a thrush infection that is irritating the nappy rash. Also, changing a baby's nappy too regularly can sometimes be harmful as the baby may be sensitive to the wipes being used.

The most usual way to deal with nappy rash is to "air" the bottom as often as is practical. After thorough handwashing, clean your baby's bottom carefully with cotton wool and warm tap water and/or emollient creams, which lubricate the skin and stop it becoming too dry, and avoid soaps or wipes. Then leave your baby without a nappy on an absorbent mat or towel for a while. When you change his nappy,

Nappy changing

Although you may feel a bit hesitant at first about changing your baby's nappies, and many babies protest strongly when having their nappy changed, you will soon master the technique and learn how to change his nappy quickly and with the minimum of fuss. The key to successful and stress-free changing is to have everything ready before you start. Choose somewhere warm and draught-free to change your baby; you may also want to lay down a towel on top of the changing mat for extra comfort.

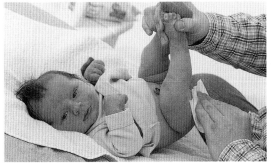

CLEANING THE NAPPY AREA: With damp cotton wool pieces, clean around the genitals and in between the leg creases. Wipe from front to back with girls. Dry the area and apply a barrier cream if necessary.

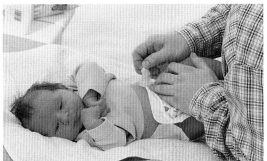

PUTTING ON A NAPPY: Slide the nappy under your baby's bottom and then bring the front up between the legs. Bring the sides over and fasten the tabs. Wash you hands before and after nappy changing.

apply an emollient or barrier cream thinly so that it protects the skin but does not prevent the nappy from soaking up urine. Suitable ointments and creams include zinc oxide or petroleum jelly. Another ointment called metanium ointment contains titanium dioxide, which seems to be effective in healing nappy rash, although it does have a strange smell and can stain fabric.

Occasionally, a moderate or severe nappy rash may be infected. In this case, treatment with antibiotics may be necessary. Also, to reduce inflammation, a corticosteroid cream may be suggested for application once a day, to reduce the inflammation of the nappy rash and give the rash a better chance to heal. An antifungal cream will also be recommended as many moderate to severe rashes are infected with the bacteria *Candida albicans*. If the rash persists after 7–10 days, the doctor may recommend an antifungal syrup to try to treat the whole bowel for thrush infection. If this occurs, you should also apply an antifungal cream to your nipples if you are breastfeeding. Although unusual, if the nappy rash still shows no sign of healing, your doctor may refer your baby to a dermatologist.

Q Should we use baby wipes or just cotton wool when changing a nappy?

Most midwives would advise that you stick to warm water and cotton wool balls, preferably organic, to clean your newborn baby when changing his nappies. Any soaps, perfumed or otherwise, or baby wipes should be used with caution as, although baby products are designed to be kinder on a baby's sensitive skin, they can still irritate the skin if over-used or not washed off and dried properly. It's best to avoid baby wipes altogether until your baby is a few months old.

Q My baby's scalp has become scaly. Is this cradle cap and what should I do about it?

Cradle cap, or seborrhoeic dermatitis, is a common condition in young babies, appearing as yellow, scaly patches on the scalp. This condition is harmless and will clear up on its own over time. However, if you are concerned that it is unsightly, gently massage some olive oil into the scalp, leave this on overnight, and then wash your baby's hair in the morning with a mild baby shampoo; most of the flakes should disappear. Don't pick at the scales as this could damage the skin and increase the chance of infection.

Q What temperature should our house be when we bring our new baby home?

Babies find it hard to maintain their body temperature. Maternity units are notoriously hot as they are dealing with babies who have just been born and are still quite wet from the delivery. Once you are home, the guidelines are to maintain room temperature at around 16–20°C (62–68°F) and you may find purchasing a room thermometer helpful. Babies are at risk of cot death (see p.276) if they become too hot due to being in a warm room or being overwrapped.

However, the room temperature is a guideline only and you should learn to check for other signs that your baby is too hot or too cold. As a guide, a baby's hands and feet feel cool and their heads feel hot as they tend to lose heat through their heads. Check his temperature by feeling your baby's chest with the back of your hand, not your fingers, as these may be cold. If your baby feels warm to touch, he is probably warm enough. If he is hot or sweaty, remove a layer of clothing or a blanket or sheet. If he is cold, add a layer. Duvets are not recommended until your baby is at least a year old, to avoid overheating.

If your baby is unwell, hot, and shivery, your immediate reaction may be to wrap and cuddle him, but this can make him too hot. Instead, remove a few layers so that your baby can cool down. Seek medical help straight away if your baby has a temperature over 39°C (102.2°F) or if he is particularly unresponsive and listless.

Q How should I place my baby in the cot?

The Foundation for Sudden Infant Death (FSID) recommends that your baby should be placed with his feet towards the bottom of the cot to prevent him wriggling under the blankets and possibly

Dressing and undressing

Your baby is likely to wear vests and sleepsuits, or babygrows. Choose vests with envelope necks that are easy to get on and off and opt for sleepsuits with front-opening poppers.

✱ Lie your baby down. Put the vest on by holding the neck opening wide and gathering the rest of the vest. Gently lift the back of his head and ease the back of the vest behind his head. Lift the front over the head, avoiding his face. Gently lift the sleeve down over the hand and arm, stretching the vest rather than pulling your baby's arm.

✱ Lay the sleepsuit out with the poppers undone. Place your baby on top, then gently insert his legs, then his arms into the suit and do up the poppers.

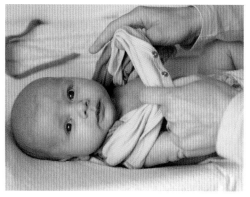

CHANGING YOUR BABY'S CLOTHES: In general, clothes should be changed just morning and night, and if any soiling occurs in between.

Distract your baby to keep him happy while dressing and undressing him – put some music on and talk to him constantly

suffocating himself (see p.276). Light cotton blankets and sheets, available in cot sizes, should be used rather than quilts or duvets, so that layers can be built up or taken off. The blankets and sheets should be tucked under the baby's arms so that your baby is less likely to pull them over his face. Swaddling is another method of wrapping your baby which some babies find comforting (see p.257).

Is it OK to swaddle our baby? There seem to be conflicting opinions.

Swaddling means wrapping your baby in a light cotton blanket or sheet, the idea being to keep him feeling warm and secure in the outside world (see p.257). The baby is so well wrapped that his arms and legs are "strapped" to his sides, restricting movement of the limbs. There are differing views as to whether a baby should be swaddled. The practice is very popular in Asian and Eastern European areas. Its popularity is also on the rise in the UK, especially since parents have been encouraged to put babies in their own cots to sleep rather than bedsharing to prevent cot death. It is also thought that the swaddling may help a baby to sleep comfortably on his back.

The FSID warns of the risks of overheating a baby so any swaddling should be done with a light cotton sheet or blanket and the room must not be too warm. On the other hand, some believe that swaddled babies risk getting cold as they cannot maintain their temperature by moving.

Should my baby wear his hat indoors?

One factor known to increase the risk of cot death is an overheated baby. Although babies lose excess heat from their heads and it is a good idea to cover a baby's head outside if it is cold or windy, the baby's hat should be removed indoors or when you enter an area that is warm, such as on a bus or going into a shop, even if it means waking your baby.

There are some exceptions. If a baby was born prematurely, had a very low birth weight, or has difficulty maintaining his temperature, then they may need to wear a hat indoors. However, once these babies are a healthy weight or able to maintain their body temperature, this no longer applies.

He screams when I undress him. What can I do?

Babies use crying as their means of communication. It may be that when you undress him, he is either protesting that he is cold or that he does not like the feeling of air on his skin, which he is unused to after been snuggled in the womb for nine months. Try to keep the changing time as short as possible, making sure he is not in a draughty or cold environment. Afterwards, comfort your baby by rocking him; swaddling and keeping him in an upright position can also soothe him.

When can we take him out?

Some recommend waiting for 1–2 weeks before going out, but this will depend on individual circumstances. When you feel well enough, you could try going out for a short walk, but bear in mind it will be the same distance to get back, so do not overdo it. You may have a local park you could visit or simply have a walk round the block – it's best to keep it simple at first until you get used to being out together. You are likely to feel rather nervous at first about taking your baby outside of the home, but, as with most aspects of baby care, once you get used to going out you will probably lose much of your anxiety. As you start to increase the distance and time away from home, make sure you have taken everything you will need to care for your baby while you are out. This will include changing equipment, and blankets, pram covers, or parasols to protect your baby from different weather conditions. The time of year will also affect how long you stay out.

Q Can he sleep for long in his car seat?

There are no laws to state how long a baby should remain in a car seat, but bear in mind that being fixed in one position for long periods of time would be uncomfortable for anyone, regardless of age. Generally, it is not recommended that babies are left for a long period of time in car seats because if they fall asleep curled up in this position it may affect their breathing, and can encourage wind to get trapped, causing discomfort. You should also take care when carrying your baby around in a car seat as they tend to be heavy and you are more prone to back injuries in the postnatal period.

Q My wife won't let me do a thing but I want to get better at it. How can I help?

Some women do feel that it is their responsibility to care for the baby, but it is well documented that a couple's relationship is strengthened when the care is shared. This involves joint decision-making and making choices regarding care together. Babies can pick up on positive and negative feelings expressed by their parents, and it is important for all concerned that both the mother and the father bond with the child. Offer to perform routine tasks in front of her to instil her confidence in your ability. This may take time, but the reward is worth it. She will also benefit from being able to take breaks, confident in the knowledge that you can cope as well as she can.

Q My friend's baby had colic and she had a miserable few months with it. Will my baby get it?

The term "colic" refers to when babies cry continually for around three hours each day and cannot be soothed (see p.274). Although obviously

Dads need to be assertive with baby care. Don't worry if you feel all fingers and thumbs at first – it will soon be second nature

distressing for the baby, it is equally upsetting for the parents to listen to their baby crying so painfully for so long. As no-one knows exactly why colic occurs, it is impossible to say whether or not your baby will suffer with it. However, there are several theories as to what causes colic. One is that the baby's intestines are immature and working too hard, causing a cramp. Another is that the bowel movements are too slow and the air in the bowel is trapped. Another theory is that the baby is eating too much, too fast, and has air trapped. None of these is proven and all we know is that colic occurs in around 10–15 per cent of babies.

Q My baby cries continually. I'm not having much success with breastfeeding – is he hungry?

Newborn babies cry on average for two and a half hours each day. Crying is your baby's only means of communication and so he cries to get you to respond to his needs, whether he is hungry, wet, or just wants a cuddle. Some babies cry more and may struggle when you try to comfort them, which can make you anxious. If you are anxious about breastfeeding, your baby may sense this and begin to cry. Sometimes, it is necessary to take a step back and try to relax. Having a warm bath with your baby skin-to-skin, sometimes called "rebirthing", can help to calm you both and may help you to relax more while feeding. Once warm and calm, your baby may try to get into a good position to feed. Ensure he latches on well and does not cause pain after the first few sucks (see p.228). Allowing your baby to feed as and when he wants is also important. As your baby gets older, the regularity of feeds will settle and feeding will change.

Other reasons why babies cry include being overstimulated (try rebirthing); being uncomfortable (try winding); being wet or dirty (change his nappy); being cold or hot (change the clothing and room temperature); wanting comfort (try swaddling); or boredom (talk to your baby, sing, and play with him).

Q My midwife says that our baby comfort sucks. I'm reluctant to introduce a dummy – should we?

If a baby has latched on well at the breast and has sucked and swallowed well during a long feed, and then settles on the breast taking small sucks and not swallowing, he is comfort sucking. Many babies like to comfort suck, not just breastfed ones. If your baby falls asleep, you may be able to gently ease him off the breast, or if you are comfortable, leave him there.

Your baby may comfort suck for many reasons. He may be stimulating the breast to increase your milk supply; he may be "cluster" feeding and is dozing before the next feed; or he may want to snuggle close. Comfort sucking is thought to steady the baby's heart rate, relax his stomach, and help him to settle.

Introducing a dummy is your choice. Some parents think they are the best way to get a baby to sleep, day or night; others think they should be used only at night, and some believe they should not be used at all. The Foundation for Sudden Infant Death (FSID) suggested in June 2007 that using a dummy can reduce the risk of cot death, but that breastfed babies should not be given one until over a month old and feeding is established. This advice is based on studies suggesting a lower incidence of cot death in babies given a dummy.

If your baby likes to suck, you can also offer him a clean finger to suck on; later on, some babies comfort themselves by sucking on their own thumb or finger

What does swaddling mean?

Swaddling is an old practice of wrapping a baby snugly in cloths or blankets so that movement of the limbs is restricted. Many midwives swaddle infants soon after birth and it is now a standard newborn care practice in many hospitals. Research has found that swaddling may help newborns to sleep as it prevents the "moro", or startle reflex – the tendency for newborns to startle themselves by moving their arms suddenly.

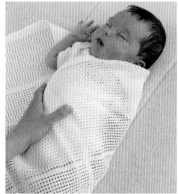 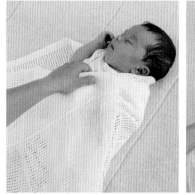 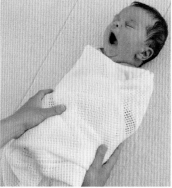

FOLDING: Fold the blanket's corner. Lay the baby with his head above the edge. Fold the side over his arms.

TAKING UP THE BOTTOM: Take the bottom corner up to his chest and tuck it underneath the top edge.

THE LEFT-HAND SIDE: Bring the left side of the blanket across your baby and tuck it underneath him.

Losing a baby
coping with a devastating loss

Q What is a stillbirth?

A stillbirth is when a baby dies in the uterus after 24 weeks' gestation before it is born. Losing a baby is very different to other losses, which may be partly due to the fact that we do not expect to lose babies in this day and age of technology and healthcare advancements. The cruel contrast between birth and death occurring at the same time and having no physical live memories of this person that you have bonded with during the pregnancy and looked forward so much to meeting is very difficult to comprehend. Parents often search for answers to questions that may be unexplainable, and this can often delay the whole grieving process. The important thing for couples who experience such a loss is to try not to dwell on the ifs, buts, and maybes and remember it was not their fault.

Q How likely is a baby to die in labour or shortly after birth?

The death of a baby during labour is known as interpartum death; this is usually caused by a lack of oxygen during labour, possibly due to a problem with the placenta, or an injury to the baby during labour and birth. However, this is extremely rare today thanks to improvements in monitoring the mother and baby during labour and dealing with signs of distress. When a baby dies in the first four weeks of life, this is known as neonatal death, which affects around 3 out of 1000 babies. Neonatal deaths usually occur in babies who are very premature who may have breathing difficulties, or in babies who have severe chromosomal or genetic abnormalities. Infection used to be a more significant cause of neonatal death, but this is now rare. For couples who lose a baby in these circumstances, it's important to accept that it was extremely unlikely to be related to anything they did or didn't do.

Q I feel like there is a big empty hole where my baby was. I'm devastated – will I get over this?

Losing a baby is extremely difficult and overwhelming. Some people say that time is a good healer, but others find it hard to make sense of it all. If you have been given a possible cause as to why your baby died, this may help you to understand that it was not your fault and to be able, in time, to move on. Keep hold of any precious memories or keepsakes you may have been given at the hospital, such as a photograph or a lock of hair, and seek support from your loved ones and counsellors, if necessary. The Stillbirth and Neonatal Death Society (SANDS) (see p.310) can offer you support and put you in touch with other families who are in a similar position. You may find that sharing your thoughts and

---

MIDWIFE WISDOM

✳ **Coping**
how to deal with the death of a baby

The death of a baby is one of the most devastating experiences. Although you will never forget your loss, there are ways to help you cope.

✳ The most important thing is to talk about what has happened, whether to your partner, family, friends, counsellor, or supportive organization.

✳ Recognize that you and your partner need time to work through your feelings and that you may not always feel the same thing at the same time.

✳ Be prepared for some people's inability to talk about what has happened.

feelings with people who have been through the same tragedy helps you to process your grief and, over time to move forwards, although of course the sadness will never leave you.

I'm so busy being a shoulder for her to cry on, but I don't know how to cope myself.

Often the effects of the loss of a baby on the father are not considered. This may be because of outdated notions about the way men react to grief, in particular by not letting their emotions show. It is also common for men to feel that they have to be the stronger party and to feel that it is not masculine to express their feelings openly. Fathers often throw themselves back into their work to take their mind off things, or distract themselves with other activities and pursuits. It's important that you recognize that this is a difficult time for both of you and that you may not be able to support each other by yourselves, particularly if you are grieving in different ways. You may need to consider counselling and approaching support groups, such as SANDS, as well as friends and family.

I want to find out more about why my baby died – how could I go about this?

Seeking answers to your questions may be a positive part of the grieving process and can help you begin to move forward. During the delivery of your baby and shortly afterwards, you may have consented to having certain tests performed. These may have included blood tests, swabs, an analysis of the placenta, and a postmortem of your baby. Once the results of these have been gathered, along with your case notes, the consultant will usually make an appointment for you to come in and discuss the results and any possible explanations as to why this may have happened. It is often the case that there are no obvious reasons as to why this tragedy has occurred. This can be both frustrating and upsetting and you may feel that counselling or a support group may be able to help you.

Talking to someone about your loss, whether to a trained counsellor or other confidante, is often the starting point in healing

The hospital won't admit they made mistakes when our baby died – where can we get help?

You are likely to be experiencing great emotional turmoil and it is extremely important that you seek as much information as you can before you take matters further. I would suggest that first you write to the Head of Midwifery and request a meeting as this may answer some or all of your questions.

If you are still not satisfied, very occasionally, parents may feel that they need to seek legal advice if they think that negligence was the cause of their baby's death. If you feel this is the case, then you could talk to the Citizens' Advice Bureau or find a solicitor to discuss your case with. Some solicitors and the Citizens' Advice Bureau offer a half-hour appointment to discuss the situation and advise whether they think your case is worth pursuing before you make a commitment in terms of time and money. If you do decide to take a case forward, you should be aware that the procedure can be frustrating, stressful, and upsetting. As before, you may also benefit from some counselling or by talking to the support group SANDS.

I never held my baby after she was stillborn. I couldn't face it and now I regret it. What can I do?

Losing your baby is a devastating experience and the grieving process can be made more difficult by the fact that you did not get to know your baby and have no memories of her to hold on to. Seeing and holding your baby after the birth and taking photos can help in the grieving process as it enables you to give your baby an identity and to visualize her, and medical staff often encourage couples to spend time with their baby to enable them to say goodbye.

However, at the time of losing a baby, there are many things that you have to deal with physically and emotionally and making decisions while you are in a state of shock and grieving is a very difficult thing to do. Try to understand this and accept that you felt unable to hold your baby after the birth, and instead think of other ways to remember and cherish her. You may have been given a keepsake, such as a photograph, a hand- or footprint, or a lock of hair to remind you of your baby, but if this wasn't possible, you could make a special box of toys, clothes that you had bought for your baby, and scan pictures in memory of her. You may also like to plant a tree or a shrub in honour of your baby, or create a special place to visit to remember her. Sometimes, writing down your thoughts and feelings in a diary can be a personal tribute to your baby and can help you to deal with your grief.

Q I feel so angry; I can't even cry. It's affecting my relationship with my wife – is this part of grief?

Yes, this is a very normal part of the grieving process, which is a natural phenomenon that helps us move forwards and can include sorrow, guilt, anger, blame, and depression. It is very common for men to show their emotions in different ways to women, often feeling it is not "masculine" to cry and that they have to be the stronger of the two. You will both be grieving in different ways and will enter and leave some or all of the stages of grief at different times, and the whole experience is likely to put a great strain on your relationship as your different emotional responses can lead to misunderstanding and resentment. You may find it helpful for both of you to see a counsellor as an independent trained person may be able to offer you the additional support that you need. You may also need some specific help to help you to deal with your anger, and an anger-management course may be suggested.

Q How long should we wait before we try for another baby?

Following the tragic loss of a baby, there is no set time when a couple should try for another baby. This will largely depend on when you both feel mentally ready. What stage your pregnancy loss occurred and how you delivered your baby may also affect how ready you are to consider trying again; often, a loss in the later stages of pregnancy can take longer to recover from. From a physical point of view, it is usually better to give your body six weeks to return to its normal state. If you had a Caesarean section, it is recommended that you wait for a year for your scar to heal before getting pregnant again. Counselling and support can help you decide when you are psychologically ready to try again. Your doctor or midwife can refer you for this.

Losing a twin
How to cope when one baby dies

Losing one twin, or triplet, is extremely hard and can be a very bitter-sweet experience. Parents who lose one twin are likely to have many conflicting emotions as they are faced with the prospect of grieving for their lost baby, while welcoming the surviving twin into the world. Some may find that they are unable to do both at once, and so the grieving process is put on hold in order to care for the other baby. This can lead to feelings of guilt and anxiety and can cause a great deal of stress. Parents may also be made to feel that the dead twin is compensated for by the surviving one and therefore may feel that they cannot express the devastation they feel at losing a baby. It is therefore extremely important that parents who lose a twin or triplet seek help and advice if they feel they are unable to cope with their grief, or need support caring for the surviving baby.

ESSENTIAL INFORMATION: NEW PARENTS

Helping and consoling
Coming to terms with loss

The death of a baby in pregnancy or, more rarely, in labour or shortly after the birth, is a devastating loss and couples who experience this will have to cope with feelings of shock, confusion, anger, guilt, sadness, and regret. It will take time to work through all of these emotions and it's important that you allow yourself this time to grieve and don't feel under pressure from others to "move on" before you feel ready. Both of you may benefit from a period away from work. For the mother, this allows time for her body to recover from the pregnancy and birth, and for both partners, this time may be needed to recover from the initial debilitating shock of losing their baby.

How can we help each other? Although you may feel that you don't have the resources to help anyone else, you and your partner can help each other by recognizing that you may be dealing with your loss in different ways. You may not be at the same stage of the grieving process as each other and may also display your emotions differently. Understanding this can help to avoid feelings of resentment building up between you. The best way to appreciate how you both feel is to keep the channels of communication open. Although grief can be an intensely private experience and it is easy to withdraw from others, talking about your shared loss can help to ensure that your relationship remains supportive.

Will friends and family help? Although having the support of family and friends is important at this difficult time, you will probably find that there are a variety of responses to your grief. You may find that close family and friends are unable to offer the level of support you need

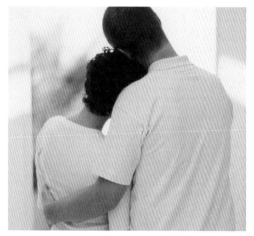

TAKING TIME OUT: The loss of a baby can put relationships under an enormous strain. Couples who allow themselves time to grieve may find it easier to work through the onslaught of emotions.

as they are possibly grieving your loss too. On the other hand, you may find that when you talk to others, they reveal their own tales of grief and suffering and are able to empathize with your loss. Sometimes people are unsure about how to respond to your loss; they may feel embarrassed and at a loss for words of comfort, or fear that they will upset you if they talk about what has happened, and sometimes may even avoid interacting with, or seeing, you. Unfortunately, this can leave you feeling more isolated and lacking in support, and emphasizes the importance of finding someone you can talk to, such as a professional grief counsellor who deals with miscarriage and stillbirth, who can help you to channel your grief. There are also plenty of support groups where you can share your experience with other bereaved parents.

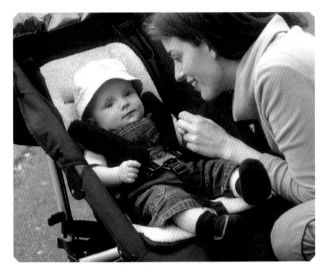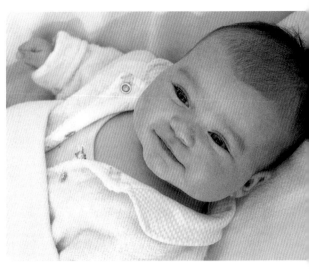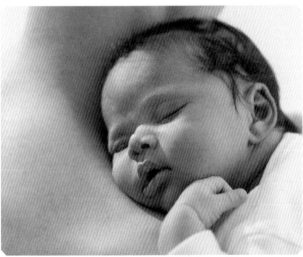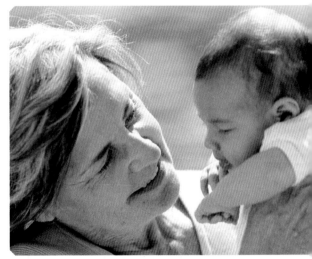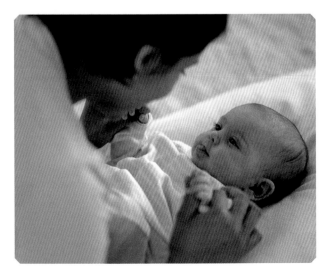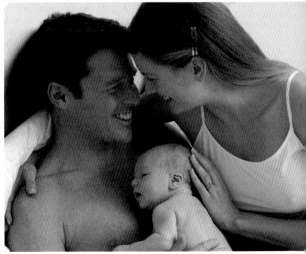

A new 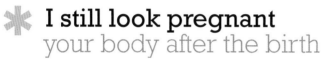life

* **I still look pregnant**
  your body after the birth

* **Sleep – what is sleep?**
  life after the birth

* **I'm feeling so depressed**
  your emotions after the birth

* **I'm sure I saw my baby smile**
  getting to know your baby

* **We're a family now**
  your new life together

* **Time out for us**
  nurturing relationships

I still look pregnant
your body after the birth

Q I've heard about "afterpains", but what exactly are they?

The term "afterpains" refers to the discomfort felt after the birth as the uterus starts to contract back down to its normal, pre-pregnancy size. These pains are often described as feeling similar to period pains. Sometimes, women having their first baby may not notice any afterpains, or they are fairly mild; they are more commonly felt by women having their second or subsequent baby, due to the fact that the uterus has to work harder to regain its usual size after being stretched on more than one occasion.

Afterpains also tend to be felt more in women who are breastfeeding their babies, as breastfeeding stimulates the release of the hormone oxytocin, which in turn triggers the uterine contractions that are felt as afterpains.

If you experience particularly uncomfortable afterpains, it is perfectly safe to take a mild analgesic or a painkiller such as paracetamol. You should find that the discomfort disappears after a few days. Taking warm baths can also be soothing.

Q I'm still bleeding heavily. How long will this last?

The bleeding you experience after birth is known as lochia, which is a heavy, bloody vaginal discharge made up of blood and tissues from the uterus and from the site where the placenta was attached to the wall of the uterus. This is how your body gets rid of the lining of the uterus that supported your baby. Most women find that the bleeding looks initially like a "period" type of blood loss, and then gradually turns to a brownish or pinkish, watery discharge. The final colour may be yellowish and the discharge quite scanty. This bleeding can last for anything from two to six weeks after giving birth. If you are breastfeeding it may finish sooner as the let-down reflex stimulates oxytocin, which in turn triggers uterine contractions.

Q Is it safe to use tampons while I'm bleeding?

It is not advised to use tampons for around six weeks after giving birth. This is because you are more vulnerable to contracting an infection during this period, so it is important to pay close attention to personal hygiene at this time to keep your vaginal area free from any bacteria, which can be introduced through the use of a tampon. So you should avoid using tampons while you have the post-pregnancy bleed known as lochia.

You can start to use tampons again for your first period after the birth, as long as this occurs at least six weeks after the birth.

MIDWIFE WISDOM

Getting enough rest
helping your body to recover

Whether you had a vaginal or Caesarean birth, you are likely to feel exhausted in the first few weeks. It's important that you don't take on too much and give yourself time to recover.

* Rather than try and catch up on chores while your baby sleeps, have a nap to catch up on sleep lost through interrupted nights.
* Avoid heavy lifting as much as possible.
* It's fine to stay indoors at first and take things at your own pace while you get used to life with your new baby.
* Don't feel you have to entertain visitors – ask them to make you a cup of tea!

Ouch! My stitches are really uncomfortable. What's the best way to ease the pain?

Stitches do cause discomfort for a few days after giving birth, so keep the area as clean as possible as this will help prevent infection and minimize your discomfort. You should wash the area with warm water several times a day and make sure you change your pad frequently. Many women find the following techniques for reducing discomfort helpful:

✱ **Using a cold pad.** You can use a cooling gel pad that has been specially designed for the purpose of soothing the discomfort caused by stitches in the perineal area. These have been demonstrated to effectively reduce swelling, briusing, and pain. Or make your own cool pad by placing crushed ice in a plastic bag and wrapping this in a dry flannel.

✱ **Taking the homeopathic remedy arnica**, which is thought to help reduce bruising.

✱ **Having a warm bath** with a few drops of lavender or camomile essential oil.

✱ **Taking painkillers** such as paracetamol or ibuprofen. Ask your doctor or midwife for advice.

How quickly will I lose the weight I put on during pregnancy?

How quickly a woman loses weight after the birth of her baby varies widely. Some women seem to get back into shape within a few weeks of the birth, while for others, losing their pregnancy "flab" can take a few months or more. Whichever category you fall into, it is important not to adopt a strict diet during the early weeks and months of parenthood, especially if you are breastfeeding. However, it is sensible to eat a healthy, balanced diet and take some exercise. You should aim to lose your "baby weight" gradually as this will ensure that you are receiving enough nutrition in the postnatal period, and will give your tummy more time to adjust its shape. Some women do attend professional sessions such as Weight Watchers, but it is important that you inform the trainer or person in charge that you have recently had a baby.

Coping with constipation
Helping your bowels to work after the birth

It's common for bowel movements to be fairly sluggish after giving birth as your abdominal muscles have been stretched during the pregnancy and so exert less pressure, which slows down the movement of faeces through the bowels causing constipation.

You may also feel uncomfortable after the birth and be anxious that opening your bowels, and possibly straining, could damage stitches if you had any. However, this is extremely unlikely. The best way to avoid constipation is to drink plenty of fluids each day, preferably water (also important if you are breastfeeding), and to eat lots of fibre-rich foods, such as fresh and dried fruits, cereals, and other wholegrain foods. Once you have recovered from the birth, gentle exercise that tones the abdominal muscles may also help your bowels to become more efficient (see pp.268–269).

How can I get rid of my stretchmarks?

Unfortunately, there is no magic way to get rid of stretchmarks, which affect a large number of pregnant women and seem to be influenced by genes as they often run in families. You will find that the marks fade over time from bright red to a paler pink, and then to a silvery colour that blends in with your skin tone. Massaging a natural oil into your skin may help them to fade.

If, after time, your stretchmarks are still troubling you, you could discuss treatment options with your doctor, which include laser treatments to reduce the redness of stretchmarks. However, you should be warned that treatments for getting rid of stretchmarks are often not completely effective and simply speed up the natural fading process rather than eradicate the stretchmarks altogether. Also you would have to pay for these treatments privately.

Q I'm losing weight fast, but my tummy is really flabby – how can I tighten it up?

This is a common problem after giving birth. The flabbiness you are experiencing is caused by the muscles and skin having stretched to accommodate your pregnancy and baby. After the birth, these muscles relax and have lost their tone. However, you should find that the muscle tone gradually returns, although it may never be quite the same as it was before your pregnancy.

You can try some gentle toning exercises (see pp.268–269) as soon as you feel able to after the birth, although you should wait for at least six weeks if you have had a Caesarean. Your midwife will be able to give you more information about what is safe to do and what is not. If you do go to a professional exercise class or gym, make sure you inform the trainer that you have recently given birth and what type of birth you had so he or she can give you appropriate advice and guidance.

Q I've still got a huge appetite – is this because I'm breastfeeding? How much should I be eating now?

This could be because you are breastfeeding, which requires an extra 500 calories each day. However, this may not equate to as much food as you think – it works out at about two slices of toast with baked beans! Your big appetite therefore isn't a problem in itself, but how you satisfy it can be! As long as you are eating a healthy, balanced diet, you shouldn't find that you gain weight (and you definitely shouldn't be trying to diet while you are breastfeeding). Ensure that your diet is providing sufficient quantities of protein and carbohydrates and plenty of fresh fruit and vegetables. Also avoid filling up on "empty calories" such as sweets, biscuits, and crisps, and instead try to snack on foods such as fruit, nuts, and seeds. This will ensure that you receive the best nutrition during such an important time, which will benefit you and your baby, and will also help you to lose any extra weight you have gained during the course of your pregnancy.

Q I've heard that breastfeeding helps you to lose the weight quicker. Is this true?

Breastfeeding can help you to lose weight more quickly after the birth as your body is using up energy to provide an adequate milk supply for your baby. Some of the 500 extra calories a day you need may be taken from fat supplies deposited in pregnancy. Often, extra fat laid down on the hips and thighs in pregnancy is lost first, providing the "fuel" required to make milk and breastfeed your baby. Gentle exercise such as walking and swimming will also help to shift the pregnancy pounds.

Q I'm not breastfeeding my baby at all – when will my periods start again?

If you are not breastfeeding, you can expect your first period to arrive any time from four weeks after the birth. Most women find that the first period is a little different from normal. It may be heavier or lighter and it may last for longer or shorter than usual. A more regular pattern should establish itself over the next few months.

Q What will happen at my postnatal checkup?

Around six weeks after the birth of your baby, you will need to see your doctor for your postnatal checkup. During this appointment, the doctor will ensure that your body is returning to normal after the pregnancy and birth. You may have your blood

Take heart – you will lose your baby weight, although not overnight. Why not try power walking with other new mums?

A balanced diet

It's easy to neglect your diet once your baby arrives, as you find that you are too tired to prepare proper meals and perhaps think it less important to watch what you eat, now that your baby is outside the womb. However, eating a healthy diet now is as crucial as ever. If you are breastfeeding, you need to eat a healthy balanced diet and drink plenty of fluids to ensure a good milk production. Eating well also gives you the energy to cope with broken sleep and the demands of your new baby. Make sure your diet contains plenty of protein and cabohydrates, as well as foods rich in calcium, such as eggs and dairy, and iron-rich foods, such as green leafy vegetables. Avoid sugary and salty foods and snack instead on fresh fruit.

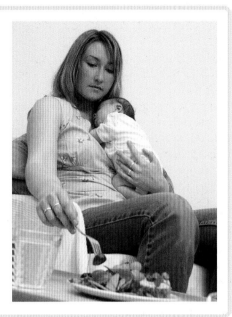

NUTRITIOUS MEALS: You may find it easier to eat little and often to keep your energy levels up. Opt for light, easy-to-prepare meals, such as salads or wholemeal bread sandwiches.

pressure checked, and you may also be given an internal examination to make sure that any stitches you had have healed and that your uterus has returned to its pre-pregnancy size. Your doctor will also ask you about your contraception plans and discuss the available options, and you may be asked about your emotional health – how you are adjusting to parenthood and whether you have any particular issues or concerns.

Q I had an emergency Caesarean – when is it OK for me to go for a walk with the baby?

Nowadays, women who have had a Caesarean section are encouraged to get up and move about as soon as possible after the operation, even if this is just to get out of bed and walk a short distance. This is to reduce the risk of problems developing, such as blood clots in your legs (known as deep vein thrombosis) or chest infections. However, it is still important that you take things slowly and don't try to do too much too soon. You should find that you are able to walk short distances within 12 to 24 hours

after the operation, but you probably won't feel like going for a longer walk outside for another few days, or perhaps even more.

Q How long do I have to wait after my Caesarean before I can drive again?

It is generally thought best to wait for around four to six weeks before driving again following a Caesarean section, although there are no specific guidelines based on research on the subject. We would suggest that you wait until you feel that you have totally recovered from the operation and that you would be able to perform driving manoeuvres such as reversing and parking, as well as an emergency stop, without experiencing pain or discomfort. You would also need to feel comfortable with the car seat belt around you, as this will be directly over the area of your wound.

You should contact your insurance company as well to check their criteria, as some do not insure women to drive within a certain period following a major operation such as a Caesarean.

ESSENTIAL INFORMATION: A NEW LIFE

Postnatal exercise
Getting into shape

You can exercise as soon as you want to after your baby's birth. The amount you do and how strenuous the exercise will depend on the type of birth you had and how much you exercised before you had your baby. Other considerations are whether you are breastfeeding and the amount of discomfort you feel. Always listen to your body as you will become uncomfortable if you do too much. Your body has just undergone an enormous change throughout the course of pregnancy and childbirth, particularly if you had a Caesarean section. There are also high levels of hormones still in your body, which can make you more supple and prone to injury. If you are breastfeeding, you may just want to do gentle exercising until feeding is established. It's a good idea to wear a supportive bra while exercising, and exercise following a feed rather than before one, which may make it more comfortable for you.

Always warm up, wear the correct footwear, and drink plenty of fluids while you are exercising. Stop and seek medical advice if you feel unwell or experience any severe pain or your bleeding increases. Although getting back to your pre-pregnancy shape is important for your wellbeing, do be patient with yourself as it will take time.

Which exercises can I do? Pelvic floor exercises can be commenced straight after the birth (see p.57). These important exercises help prevent you from leaking urine when you laugh, cough, or sneeze. The exercises involve drawing up and holding the pelvic floor muscles, tightening around the back and front passages, and then letting go. Make sure that you are tightening the pelvic floor (not your buttocks, thighs, or tummy muscles). Keep breathing and relax your other muscles.

Exercises for 0–6 weeks

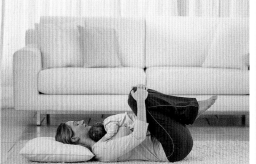

ABDOMINAL EXERCISE: Lie on your back with a cushion supporting your head; bend your knees and place your feet on the floor. Draw your knees up to your chest, holding them with your hands. Breathe deeply into your abdomen.

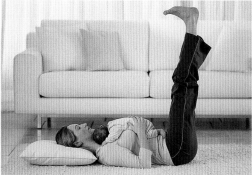

ADVANCED ABDOMINAL EXERCISE: If you are able, lift your legs up towards the ceiling. You can keep the knees slightly bent, or straighten them if possible. Focus on your breathing and pull up your pelvic floor muscles in time with your breaths.

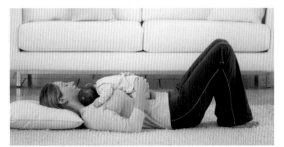

RELAXATION POSE: Lying flat on your back with your knees bent and your head supported by a cushion is extremely relaxing for your lower back.

Pelvic floor exercises can also be done lying on your side or back with the knees bent and slightly apart.

Other gentle exercises, like lying on your back with your knees bent and doing pelvic tilts (pulling your belly-button in and upwards towards your spine), are recommended in the first few days after the birth (not if you had a Caesarean). Your abdominal muscles may have separated in pregnancy, so doing these gentle exercises will help them to reunite. The exercises below will help strengthen abdominal muscles (avoid after a Caesarean and follow the exercise advice given by the hospital). Build up exercises gradually, starting with one cycle and then repeating this as many times as you feel comfortable. Always breathe normally. Walking and swimming are excellent ways to build up your fitness levels once you have stopped bleeding.

What should I avoid in the first six weeks? Full impact and resistance exercising should only be done about six weeks after the birth, to prevent any strain on the pelvic floor area. Ask your fitness instructor for advice and gradually increase your exercise. Always let your instructor know that you have just had a baby, so exercises can be tailored to your needs. If you had a Caesarean, your hospital will have given you a leaflet describing the sort of exercises you can do safely, and before you carry out abdominal exercises, such as sit-ups, check with your doctor first; these are usually safe to do around 6–8 weeks after the birth. You can gently introduce single leg-raises while lying on your back once you feel ready, probably after about a month.

Exercises for 6–16 weeks

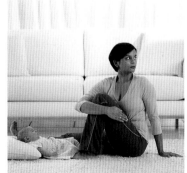

SITTING TWIST: Sit upright; bend your left knee, your foot flat on the floor. Place your left hand behind you, then exhale and turn your torso. Repeat the other side.

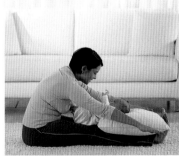

EASY FORWARD BEND: Sit with your legs straight in front of you. Raise your arms, then exhale and reach forwards, extending from the hips.

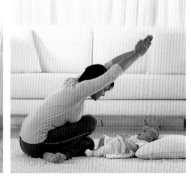

TWISTING FORWARD BEND: Cross your legs with the right knee resting on the left knee. Lift your arms, palms joined, and stretch forwards, your back straight.

Q I developed piles at the end of my pregnancy – will they go now the baby has been born?

Piles, or haemorrhoids, are swollen veins in or around the anus. They are fairly common in pregnancy and after childbirth due to the weight and pressure of the baby's head pressing down. Most women find that haemorrhoids disappear within a month of giving birth, although a very small minority of women are not so fortunate and will need to discuss treatment options with their doctor. In the meantime, if you are finding the haemorrhoids uncomfortable or itchy, there are a few things you can try. Applying a maternity cool pad to the area can be soothing (you can make your own by freezing a folded wet flannel), or your doctor or pharmacist may be able to recommend a cream that can ease the discomfort. You should also try to avoid becoming constipated as straining to go to the toilet will make the piles

worse, so drink plenty of water and eat lots of fresh fruit and vegetables as well as wholegrains.

Q I had an episiotomy and am terrified of going to the loo. Do you have any advice?

Many women who have had a cut or tear to the perineal area experience discomfort for a while after the birth. There may also be some pain or "stinging" when passing urine or opening the bowels, but this should last only for a few days. You may find it helpful to tip a jug of warm water over the area when you pass urine, as this helps to dilute the urine and reduce the stinging sensation acidic urine can cause. If your loo is near the shower, you may be able to use the shower head over the toilet. A bidet, of course, is ideal, though not many people have these. Drinking plenty of fluids will also help to dilute your urine.

It is normal not to open your bowels for a day or two after the birth. Many women feel anxious the first time they pass a bowel motion, but it is very unlikely that this will damage your stitches. However, if you become constipated, this could cause discomfort. Make sure you drink plenty of water, and eat fresh fruit and vegetables to help prevent this. If you find that you are still feeling constipated, your midwife can give you a mild stool softener if necessary.

After an episiotomy
How to ease the discomfort of stitches

If you had an episiotomy, you may find that your perineum is quite uncomfortable after the birth, as the surrounding skin can swell, causing the stitches to become tighter, and sitting down becomes increasingly difficult. Here are some ways to relieve this discomfort.

✻ Sit on a rubber ring to take the pressure off your stitches and enable you to relax.

✻ Apply a cooling gel pack to the area, or ask your midwife or doctor to recommend an anaesthetic cream or spray.

✻ Try squatting over the toilet seat when you pass urine as this helps prevent acidic urine running over your stitches. Gently wash and dry the area after going to the toilet.

✻ A warm bath or shower can be soothing. After washing, dry the area carefully by patting the area gently with a towel.

Q I had a long delivery and I'm worried that my vagina has stretched. Will it get back to normal?

Try not to worry. Although at first you may notice changes to your body as a result of the pregnancy and birth, a woman's body is designed to give birth and return to normal afterwards. To help the muscles around your vagina to tighten after the birth, do some pelvic floor exercises as you did in pregnancy (see p.57). These involve identifying which muscles you need to exercise by tightening the muscles around your vagina and back passage and lifting up just as if you were trying to stop yourself passing urine and wind at the same time. You should practise 5–6 at a time, ideally several times a day. If at first you are not able to hold the muscles tight for 5 seconds, just do what you can and keep practising. You can also try faster contractions where you tighten and lift the pelvic floor muscles quickly and hold for one second, then relax for one second, and repeat.

Q It's four weeks since the birth and I feel such a mess still – how can I get my self-esteem back?

When you have had a baby, your body will (at least at first) look and feel different from usual; you may feel sore from stitches, have hard leaky breasts, and will be extremely tired! In addition, you are learning how to care for, and bond with, your new baby and still keep your other relationships intact – that's quite a lot to deal with. It can take anywhere from a few weeks to a few months for your body to return to normal. How you feel will also depend on the type of birth you had, whether you are breastfeeding, and how healthy your lifestyle is in terms of diet and exercise. In the meantime, there are a few things you can do to improve the way you feel about yourself:

* **Take time out for yourself.** Whether you have a bath, wash your hair, or do your nails, regularly having even just half an hour to yourself each day can really help you to relax and feel good.

* **Go to the hairdresser.** Even if you're not happy with the way your body looks, having a haircut can be a real boost.

* **Invest in a few new items** of clothing if you can afford to. During the early period of parenthood, maternity clothes are too big, but your usual clothes may be a little tight. Having clothes that fit you properly will not only feel more comfortable but will look good too!

* **Get some gentle exercise.** Go for a brisk walk pushing the pram. Your baby will benefit from the burst of fresh air and the exercise will give you an energy lift too.

* **Keep reminding yourself** that you have done an amazing job bringing your baby into the world, and are now doing another amazing job nurturing and caring for him each day. There's no job quite as exhausting as looking after a newborn baby, but equally nothing that is quite as rewarding!

Carve out some "me" time each day: a warm soak, or a lie down. Taking care of yourself helps you give your best to your baby

Q My feet are still swollen after the birth – is this normal?

Swelling in your feet and legs is an unpleasant side effect of pregnancy. After the birth, the pressure on your veins decreases and your blood flow returns to normal, so excess fluid is no longer pushed into the tissues. You will excrete the extra fluid that your body collected and so may urinate a lot at first. This can take a while and the swelling can linger for at least a week, which is normal. You can relieve swelling by resting on your left side; sitting with your legs raised; drinking lots of water; urinating often; stretching your legs and feet; not standing for long periods; taking gentle exercise, such as walking; and eating healthily.

Q I've had a headache since the birth. Is this due to the epidural?

Headaches after childbirth are common and causes include tiredness, dehydration, stress, and lack of fresh air and exercise, as well as the upheaval in your hormones after delivery. After an epidural, you have a 1:100 to 1:500 chance of developing a "post-dural puncture" headache. This occurs between one day and one week after the epidural, is worse when sitting up or standing, and is relieved by lying down and taking pain-relieving drugs, such as paracetamol. Drinking fluids and avoiding lifting can also help. If this is thought to be the cause, the midwife or doctor may refer you back to the anaesthetic team for treatment. However, it's most likely that your headache is not related to the epidural.

MYTHS AND MISCONCEPTIONS

Is it true that...

 ### Crying is good for your baby's lungs?

Don't listen to this well-meant but misguided advice – if your baby is crying there is usually a good reason. As any mother knows, a baby's cry can mean, "Feed me!", "I'm lonely", "I'm over-tired", "I'm in pain", "I'm wet and need changing", or even "I've been over stimulated, leave me alone." Crying is your baby's way of communicating something to you, and it is natural and healthy to respond to it.

You can become addicted to pills for postnatal depression?

Don't worry about getting addicted. Postnatal depression is serious and distressing, but it is treatable. Anti-depressants (usually prescribed alongside other talking therapies) are not thought to be addictive, and you will be able to discuss any concerns with your doctor. However, you are recommended to take them for six months and not to stop taking them abruptly.

Babies can be spoiled if held too much?

Unlikely. During your baby's first few months, holding him makes him feel loved and secure. While some babies don't seem to need much close physical contact, others want to be held all the time. If your baby needs a lot of holding, you can try a baby sling, which allows you to keep him close to you while leaving your hands free for other tasks (but take care if handling hot water, and avoid standing on chairs). But when your baby is quiet and calm, do let him entertain himself or fall asleep on his own.

Sleep – what is sleep?
life after the birth

Q Why do babies cry?

All babies cry – even entirely healthy newborns will cry for somewhere between one and three hours each day – as crying is a baby's only way of communicating its needs. As a new parent, it can be difficult to work out what your baby is telling you: is she hungry, cold, hot, thirsty, wet, bored, looking for a cuddle, tired, or over-stimulated ? However, you will gradually begin to recognize your baby's different crying patterns and anticipate her needs. As babies grow, they learn other ways to communicate, such as making eye contact, noises, and even smiling, all of which reduce the need to cry.

Q My baby is two weeks old and cries all the time. I'm feeling so tired. Will things get better?

You will almost certainly find that things improve with time – babies grow and change and you will also grow in confidence as a parent. However, you need to know how to cope with, and hopefully enjoy, life at the moment and you may need some additional help and support to manage this.

Until your baby is 28 days old, you are still officially under the care of a midwife, even if you are not having visits any more, which usually stop after about two weeks if she is happy that you and the baby are fine. It's fine to give your midwife a ring so that she can advise you over the phone about feeding and settling your baby. Your health visitor may visit you at home and will also be able to offer advice and support if you explain the problems you are having. In addition to this, it is important to have someone (your partner, close friend, or mother) who can give you a hand with practical chores, such as cleaning and cooking, while you care for your baby. They can also take the baby out for a while so that you can have a much needed rest.

Q When will the health visitor come to our home?

This varies from area to area, but the first visit the health visitor makes to your home is usually around two weeks after the birth. Officially, you are under the care of community midwives until your baby is 28 days old. In some areas, the health visitor, who is usually linked with your doctor's surgery, will make contact with you during your pregnancy. Your health visitor will give you information about the local baby clinic. These clinics are usually held at your doctor's surgery on a weekly basis and are an opportunity to meet other mums and babies, have your baby weighed, and chat to the health visitor about any concerns you may have.

Q The screaming is getting on my nerves – what should I do?

Most of the time, a baby who cries a lot will not do herself any harm, but may cause stress and worry for you. If your baby seems to resist every effort you make to calm her down, it can be hard not to feel rejected as well as frustrated. Parents sometimes blame themselves, feeling they are doing something wrong. If you know that your baby's needs are met, she is not ill, and you've tried everything you can think of to calm her but nothing has worked, it's good to have a coping strategy in place for how to deal with situations when you feel overwhelmed. Here are a few suggestions:

* **Take deep breaths.**
* **Put your baby down** somewhere safe, in the cot or Moses basket, leave the room, and let her cry for five minutes out of your hearing until you feel calmer.
* **Play your favourite music** and let yourself relax for 10 minutes.
* **Call a friend or relative** to take over while you take a break.

✱ **Talk to your health visitor** about local support groups or mother-and-baby groups where you can share your feelings and experiences and discuss ways of coping with your baby's crying with other new parents.

✱ **Sometimes taking your baby out for a walk** in the fresh air may help to calm her and give you a clearer head.

✱ **If it all gets too much**, call one of the telephone helplines. The CRY-SIS helpline (see p.310) is for parents of babies who have sleep problems and/or who cry excessively. The helpline is open 24 hours a day, seven days a week, for support and advice. Crying is your baby's way of expressing herself, and no matter how tired and low you are feeling, never blame yourself for the crying.

Q Should I pick my baby up every time she cries?

Although this is a matter of personal choice, you should never feel you are "spoiling" your baby by attending to her cries, or by giving her plenty of cuddles and carrying her around with you if this comforts her. Crying is initially a baby's only method of communication. It is meant to get your attention and is designed to affect you so that you will quickly find out what is needed. However, as long as you have met her basic needs and you are happy that she isn't hungry, thirsty, too hot or cold, bored, wet, or ill, there is no harm in leaving your baby to cry for a few minutes. Some babies learn to comfort themselves, while some parents find any cry too distressing and quickly go to their baby. You have to trust your own judgement and decide what is right for you. However, do try to make sure that you and your partner are consistent in how you respond to your baby's cries.

Q My baby cries for hours every evening. Could this be colic and is this serious?

Colic is fairly common in newborn babies, affecting around 10–15 per cent of infants, and usually appears in the first few weeks after the birth (see below). Babies suffering with colic may lift their head, become red in the face, draw their legs up in pain,

What is colic?

The definition of colic is uncontrollable crying in an otherwise healthy baby. To be termed "colicky", a baby needs to cry or fuss for more than three hours a day, for more than three days in any one week. Although colic can occur at any time of the day, it is more common between six in the evening and midnight and is traditionally worse at around three months of age. Unfortunately, around 10 per cent of babies suffer with colic of varying degrees. There are several theories as to what colic is, why it happens, and the courses of treatment. It is more common in boys, bottlefed babies, and in first-borns, and it generally starts at around two to four weeks and can continue for as long as three months. If it has not settled by five months, you should see your doctor. For the very unlucky, it can continue for six to nine months.

LIVING WITH COLIC: Dealing with a colicky baby can be exhausting and upsetting. Keep reminding yourself that it will pass eventually.

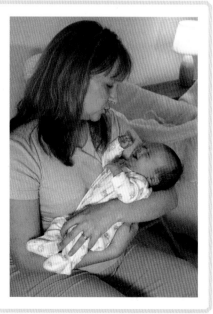

and pass wind. There are many theories as to what causes colic, such as swallowing air when feeding or crying, or gas in a baby's tummy, but none of these is proved. The condition usually lasts for three to four months. Colic is not a serious condition, and research shows that babies with colic continue to eat and gain weight normally, despite the crying, but it can have a big impact on the family as the crying is very exhausting. There are plenty of remedies that may ease the symptoms.

✳ **If you are bottlefeeding your baby,** you could try switching to a different brand of formula to see if another type is less irritating to her.

✳ **If you are breastfeeding,** you could try not drinking cow's milk for a few days, as some believe this can cause colic. Also, some mothers swear that their baby is calmer when they abstain from spicy foods, caffeine, or alcohol, and you could try omitting these from your diet one at a time to see if this helps your baby to settle.

✳ **Trying different teats or bottles** may help.

✳ **Winding your baby regularly** during and after feeds may help to relieve pressure in her tummy if she swallows air.

✳ **Colic drops** containing a substance called simethicone may help break down bubbles in milk feeds in the stomach, allowing swallowed air to be brought up more easily by the baby.

✳ **Homeopathic colic granules** are available from pharmacies, or you may prefer to visit a trained homeopath.

✳ **A dummy** may satisfy your baby's need to suck and reduce the level of crying.

✳ **Gentle massaging** over your baby's tummy, in a clockwise direction with a little almond oil, can be comforting for your baby and may relax the parents a little, too!

✳ **A warm, relaxed environment** in the evenings may help to induce calm in your baby, whether you are bottlefeeding or breastfeeding.

✳ **White noise,** such as the rhythmic sound of the washing machine, and gentle movement, such as pushing the pram around the block or having a drive in the car, can also help to calm your baby.

> Attending to your own needs is good parenting. If it all gets too much, put your baby in her cot and take a five-minute breather

✳ **Arranging for some extra help** in the evening when you are tired and stressed will offer you relief.

If your baby's crying is becoming very scary and stressful for you, contact your doctor or health visitor for advice. The CRY-SIS helpline also offers support and advice (see p.310).

Q My friend fed her newborn every three hours to establish a routine. What do you think of this?
Although this is your baby and you must decide how you want to care for her, the recommended way to feed your baby is to feed on demand, whether you choose to breast- or bottlefeed.

A baby needs to take in sufficient calories over a 24-hour period to grow and develop. If you restrict your baby's feeds during the day to every three hours or so, then she will need to wake more often during the night to take in the calories she has not taken during the day. It's often best to accept that life with a newborn baby is very tiring. At this early stage, if you concentrate on feeding your baby when she wants, you will probably find that she will develop a routine naturally over the next few weeks and will eventually sleep through the night. If you do decide to regulate your baby's feeds at an early stage, you will also need to think about how you will deal with a crying baby who wants to feed earlier than she should according to the regime you have established. You could try discussing this with your friend as well as asking your midwife and health visitor for their advice.

ESSENTIAL INFORMATION: A NEW LIFE

Safe sleeping and SIDS
Protecting your baby

There has been much research into sudden infant death syndrome (SIDS), or cot death, to try to find out why babies unexpectedly die. Several simple measures can be taken to reduce the risk.

How can I reduce the risks? The Foundation for the Study of Infant Death (FSID) and the Department of Health suggest the following:

✱ Don't let anyone smoke near your baby.

✱ Do not smoke during your pregnancy, and encourage your partner not to smoke.

✱ Place your baby on her back to sleep (and not on the front or side).

✱ Do not let your baby get too hot, and keep your baby's head uncovered.

✱ Place your baby with her feet to the foot of the cot, to prevent her wriggling under the covers.

✱ Never sleep with your baby on a sofa or chair.

✱ The safest place for your baby to sleep is in a crib or cot in your room for the first six months.

✱ Settling your baby to sleep (day and night) with a dummy can reduce the risk of cot death, even if the dummy falls out while your baby is asleep.

✱ Breastfeed your baby. (Establish breastfeeding before starting to use a dummy.)

✱ If you do take your baby into your bed, be aware that it is dangerous for your baby if you (or your partner) smoke, even if you never smoke in bed or at home; have been drinking alcohol; have taken medication or drugs that make you drowsy; feel very tired; if your baby was born before 37 weeks; weighed less than 2.5kg (5lb) at birth; or is less than three months old. Also, accidents can happen: you might roll over and suffocate her; your baby could get caught between the wall and the bed; or could roll out and be injured.

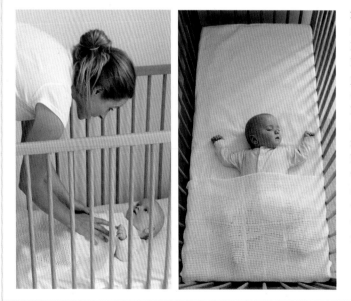

FAR LEFT: Light cotton sheets and blankets, or a suitably sized baby sleeping bag, are sufficient bedding for a small baby, preventing her from becoming overheated. If you feel she is too hot or too cold, you can take away or add a layer as necessary. **LEFT:** Placing your baby in a "feet to foot" position, with her feet at the bottom of the cot, ensures that she will not wriggle down under her blanket during the night and therefore reduces the risk of suffocation.

Q I want to feed my baby on demand. My mum says I'm making life harder – is she right?

Demand feeding is the recommended way to feed your baby. This method of feeding simply means that you feed your baby whenever she signals that she is hungry and wants food – usually by rooting, crying, or sucking on her hands – rather than according to a schedule set by you. Over time, parents start to recognize the signals more rapidly and know when their baby wants to be fed.

In the early weeks of breastfeeding, you may feel as though your baby feeds constantly. However, bear in mind that newborns have tiny stomachs – about the size of their fist – and so can only hold a certain amount of food. Easily digested breast milk quickly fills a baby's stomach and is easily absorbed, so she will need to eat again relatively soon. For the first six weeks, breastfeeding is being established and it is important to totally demand feed during this time. This means that your baby regulates the amount of milk you produce by feeding more to produce more. When she has let your body know how much she needs, she will sleep better between feeds and only demand more when she needs more. If your baby seems hungry soon after eating – for example, she may be fussy, sucking on her fist, or rooting at your breast – go ahead and feed her again as this will boost your supply. Bear in mind, too, that babies are just hungrier on some days. It's also important to make sure that your baby empties each breast, as the hindmilk at the end of a feed contains more fat and nourishment and so babies feel fuller and satisfied for longer.

If you feed her on demand, she will also begin to sleep longer at night. This way, you don't need a feeding programme; you can just give your baby whatever she asks for and continue to do this until she begins weaning.

Q How long should our new baby sleep for?

Although young babies sleep for around an average of 16 hours each day, usually taken in short stretches, all babies are different, so it is impossible to say exactly how long a newborn baby should sleep for. Initially, many babies are extremely sleepy and it can feel like they sleep for much of the time. However, as long as they are woken regularly for feeds, this isn't a problem. Other babies seem to be more unsettled from the beginning, sleeping only in short bursts. Ideally, a new baby will sleep whenever and wherever she needs to as long as she isn't feeling hungry, too cold, too warm, or otherwise uncomfortable.

You will probably find that once your baby is a few weeks old, she will be spending more time awake and alert and will start to take more of an interest in what is going on in the world around her. You may also begin to notice a pattern forming in your baby's sleep habits by about six weeks, which will continue to evolve, and by around four months your baby will probably be sleeping for twice as long during the night as she does during the day. Generally, if your baby seems on the whole relaxed and contented, and is feeding and growing and developing well, then she is most likely getting enough sleep.

Q Our baby only settles if lying on my partner or me. We allow this as we want a rest. Is this wrong?

Although this is not wrong – getting a rest is important – there is a safety aspect to consider. Bed sharing, or even sleeping on the sofa together, is not advisable unless the adult is awake, so never fall asleep with your baby on a sofa or armchair.

If you have met her basic needs and she isn't ill, you could try other methods to calm your baby, such as putting her in a sling, going out in the car or with the pram, or singing to your baby. When she is sound asleep try to move her to her sleeping place.

Q Is it OK for our baby to share our bed? I'm confused about the advice.

Bed sharing while feeding or relaxing when the adult is always awake is enjoyable and can also benefit breastfeeding. However, there are dangers in bed sharing if you are asleep, including accidents involving suffocation and falls. The clear message from health professionals is that the safest place for your baby to sleep, night and day, is in a crib or cot in a room with you for the first six months of her life. The Foundation for the Study of Infant Deaths (FSID) and the Department of Health outline steps to reduce the risk of cot death, which include not sharing a bed with your baby under certain circumstances (see p.276). If you want to keep your baby close by, there are cots available that butt up close to the side of the bed.

Is it OK to rock our baby to sleep, or are we making life more difficult for ourselves?

If this is acceptable to you and your partner then it isn't a problem. However, you should be aware that babies tend to be creatures of habit, so if you use a certain technique to get your baby to sleep in the daytime, she probably won't settle at night without the same technique. So avoid rocking her, walking her up and down, or taking her for a drive in the car unless you're happy to repeat these things in the early hours of the morning!

If you find that sleep problems are beginning to dominate your life, there are techniques to encourage your baby to sleep (see p.280). However, these are not really recommended until your baby is a few months old, although if you are desperate for your baby to sleep in the evening, you may want to try one a bit earlier. All sleep solutions rely on

> Learn to trust and follow your instincts. These are often spot on and are the signposts that guide you on this unfamiliar journey

consistency, as well as being sure that your baby can cope on her own. Before you start a routine, make sure that you and your partner agree it is the right thing to do and will support each other during the first few difficult nights.

Is it a bad idea to carry my baby around in a sling at home? It really calms her.

You are not spoiling your baby at all if she enjoys being carried close to you. An American study observed that the young of animals fell into two categories – cache or carry. Either they were meant to be left for long periods of time in the nest while their parents were out hunting for food (cache), or they were meant to be carried all the time while the parents hunted (carry). The study concluded that humans fell into the carry category. The researchers based their conclusion on the fact that human breast milk is low in protein, so human babies need to be fed fairly frequently, around every two to three hours, and that a human baby has reflexes that represent clinging and attachment.

My mum says babies sleep better on their tummies. Is she right?

Your mother is mistaken on this and nowadays it would not be advised by health professionals. A key piece of advice from FSID and the Department of Health is to place babies on their backs to sleep. In 2006, FSID introduced a campaign to help parents to remember the importance of putting sleeping babies on their backs to avoid the risk of suffocation, but allowing them time on their front or sitting up safely when they are awake to help their head control and healthy development.

Depending on your mother's age, the advice may have been to put babies on their tummies when you were young. Also, many grandparents state concerns about babies vomiting while on their backs, but in reality babies turn their head if they are sick. If you are still concerned about this issue, discuss it further with your midwife or health visitor.

ESSENTIAL INFORMATION: A NEW LIFE

Sleeping and routines
How patterns emerge

In the early weeks, there is unlikely to be any set pattern to your days. Feeding on demand helps to establish successful breastfeeding, so it is best to simply "go with the flow" at this stage. By around six weeks, patterns will start to emerge, and you can think about introducing some routines.

Can I introduce a routine from the start?
One school of thought is to impose a strict routine of four-hourly feeding. However, this is not the ideal way to establish breastfeeding. Your baby has a small stomach and needs to feed "little and often". As she sucks, your breasts are stimulated into making more milk – so feeding on demand boosts your milk supply. Equally, in these early days, there is no structured sleep pattern – so it really is too early to impose any sort of routine.

When should I consider a routine? By about
six weeks, you will see a broad pattern emerging in which your baby will probably feed for longer and sleep for longer at night. You can start to help your baby become a good sleeper during the night, for example by teaching her the difference between night and day, encouraging her to be more active during the day, and by responding to

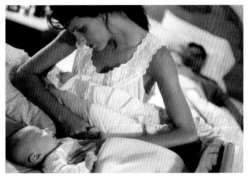

WAKING IN THE NIGHT: When your baby wakes in the night, quietly see to her needs, then put her back down with as little fuss as possible.

night wakings with minimal fuss in a darkened room, which will encourage her to settle herself back down to sleep.

What should a routine consist of? Regular
times for playing, feeding, and sleeping can be beneficial for you both. A pre-bedtime routine could include a warm bath, a massage, a feed, and then putting your baby into the cot drowsy but awake. You don't need to be rigid, but try to follow the same sequence each evening.

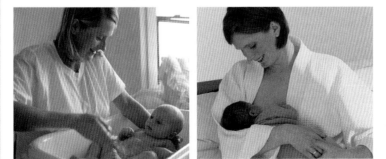

FAR LEFT: An evening bath can become part of your baby's bedtime routine. **LEFT:** Once your baby is changed and ready to be put down, a bedtime feed will help her to settle contentedly. .

Q My friend sleep-trained her baby within three weeks. How early can you start?

All children have different sleep patterns and differ in the amount of sleep they need. Problems begin when the baby prevents either parent getting the sort of rest they need. It is important to establish what your sleep expectations are for your baby, bearing in mind that one in three children wake regularly in the night at 12 months. You could talk to your friend about her technique and when she started it. However, generally sleep-training techniques aren't started until a baby is several months old. If you try a sleep-training technique, you must continue it faithfully for at least a week, although after two or three nights you should see an improvement.

A popular method is "controlled crying". With this method, you leave your baby to fall asleep alone but visit her briefly after 5 minutes, then after 10 minutes, and again after 15 minutes, if she is still crying. Pat her back, say a few words, and tuck her in; don't cuddle her or pick her up. The first few times she may cry for a while. If she wakes at night, follow the same routine. Another technique is to move away gradually from her cot. First sit by her cot and hold her hand for a few nights until she falls asleep. Then move further away each night until you sit just outside her door where she can still see you until she falls asleep.

Q Can you use a baby sleeping bag for a newborn?

These are safe for a newborn provided you are using the correct size, although some manufacturers suggest waiting a few months before using one. They are suitable for babies from approximately 3–4.5kg (7–10lbs) and have different tog values (like a duvet) for different times of year. They are worn over a sleepsuit and it is important you follow the instructions on sizing and tog values. The ideal room temperature for your baby is around 16–20°C (61–68°F). If the room is warmer or colder, adjust the level of clothing or the tog of the sleeping bag. Sleeping bags prevent overheating by using too much bedding and reduce

A man's natural instinct may be to hold back and let someone else pick up the baby, so be inclusive when caring for your baby

the risk of bedding going over a baby's head; there is also less chance for a baby to become tangled in covers or kick them off in the night. If you use a sleeping bag, it needs to be hoodless with the right size opening at the neck so your baby won't slip down. Sleeping bags must never be used with a duvet or quilt. They can be used in a Moses basket, car seat, or buggy.

Q My partner never wakes when I'm pacing the floor with the baby. How can I get him involved?

You need to find time when your baby is settled to discuss this issue calmly with your partner. It is possible he is unaware of how you are feeling, or he may be a particularly heavy sleeper. Sometimes partners feel inferior as they think that the mother is better tuned in to their baby's needs. Also bear in mind that your partner may need to function at a different level if he is working during the day and may therefore need a fairly full night's sleep. Perhaps you could suggest that he takes over one night at the weekend to try and let you get a better night's rest. Or you could organize a "lie-in" morning at the weekend, so one day you get up and let him have extra sleep and then swap the next morning. You could encourage your partner to help out in other ways too, with nappy changes or feeding, or taking the baby for a walk, so you have time to do something for yourself. The more you encourage baby and father interaction, the more inclined to help out he may become. Try and remain calm and hopefully you can resolve this issue together.

I'm feeling so depressed
your emotions after the birth

Q What are the third-day blues?

The third-day blues or "baby blues" is a term used to describe the bouts of weepiness many women experience around the third day after delivery. It is thought that half of new mothers experience the blues. They are due to the enormous physical, hormonal, and emotional changes your body goes through as you adapt to a non-pregnant state. When this is combined with a lack of sleep, tender breasts, and changing hormone levels as milk begins to be produced, and the physical discomfort of stitches and bruising, many women feel down and find themselves weeping a few days after the baby is born. The treatment for these temporary blues is plenty of support and love, along with as much rest as you can possibly get.

Q How long do baby blues last?

The baby blues are the least severe postnatal illness. They don't usually last very long – sometimes just hours, starting from around the third day after the birth and lasting no longer than the tenth day. During this time, you may feel tearful and irritable, but no medical treatment is needed. Although most women rapidly get over the blues, a few go on to develop more serious postnatal depression. If you find that you are feeling low and weepy after the first week, you should talk to your midwife, health visitor, or doctor as soon as possible.

Q I had my baby three weeks ago and I'm feeling really low – is it just my hormones?

You may find that the weeks and months after your baby is born are not the happy time you expected. If you are feeling tired, confused, and unable to cope, you may be suffering from postnatal depression (PND). Current medical opinion suggests that PND occurs in around 1 in 10 women, with different degrees of severity. PND has many symptoms, which can vary between individuals, but includes some or all of the following:

* **Lethargy and exhaustion**.
* **Being unable to bond** with your baby.
* **Feeling unmotivated** and unable to perform everyday tasks; even looking after yourself and the baby may seem an impossible chore.
* **A sense of isolation** from your partner, family, and friends.
* **Anxiety and panic attacks**.
* **Feeling that your life is drained of pleasure**.
* **Thoughts of self-blame and insecurity**.
* **Feeling at risk of harming yourself or your baby**.

PND is an illness, so professional help is needed if the sufferer is to regain health and peace of mind. If you think that you may be suffering from PND, it is important that you seek help as soon as possible. Talk first to your doctor or health visitor. Anti-depressants often form a part of the initial treatment. Although some women feel unhappy at the prospect of taking pills, these can play an important role, helping to lift your mood while the possible causes of the depression, such as feelings of isolation, anxiety, and guilt, are tackled. Most anti-depressants are non-addictive, and some can be taken safely while breastfeeding (advise your doctor if this is the case). Your doctor may also refer you for counselling sessions to help you to unravel the causes of the depression, allowing you to come to terms with your problems. Also, the Association for Postnatal Illness (see p.310) is an organization specifically run to help women with postnatal blues and depression. As well as offering advice, sympathy, and information covering all aspects of postnatal depression, it also arranges one-to-one support from its network of volunteer counsellors across the UK.

Self-help measures

Following the birth, it's often the case that the attention that was focused on the mother during pregnancy shifts to the baby and, as a consequence, the mother's emotional needs may be neglected. There are steps you can take to help avoid postnatal depression, or to deal with it quickly if you think you are becoming depressed.

* Don't have unrealistic expectations of how you should be as a mother. Accept that you will make mistakes and that this is OK.
* Get out of the house each day: walk to the park, go to the baby clinic, join postnatal groups, or arrange to meet friends or family.
* Tell your partner and doctor how you are feeling. This will help you feel supported and your doctor may prescribe anti-depressants.
* Get some exercise and eat healthy, regular meals.
* Arrange some time off, either alone, or to go out with your partner.

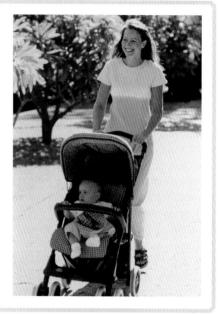

KEEPING ACTIVE: Making sure you get out of the house during the day helps to lift your spirits and provides a focus for the day.

My mum had postnatal depression. I don't want to get it too. What can I do to help myself?

The fact you have an awareness of PND is a major help. You should mention its existence in your family to your doctor so that he or she is aware of it as a potential problem. Being prepared for life with a new baby may help you to avoid depression. For example, before the birth get ahead of domestic chores and have a well-stocked kitchen with easy-to-prepare, nutritious meals. Talk to your partner, friends, and family to see if they can help out, maybe by preparing a meal or buying bread and milk. If it is thought that you are at a higher risk of developing PND, for example if you felt depressed in pregnancy, have a history of depression, or had a traumatic birth, you could talk to your doctor about other preventative measures. Sometimes, high doses of progesterone are given after labour and in decreasing doses for eight days by injection. The mother then uses progesterone pessaries until menstruation starts. This treatment is as yet unproven, but early results indicate that it can sometimes be helpful. Or anti-depressants can be taken in late pregnancy. Views on this are mixed, with many doctors feeling that exposing the baby to anti-depressants in pregnancy is not ideal, while others feel that the benefit to the mother outweighs the risk to the baby.

I've heard that postnatal depression is more common in mothers of twins. Is this true?

It is the case that mothers of twins or more are more vulnerable to PND simply because they are likely to be more exhausted and possibly struggling to cope. It's therefore important for couples expecting twins to think about their support network before the birth and try to arrange for extra help. After the birth, it's important not to dismiss feeling low as simply being down to the extra workload of twins.

We had our baby after IVF and were elated during pregnancy. Now I feel so low. How can this be?

After the emotional and physical turmoil of what could have been several years of trying to conceive, the reality of life with a newborn is bound to be a shock. Both you and your partner have been through a tremendous experience – not just the pregnancy but the process of becoming pregnant. Although all your anticipation and worries are hopefully replaced by caring for a baby and developing a new family life, that is not without its stresses. Feeling low in the week after birth as a result of changing hormone levels is common (see p.281). Sleep deprivation also causes stress and extreme tiredness. Feeling low is particularly distressing when you have looked forward to having your baby and had to endure a lot to conceive him. You may feel guilty for feeling like this, or even feel that you can't cope with being a mother.

Having been through the process of IVF, your expectations were probably very high and you may not have been prepared for the tiredness and hard work that is the reality of having a baby. Rest assured that things will settle down after about six weeks, as your baby starts to develop some sort of routine and you become more used to your new role as a mother and start taking pleasure in being with your baby.

If you continue to feel low after a week or two and are feeling tired, confused, and unable to cope, you may be suffering from PND, in which case it is extremely important that you seek help as soon as possible. Talk to your doctor or health visitor and try to enlist the support of family and friends as mild PND can be helped by increased support.

How is postnatal depression treated?

If you think you have PND, talk to your doctor, midwife, or health visitor. There are a number of different forms of help available, including talking therapies, such as counselling, and anti-depressant medicines. The most important step in treating PND is acknowledging the problem and taking steps to deal with it. The support and understanding of your partner, family, and friends also plays a big part in your recovery.

Your doctor can arrange counselling – some practices have a counsellor on site. Psychological treatments include cognitive behavioural therapy (CBT), which aims to reduce unhelpful thoughts and behaviour; cognitive therapy (CT), based on

the idea that certain thoughts can trigger mental health problems; and interpersonal counselling, which focuses on your past and present relationships. Many trusts offer "listening visits" and some areas run therapeutic groups. Health visitors provide practical support and sharing your experiences with other mothers affected by PND can help.

You could seek social support by contacting the Association for Postnatal Illness (see p.310), which offers advice and one-to-one support. Another organization, MIND (National Association for Mental Health) (see p.310) has over 200 branches across England and Wales, most of which offer counselling services for depression. Some areas will have specific support for PND. Drug treatment with anti-depressants is another option. These ease symptoms such as a low mood, irritability, lack of concentration, and sleeplessness, allowing you to function normally and to cope better. Anti-depressants can take two weeks to work and should be taken for six months after you start to recover to help prevent PND recurring. It's possible to continue breastfeeding on certain anti-depressants. Some herbal preparations, such as St John's Wort, can relieve symptoms, and the homeopathic remedy *Pulsitilla* may be helpful. Some research has also indicated that baby massage helps women suffering with PND to bond with their babies.

Practical measures, such as help with childcare and having time off, can be useful. It's important to get as much rest and support as possible. Some women get better over time without treatment. However, this can mean suffering for longer, which

Meeting the demands of a baby can be draining. Be aware of this and remind yourself that no-one is a perfect parent means a greater likelihood that PND will disrupt your experience of motherhood, and strain relationships. It's important to get help as soon as possible to relieve the depression, help your relationships, and to help your baby's long-term development.

Q We had a baby six weeks ago and my girlfriend seems so down. How can I help?

It is good that you are aware of your girlfriend's mood and are motivated to help her. If your girlfriend is suffering with PND, there is no instant solution, but there are things that you can do to help her, such as simply being there for her and listening to how she feels. Take some pressure off her by helping out with babycare chores, and welcome family and friends who are willing to do something practical, such as ironing, walking the baby, or a supermarket shop. Your health visitor will be experienced in dealing with PND and will be used to supporting women and their families through such difficulties, so you can ask her for further advice.

It's important that you encourage your girlfriend to see her doctor – perhaps go together – as PND is an illness that usually needs professional intervention if the sufferer is to regain their health and peace of mind fairly quickly. You could also seek support by contacting the Association for Postnatal Illness or other organizations (see p.310) that are run to help women with PND.

Q My partner is so depressed. Do dads get postnatal depression?

Although PND is mainly a problem for mothers, it is recognized that new fathers can become depressed too, and it is thought that as many as 1 in 25 new fathers are affected. Having a baby is a major life event for men too, and as such it can be a factor in the onset of depression. The pressures of fatherhood, such as extra responsibility, increased expenses, a change in lifestyle, and the tiredness, all increase the risk of depression. New fathers are more likely to become depressed if their partner is depressed, if they aren't getting along with their partner, or if they

> Feeling low and anxious at times is normal. However, don't let this go on for too long and don't be afraid to ask for help

are unemployed. If your partner is depressed, this will affect you too and may have an impact on how your baby develops in the first few months. Anyone suffering from symptoms of depression may find talking about their feelings with friends or family helpful. Professionally, few services exist for men, although your partner's doctor or health visitor may be able to offer treatment or counselling, but you may need to go together if your partner is reluctant.

Q I had an awful birth and I can't stop thinking about the details. How can I get over it?

It is important you try to resolve your concerns, as after a traumatic birth many women are frightened of getting pregnant again and going through another birth. Some women take steps to avoid pregnancy, such as avoiding sex, using multiple forms of contraception, or getting sterilized. Post-traumatic stress disorder (PTSD) that occurs after childbirth is a real problem, and if you are suffering from this you may benefit from treatments such as psychotherapy. Extreme fear of pregnancy and birth is called okophobia. The important thing is to examine your fears, look at how likely it is that the same thing will happen again, and look at steps you can take to reduce this likelihood. Many women say that before a traumatic birth they wanted more children, but the experience stopped them planning another pregnancy.

A debriefing session with the obstetrician may be helpful. Prepare a list of questions as it can be an emotional consultation. Going through your notes can help you understand why things happened and may resolve some of your concerns. It may be worth contacting your midwife too.

Q My partner has "flu" every other day and wants me to look after him. Is he jealous of the baby?

There may be several reasons for this, one of which could be jealousy. Talk to him without being critical. Does he need to feel more involved in the care of your baby? Suggest things he could do so he doesn't feel excluded, such as bathing the baby or taking him for a walk. Spend time with him as well as with the baby, as for both of you the focus of attention has shifted and this could feel like a loss. Also, dads present at the birth witness the pain of their partner; the feeling of helplessness for someone they love can be upsetting and this could be affecting his behaviour. Tiredness may be a factor as disturbed sleep is exhausting, especially if he has returned to work. Your partner may be suffering from depression, which can occur in men after the birth of a baby (see left); it may be worth visiting his doctor together if he is willing. Communication is vital, so make time to talk.

Q We're over the moon and want to spend every minute with our baby. Does everyone feel like this?

Parenting ought to be an idyllic experience, but may not be once the realities of physical and emotional stress take their toll. However, many new parents do experience a sense of euphoria, which can be brief or last for a while. All of us have unique reactions to becoming a parent and expectations from childhood, family, and friends influence this, as does your experience of pregnancy. For families who don't feel as positive, there are ways to enhance the experience of parenthood, such as giving your baby a massage, having family walks, and enjoying time together. Unfortunately for you, the need to return to some pattern of pre-baby life will probably arise, due to the necessity for one or both of you to go back to work. Try and timetable family time into your lives so you can continue to delight in your baby.

Highs and lows
Your changing moods after the birth

You may not feel constantly low or always happy, but it is true that having a new baby and coping with the changes this brings can give you intense highs and terrible lows, as you swing between feeling ecstatic about your new baby one moment to feeling unbelievably exhausted the next.

The best advice to new parents is to be realistic about what parenthood involves. If you approach life with your new baby aware that you are both likely to be incredibly tired, that you will have far less time to yourselves, and that the structure of your life will change enormously, then you will be better placed to take the highs and lows of parenthood in your stride. Accepting that you are not "perfect" parents can help you view parenthood as a constant learning curve, and to enjoy this enriching experience. You and your partner can help each other deal with the demands of parenthood by being patient with each other and helping each other with the daily care of your baby. You can also make sure that you allow each other some regular time off to do something for yourselves, such as meeting up with friends or getting some exercise.

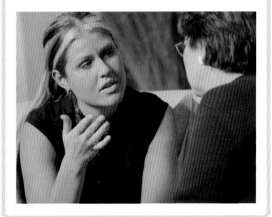

I'm sure I saw my baby smile
getting to know your baby

Q I heard that babies don't smile until six weeks. I'm sure she smiled at two weeks; is this possible?

A baby's first social smile is thought to happen at around four to six weeks, although it may be seen earlier and dismissed as wind. However, from an early age a baby can imitate the facial gestures of parents by, for example, moving her tongue and widening her eyes, which may make parents think that she is smiling.

Most parents say they see their baby's first smile between six and eight weeks. This is an important milestone as it means they have interacted with their baby, which is very rewarding. Psychologist Steve Biddulph suggests that newborn boys make less eye contact and smile less than girls. This means that we have to make an extra effort to interact and chatter with boys, so that they grow up to be toddlers who can talk as well as girls. If your baby does not smile by the time she is three months old, you could talk to your doctor and health visitor.

Q What is the bonding process and how can I encourage it?

Bonding is the attachment that develops between both parents and their baby. It makes parents want to shower their baby with love and to protect and nourish them, helps parents to get up in the middle of the night to feed their baby, and makes them attentive to their wide range of cries. It is beneficial for babies in promoting their security and self-esteem and is also believed to help a child's social and cognitive development. Bonding is easier if you aren't exhausted and, as at first, caring for a newborn can take all of your attention and energy, especially for a breastfeeding mother, it's helpful if fathers or friends can give a hand with everyday chores, as well as offer emotional support.

Breastfeeding can help with the bonding process, but there are lots of ways apart from breastfeeding to bond with your baby. Touching and stroking your baby develops a bond, and talking and singing to her during feeding and playtime encourages your baby to respond to you, which helps you to feel closer. Whether you're breast- or bottlefeeding, make eye contact during feeds and hold your baby close while you feed her. In some cases, for example if your baby is in a special care unit, you may worry about not being able to bond. However, the staff will encourage you to touch and hold your baby and be involved in her care. If you are finding it hard to develop "feelings" for your baby after a couple of months, tell your health visitor or doctor as you may be experiencing postnatal depression (see pp.281–285) and probably need professional help.

MIDWIFE WISDOM

Bonding over time
allowing your feelings to grow and develop

If you don't feel instant love for your baby, rest assured that bonding is a process and not something that has to happen straight after the birth.

* For many parents, bonding is a result of everyday caregiving.

* You may not realize you have bonded until you observe your baby's first smile and suddenly realize that you are filled with joy and love.

* Enjoy and cherish your growing feelings; bonding with your baby, whenever this occurs, is one of the most pleasurable aspects of babycare.

ESSENTIAL INFORMATION: A NEW LIFE

Baby bonding
Your feelings for your baby

"Baby bonding" is a phrase often used to describe the strong emotional feelings you have towards your newborn, and the overwhelming sense of wanting to love and protect her. Research shows that babies need this emotional interaction with you to help their development.

Will I bond with my baby immediately?
While some parents feel this bond straight away, bonding can often be a gradual process that develops as you get to know your baby. Holding her as soon as possible after birth, especially skin-to-skin, can help form an early bond. Your baby will already know the sound of your voice and will immediately respond to you, so talk to and smile at your baby as much as you can.

How does breastfeeding help bonding?
Breastfeeding is an ideal way to enhance the bonding process. It's a wonderful opportunity to be close to your baby while giving her essential nourishment. Also, breastfeeding releases oxytocin, known as the "love hormone", so is nature's way of creating a bond between you and your baby.

Are there other ways to bond? Bottlefeeding can also be a special time to be close to your baby, giving you a chance to hold your baby close and make plenty of eye contact. Bathing and nappy changing, as well as being practical tasks, are good opportunities to interact with your baby, helping you to feel close to your baby and providing her with reassurance, and baby massage is a good way to feel closer to your baby. As your baby grows, she will start to interact more with you, responding to your voice and smiles with smiles and coos of her own. This is a perfect time to start having "conversations" with your baby – talk to her in a sing-song voice and then pause to wait for her "reply". Through caring, nurturing, and interacting with your baby, you will be building a bond that will last a lifetime.

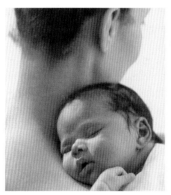
SKIN-TO-SKIN: Your baby will feel comforted by close contact and the warmth of your skin.

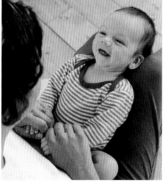
"TALKING" TOGETHER: As your baby grows, you will be able to interact more and more.

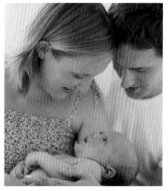
LOVING GAZE: Looking into your baby's eyes helps to strengthen the bond of love between you.

Q My partner doesn't feel as if he has bonded with our daughter yet. What can he do?

Although dads frequently yearn for closer contact with their babies, bonding frequently occurs on a different timetable for dads, partially because they don't have the early contact of breastfeeding that many mothers have. As a result, some men find that as your confidence grows, so does their uncertainty about their relationship with their baby. On a positive note, men today tend to spend significantly more time with their children than fathers of past generations did.

Talk to your partner about what he would like to do with your daughter. It's good for fathers to realize that bonding with their baby isn't a matter of being another mum and, in many cases, dads share special activities with their infants and develop their own unique relationships, offering fatherly qualities that the mother cannot provide. Both parents benefit greatly when they can support and encourage one another. Early bonding activities that you could encourage your partner to get involved in include bottlefeeding your baby (doing a night feed can help give you a rest); nappy changing; bathing and massaging your baby; going out for a walk with either a baby carrier or a pram; or simply enjoying some playtime with your baby. Bonding is a complex, personal experience that takes time. As long as a baby's basic needs are being met, she won't suffer if a bond isn't strong at first. If you're still concerned, ask your health visitor for more advice.

Taking time to get to know your baby – talking, touching, and caring for her – slowly helps to cement a lasting love

Q We've had so many visitors I feel I haven't got to know my baby yet. What do you suggest?

Perhaps if you have been inundated by visitors things may start to calm down. If not, then either you or your partner need to be politely assertive and explain that you are tired and can the visit just be for 10 minutes or put off until the weekend, or a more convenient time. It is not rude to ask for some space. Then shut the door, ignore the telephone, and enjoy some time with your baby.

Apart from crying, your baby's first attempts to communicate are in the form of eye contact. Look into her eyes from about 20cm (8in), the best distance for babies to focus. Touch her gently, stroke her, smile at her, and chat or sing to her. Look at her movements, listen to each sound she makes, and give her your full attention. You will teach your baby to make sense of the world by these early communications. Often, the best time to communicate is after a feed when your baby is relaxed and content. Pleasurable activities also include sharing a bath, going for a walk, singing to your baby, or giving a massage. Anything that both the parents and baby can enjoy. It may be nice to devote an evening each week for "family time", when you spend time all together. But try to keep the commitment and avoid interruptions.

Q What is baby massage?

Baby massage involves lightly stroking your baby's skin in a gentle, soothing rhythm (see opposite). Babies love to be touched and it's an important part of their growth and development. Baby massage is a great way to bond with your baby and is also thought to help to soothe common baby ailments, such as colic and dry skin.

Researchers from Warwick Medical School and the Institute of Education at the University of Warwick found that massage helped lower stress levels in babies, which in turn helped them to sleep better. Also, massage provides a good source of sensory and muscle stimulation, which is beneficial to all babies, but may be particularly good for babies with special needs, such as Down's syndrome, and

How to massage your baby

You can incorporate a massage into your baby's daily routine. Massage him in the morning, before you dress him, or make this part of his bedtime routine, massaging him after his bath, or before you get him ready for bed, which is a perfect way to settle him before bedtime. Rub an oil, such as sunflower oil, into your palms and massage him with gentle strokes. Make sure the room is comfortably warm.

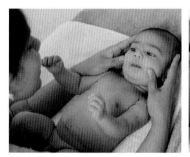

MASSAGING THE HEAD: Stroke his cheeks and forehead from the middle to the sides.

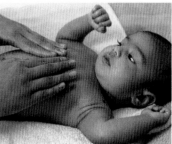

TUMMY AND CHEST: Very gently, stroke down his chest and then make circular movements over his tummy.

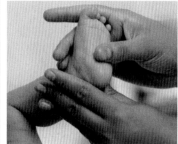

FOOT MASSAGE: Use your thumb to stroke from the heel to the toe, and then gently massage each toe.

there has also been evidence that premature babies in special care units who are touched more put on weight more quickly and are ready to return home earlier than babies who are not touched as much. Baby massage can also give you more confidence as a parent as it helps you to communicate with your baby. Ask your midwife or health visitor for information on baby massage classes in your area. There are also plenty of websites that offer guidance. The International Association of Baby Massage (see p.310) is a good source of information.

Q My baby cries continually and I'm really finding it hard to enjoy time with her. Is this normal?

Bonding is the attachment that develops between parents and their baby and this can sometimes be affected if you are worn down by constant crying. Although your baby is not doing herself any harm, this can be stressful and worrying for parents. If your baby cries continually despite your best efforts to calm her down, it's easy to feel rejected. It may help to remind yourself that bonding is a process, and not something that has to happen within a certain time period after the birth. If you are worried that the bonding process is being affected, try to recruit some extra support from your partner, friends, or health visitor to improve your situation. Some practical methods to try and reduce the crying and promote the bond between you include getting in the bath together; walking using a baby carrier (even around the house); or baby massage. The CRY-SIS helpline offers support for and advice to parents of babies who have sleep problems or who cry excessively (see p.310).

Q Is it too early to play "games" with my month-old baby?

In the first month, your baby sleeps for around 16 hours a day. Although this doesn't allow for much play time between feeds, changes, and baths, it doesn't have to mean you don't play with your child at all. There are plenty of ways to combine play with the everyday care of your baby. For example, you can sing to her while you change her nappy or play peek-a-boo – put your hands in front of your face, then take them away quickly and say "peek-a-boo" (by eight to ten weeks she'll start to remember what happens, and will gurgle with delight). Listening to music together is fun – try rocking and patting in time to the beat; and babies like to play with different textures – stroke different fabrics against her hands and arms and see her responses. When you are out and about, add a mobile or suitable toy to the pram.

At about eight weeks, your baby starts to make more sounds, such as coos and chuckles, and you can start to have a "conversation" together. Also, it's never too early to join a postnatal group or mother-and-baby group, which promotes play and allows you to spend time with your baby and meet other mums.

When should I put my baby on her tummy?

Even as a newborn, you can let your baby spend time on her tummy when she is awake to help strengthen her neck and shoulders and help her head control. It's important that your baby doesn't spend all her time lying on her back, as over time this can cause the head to become misshapen and "flattened" on one side. When she is older, lying on her front will help her to learn to crawl. Supervise during "tummy time" and be ready to help if she gets tired or frustrated; she will gradually get stronger. However, never put your baby on her tummy to sleep as this could increase her risk of cot death (see p.276).

How can I help my baby learn?

As your baby becomes more able to explore her surroundings and interact with people, you can provide opportunities and a safe environment for her to learn and develop. For example, if you respond to your baby's gurgling sounds with sounds of your own, she will be encouraged to keep using her voice for expression. Providing plenty of stimulus in the form of rattles, toys, and singing is also beneficial. Your baby's sense of touch is developing and it's a good idea to provide objects that have different textures, shapes, and sizes for her to explore. You

can introduce a baby gym with interesting objects that dangle for your baby to swat at. Your baby's sight develops quickly, so providing plenty of visual stimulus helps her to develop and learn. Spending time on her tummy also helps her to see the world from a new perspective (see above).

Be aware that there are times when your baby will have had enough stimulation and that some babies prefer more stimulation than others. It's important to recognize the signs and let your baby take a break.

How far can my two week old see?

A newborn is near-sighted and can see only blurry shapes in the distance. Perfect vision is considered to be 20/20, and a newborn has 20/400 vision. This means your baby can focus on your face from her feeding position at about arm's length (shoulder to elbow) but can't see much beyond that. Your baby's sight develops quickly. At about two weeks, she will pay more attention to your face, and any sudden movement may attract her gaze. By three months, she can recognize the outline of your face as you enter a room. Human faces are one of a baby's favourite things, especially a parent's or their own face. Placing a mirror at your baby's eye level can be a great toy. As her eyesight develops, you may catch her gazing out of a window or at a picture on the other side of the room. At about six to eight months, she will see the world almost as well as an adult does.

Can a newborn see colours yet?

Babies may see colour from birth, but have difficulty distinguishing similar tones, such as red and orange. As a result, they often prefer black and white or high-contrast colours for the first few months. They're attracted to bright colours and sharp outlines, whereas soft pastel colours are hard for them to appreciate, so keep this in mind when buying toys and books. Between two and four months, colour differences become clearer, and your baby starts to distinguish between similar shades. She'll probably show a preference for bright primary colours and more detailed designs and shapes.

MYTHS AND MISCONCEPTIONS

Is it true that...

✳ Babies are brought by the stork?

This myth comes from the so-called "stork beak marks", which are very common on the skin of newborn babies. These marks (otherwise known as stork bites or capillary haemangiomas) are due to the distension of tiny blood vessels in the skin, but they don't hurt, and your baby won't even know she has anything there. These marks tend to fade gradually without treatment.

✳ Breastfeeding babies need extra vitamin D?

Not true! Except in extraordinary circumstances (for example, if the mother herself was vitamin D deficient during the pregnancy). Babies store vitamin D during the pregnancy, and a little outside exposure on a regular basis should give a baby all the vitamin D she needs.

✳ You should wash your nipples before feeding?

This isn't true. Washing your nipples before each feeding makes breastfeeding unnecessarily complicated and washes away natural, protective oils. Don't wash your nipples too often – daily bathing is enough – and expose them to air whenever possible.

We're a family now
your new life together

Q I was in foster care when I was little. I can't believe I'm part of a family now. How will I adapt?

The whole process of having a baby can throw up many emotions and cause us to re-evaluate our lives and upbringing. Most parents, whatever their backgrounds, want a good life and opportunities for their own children. Although your childhood experiences have shaped you as a person and will obviously influence how you feel about having a child of your own and extending your own family, being honest and exploring your feelings and expectations with your partner, and maybe with your midwife and health visitor, can help you to adapt to your new life. It is important to try and maintain a healthy perspective on family life and although you are bound to want to be a superb parent, don't be too hard on yourself or have unrealistic expectations. You could consider looking into parenting courses as these may help you to increase your confidence and be comfortable with your new role, and contact with other parents can be mutually beneficial for you and your baby. Above all, try to enjoy your time with your baby rather than spending time worrying.

Q I'm in my pyjamas all day and haven't got on top of things since the birth two weeks ago.

After the initial excitement of the birth and bringing your baby home, the practicalities and exhaustion can start to take their toll. By two weeks, many partners have returned to work, visitors are waning, and life with a baby can seem relentless. Indeed, you may find that the weeks and months after your baby is born are not the happy time you expected. It can help to create a focus for each day, such as visiting a friend, doing a food shop, or walking to the park, so that you have a goal to motivate you to get ready.

Many mothers find that they have to get dressed as soon as they get up or it can be too difficult to find time to dress later in the day. You could make use of the time before your partner goes to work to have a moment to yourself to shower and get dressed.

If you are really finding it hard to motivate yourself and are feeling tired, confused, and unable to cope, you may be suffering from postnatal depression (see pp.281–285) and should talk to your doctor and health visitor.

Q I'm helping my wife with the baby at night but am feeling shattered at work. What can I do?

This is not an uncommon scenario and you may benefit from discussing this with you employer and human resources department if possible. Before talking to your boss, think about what you want and find out about your options: do you want time off, greater flexibility, or just a bit of slack? Do your requests affect your job, or other employees or your performance? Remember that the exhaustion is unlikely to be a permanent problem, so perhaps negotiating options for a month at a time may suit your employer. If you worked for your employer before your wife's pregnancy, you probably have the right to paid paternity leave (see p.65) if you haven't already taken this. Parental leave may be worth considering too. Within certain criteria, a parent of children under five, or disabled children under 18, has the statutory right to take unpaid time off work to care for them (see p.64). But consider too that most of these options will affect your salary and your wife may be on maternity leave or have stopped working.

Negotiating a "lie-in morning" with your wife is another option, so that, for example, every Saturday you get a lie-in and she gets one on a Sunday, no

Your new roles
getting used to family changes

The arrival of a baby inevitably brings with it a period when you, your partner, and other siblings need to adapt to a new family structure and learn to feel comfortable in your changing roles.

✳ Try to accept that this is a time of great change and there may be teething problems along the way as you accept your new roles.

✳ Don't be hard on yourself or your partner – being parents is a big responsibility and it's best to accept that it's a steep learning curve. Don't fret that you're not perfect parents. By loving and caring for your baby you will be doing the very best for him.

matter what sort of night you had. Also, at the weekends, there is no harm in having a nap when your baby does during the day.

My mother-in-law lives close by and helps a lot, but offers a lot of "advice". How do I deal with this?

This is not an unusual situation and never easy to deal with. It requires a calm, tactful discussion if at all possible, taking care not to damage your relationship. Everyday childcare has developed and changed over the years. Although having a grandparent close by means that you may have a willing babysitter or emergency helper close at hand, sometimes a grandparent's support can be seen as interference and their advice becomes unwanted. This can leave a grandparent feeling rejected and helpless, and parents feeling judged.

It's important to discuss your preferences and routines for your baby with your mother-in-law. This can sometimes be more difficult with in-laws than with your own parents, as you may feel more comfortable with your own parents' involvement and

be more likely to feel that you can comment when you feel uncomfortable. As your mother-in-law is local, perhaps she could attend a baby clinic with you or you could spend a day together so that she can witness your methods. Discuss how things were for her as a parent in a lighthearted way. Also try to explain the rationale for your care – such as reducing the risk of cot death by placing a baby to sleep on his back or delaying weaning until a baby is six months old. You could also have a look out for a book about being a grandparent and give this to her as a present from the baby. Some books contain practical advice, from recipes to play, plus tips on how not to tread on the daughter-in-law's toes.

We used to be equals. Now I'm at home and have nothing to talk about except the baby.

Life as a parent can mean a life that is dictated by the demands of a small person. Adjusting to being a family is hard and you may have changed your role completely. Many couples find that they need to talk about the differences between their lives before and after parenthood, and to help one another understand that each has probably had to give up a lot of time that they used to take for granted. Good communication is the key to dividing household and childcare duties. Try to find one hour a week to talk. It may also help to find extra things to do with your day, such as joining mother and baby groups, or going to the library or leisure centre.

I'm not sure when would be the best time to return to work. How do I decide?

Deciding when is the right time to return to work after having a baby is often an extremely hard decision for women to make. This is very much an individual decision and there is no right or wrong time. It will depend on how you are feeling, your employment conditions, as well as financial implications and childcare arrangements. You could make a checklist of all the things you need to consider before deciding which date to return. The main issue is likely to be childcare. Some mothers have a support network of grandparents or older relatives to care for the baby, while many couples need to arrange care with childminders, nannies, or nursery day care. Depending on how early you return to work, you may also need to think about how your baby will be fed when you are at work. Will he be fed bottled expressed milk or be given formula milk? Returning to work after having a baby can be tiring, particularly as your baby's sleep pattern may not be established yet, so you may be going to work having had very little sleep. You may want to discuss your options with your employers. For example, you may be able to work reduced hours and gradually build up to your usual working hours, or consider working part-time initially.

Q My mum says she will do all the childcare for us. Does that work well for most families?

You are fortunate that your mother is able to offer support as many couples do not have this option. Every family is different and only you can decide if this is a good option. Some women may feel that their mother is taking over and giving unwanted advice. Others may feel this is just what they need, especially in the first few months. Your mum obviously wants to be involved in her grandchild's upbringing, and to give you all the support she can. However, looking after a small child is not easy for anyone, so it would be wise to clarify with her exactly what she is offering and to have a serious discussion with your mum to agree what you both want and expect. Here are a few things to consider:

✱ **Should I offer my mum a small payment** or a gift of thanks?

✱ **How many hours a day** will this be for?

✱ **Will it be every day?**

✱ **Is my mum also offering to be a babysitter** when I want to have an evening off and maybe spend quality time with my partner or friends, or even alone?

✱ **How will we handle disagreements** about the way things should be done?

Q Are nurseries a bad thing for small babies? We can't afford a nanny.

Choosing the right sort of childcare for you and your baby is never an easy decision for families and is an area that you will need to spend a lot of time focusing

Time for siblings

It's important, with the anticipated arrival of a new baby, that you spend some time thinking about how to prepare your older children. It's common for siblings to display feelings of jealousy when a new baby arrives and you will need to deal with this. Talk to your other children before the birth about the new baby. Let them know how important they will be in the baby's life and how they will be involved. Once your baby arrives, it can be easy to become engrossed in looking after his needs, but it's important that you don't neglect to give older children attention too. Ensure that you have individual time with each child and that you continue their routines, so that they can see that all your time doesn't revolve around the new baby.

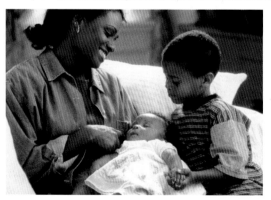

FAMILY TIME: Making sure you include older siblings and allowing them to develop their own special bond with the baby will help them to accept and love their new sibling and value their relationship.

on. It is very important that you are comfortable with whichever childcare arrangements you go with. There are pros and cons to all types of childcare and you will need to weigh up what suits you and your baby best. Some babies do very well in a nursery environment and many parents feel that their baby benefits from socializing with other children. Most nurseries have rooms specifically for babies and the appropriate staff and equipment to ensure they are well looked after. All nurseries have to be registered with Ofsted Early Years and registration includes a criminal records check on everyone involved in providing childcare at the nursery, and an inspection of the premises to look at health and safety and educational welfare issues. However, research also suggests that babies do best in nurseries once they are over a year old; before that time, they benefit from a more homely environment.

Childminders and nannies must also be registered by Ofsted. Nannies are usually the most expensive option, but your baby receives one-to-one care in his own home. Childminders tend to be less expensive than a nursery or nanny. The care is likely to be in the childminder's home and the childminder often cares for more than one child.

Q Our toddler is so jealous of the baby. I'm scared to leave them alone for a second. What can we do?

It is not unusual for a toddler to be jealous of a new baby in the home, so your child is behaving in a way that is normal for many children. Children are often confused about how the baby arrived, why he makes the sounds that he does, and why so many people seem to want to look at the baby and hold him. It is a very strange time for your toddler, as you will be giving a lot of attention to the new baby. However, it is important to address your toddler's bad behaviour, to try to understand why he is behaving this way and to make him understand that there are boundaries and that certain behaviour is not acceptable. Try not to react with anger, but to be firm and kind. In the child's mind, he may be thinking that life without the new baby was better than it is now and he may want

> Older children may worry that they will lose your love when a baby arrives. Reassure them that your love is constant

to send the baby back. If you see your child hurting the baby, even if it is not intentional, he should be stopped immediately and told why his actions are not nice. Try not to leave your child with the baby unsupervised until you feel that it is safe to do so.

Depending on your child's age, talk to him about the baby. Finding ways for him to "help" with the baby may encourage him to feel involved, but don't make him feel that he has to help. Some mothers give older siblings the job of choosing the baby's outfit each day, or at least the colour. Explore what your child is willing to do to help with the baby. Make a conscious effort to notice when your child is being helpful and praise him for the good things he does. It's important too to try to find some quality time for both you and your partner to spend alone with your toddler – perhaps he could have a special outing with dad, or you could do a favourite activity together.

To help you gain perspective, talk to other mums and dads about their experiences, as one of the best sources of help for parents is other parents. You will not be the first to encounter this problem and may find talking to other mothers useful.

Q My husband has older children from a previous marriage. I don't want them to feel left out.

Step families are very common now, with over 2.5 million children in the UK being part of a step family, either living with the step family or visiting them. Children will obviously be affected by changes within a family, and no matter what age your step children are or how often you see them, they will be affected by the arrival of a new baby. You and your partner will need to share responsibility for making the introduction go as smoothly as possible and any preparation and involvement before the birth will help them feel involved. This is a time to give them lots of extra hugs and attention and involve them every step of the way with the new baby to help them feel important and excited: a family get-together to discuss names for the baby is a good idea. Involving them once the baby arrives can also be beneficial, but be aware they may want to have some space too. Try to keep the communication channels open and consider that your husband may need to spend extra time with them.

Q I'm 18 and me and my baby live with my mum and dad. How can I become more independent?

This is something you need to sit down and talk about calmly with your parents. It may help to organize your thoughts in a list as this can be a very emotive subject. Think about your life with your baby, whether you want to continue studying or working, and how you might achieve this. There is financial support available for young parents who want to continue their education, or start training, and need help with the childcare costs. Ask your health visitor about government funding. Resuming training may also be viewed positively by your parents and will help to improve the prospects for you and your baby's future. You could perhaps use this as a bargaining tool to see if you could negotiate an evening a week when your parents babysit and you have an independent social life – this may need to be a rigid arrangement or they may prefer more flexibility. Also, is the baby's father involved in your lives? If so, could he or his family spend more time with your child so you can have a couple of hours each week to pursue your own interests? Attending a mother-and-baby group or a parenting course can be a good way to meet other mums and develop your social life, and it's good for your baby to mix with other babies. Again, ask your health visitor for information on local groups.

Where to get advice
Who to turn to for information and support

Having a baby is a life-changing event and you may find that you have to reconsider major parts of your life, such as where you live and how you structure your work or studies to fit around your baby. Whatever your situation, it's likely that at some point you will need advice and information to help you make decisions or access support.

✱ Your health visitor is often the first person to turn to for information and will be able to offer advice on a range of issues from childcare to goverenment funding.

✱ Your local education authority provides information on training and education, including services such as crèche facilities.

✱ The Citizens' Advice Bureau offers free advice and information on a range of issues including benefits and housing.

Q Can social services take my baby away – I've got a drug habit and I feel terrible about it?

This is not a question I can give you a straightforward answer to, as policies vary across the country and individual circumstances must be assessed. In some areas, a substance misuse habit, whether this is drug- or alcohol-related, does not mean an automatic referral to the Social Services, whereas in other areas, drug use is an automatic reason to refer patients immediately to the Social Services. If this is the case in your region, a detailed assessment of your situation would follow, as removing a baby from his home is not a decision that is undertaken lightly and it is always thought preferable to offer extra support and services to keep a family together wherever possible.

Having said that, the health and safety of your baby is vitally important. You must be as honest and open as you can with all the agencies involved in your care to demonstrate your responsibility for the welfare of your baby while you are pregnant, and participate in the planning of the delivery and care of your baby. Attending all your antenatal and postnatal appointments is important. Other factors to consider are which drugs you are using, whether you can reduce or stop their use or participate in a drug rehabilitation programme, and how much help and support you have and may need for life with a baby. The physical and emotional effects of having a baby are enormous, but there are also social and financial implications to consider. A positive step would be to see your baby as a reason to alter and improve your life. Many areas of the country have a specialist service for pregnant mothers with drug problems and you may find this beneficial. Ask your midwife or health visitor for details.

Q Our flat is much too small and I want to move right away.

Having a baby often makes you re-evaluate your current situation and babies will have an impact on available living space. You may be keen to move up the housing ladder and starting a family is of course an obvious time to do this. However, moving house is an expensive and time-consuming commitment, so it would be advisable not to rush into this. Although your baby may need more room as he grows and you may be thinking of having more children, while he is young your baby doesn't actually need a great deal of room, so consider your options carefully before you rush into any decisions. It's also wise to allow yourself time to recover from the birth and to spend some stress-free time with your new baby before taking on a major project such as moving.

If you are in council accommodation, having a baby is not an automatic right to obtain a larger property, especially as recommendations are for a baby to share a room with his parents for the first six months of his life. However, living in a flat may be problematic depending also on the level you are on, the presence of lifts or security systems, and how accessible it is with buggies. You should make sure

that the local authority knows if your circumstances change, for instance when you have a new baby, as soon as possible. You could speak to the Citizens' Advice Bureau for advice (see p.310).

Q We have a cat and a dog. Are they a danger to our baby?

Cats and dogs can become stressed and unhappy when a new baby arrives in the home, which can cause problems. Dogs that show unrest because of the new arrival often feel threatened. Attacks are rare and if they do occur it is usually because of mixed signals, hunter instincts, or a defensive reaction. Cats may withdraw into a quiet area or mark their territory, perhaps very close to the baby.

Ideally pets should be prepared while you are still pregnant, by training them to be in certain rooms only. Pets need routine, so try not to alter their routines drastically. You will probably spend less time with your pets, but try to have some quality time with them if that is what they are used to. Your pets may want to get close to the baby. This must be avoided, especially if there is not an adult in the room. Even if your cat and dog are known to be passive, their reaction to the baby could be unpredictable. Also do not let your pets lick your baby's face. An American study found that 28 per cent of children with cats in the house developed eczema at one year in comparison to 18 per cent in households without cats. However, children with two or more dogs in the house had a slightly increased protection against developing eczema or other allergies.

Having a baby can change your life in many ways. Try not to make decisions too hastily and consider all your options carefully

Time out for us
nurturing relationships

Q I used to dress sexily but seem to have lost interest since having my baby – am I losing it?

Having a baby and caring for her is a full-time job, which can mean that you probably don't have much time to spend on yourself. Many women struggle to find time to do their hair and even put on make-up in the first few weeks and months. However, your baby will soon get bigger and develop a routine that you can work around. So whether you want to get back into a dress for an evening out, or fit into your old jeans, this will happen in time. Although having a baby means you have taken on a new role in life and it involves a lot more responsibility, it shouldn't mean that you have to lose who you were before the birth.

Claiming some time for yourself every now and then can help you to start to take an interest in yourself again. Booking a hairdressing appointment, or treating yourself to a massage or a manicure, will help you to feel good again about the way you look.

Q We've been invited to a party. Is it a good idea to take our new baby with us?

In the early days this is fine as long as there is a safe, quiet place for her to be and this may be an easier option than leaving her with a babysitter if you're breastfeeding. Later on this becomes more difficult as most older babies like routine, so are likely to be more unsettled in a new environment, particularly if it is noisy. However, if it is a dinner party, your baby is unlikely to be so disturbed. On the other hand, babies are often capable of sleeping through quite a lot of noise, and young babies are very transportable, with the help of a Moses basket or travel cot.

You need to decide if your baby would be more settled at home cared for by a relative, friend, or babysitter, or whether she would be happier staying with you, even though the environment may be very different. Ideally your baby should be cared for in an environment that allows her to keep to her routine. You should not feel guilty about having time away from your baby and enjoying yourself. If you haven't left your baby with a babysitter before, whether a family member or paid sitter, you might want to arrange for a babysit for a couple of hours before the date of the party to see how this works out.

Q My partner is so worried about germs she won't visit my less house-proud sister. What can I do?

I can understand your partner's concern for the baby, as there is a lot of public awareness around bacteria and germs and we are constantly bombarded by the media with information on germ-busting products such as disinfectants and bleach solutions. However, if we create too sterile an environment, we are also killing good bacteria that can actually help us. Also, exposure to microbes and getting infected with some of them strengthens the body's natural immune system against allergies. An immune system that has little exposure to germs is more likely to see dust and pollen as dangerous invaders and respond in a way that causes asthma and allergies.

Human immunity is a marvellous process that works from birth and can protect even the tiniest of babies from illnesses

Babies begin preparing for the germs they will encounter at birth while still in the womb as, although the placenta acts as a filter, it lets through small amounts of allergens and microbes. It is thought that by three years, a child's body has learned all it needs to know to fight against germs. However, it is advisable to try to keep newborn babies away from people who have colds, as very young babies have difficulty breathing through their mouths, so if they have mucus in their nose this will make them very snuffly. Breastfeeding provides babies with some immunity from infections.

Babies will continue to come into contact with germs despite parents' best efforts to avoid them, and it is not really possible or desirable to live in a germ-free world. So try to reassure your partner that even though your sister may not be as house-proud, a visit to her home is unlikely to harm the baby. One exception, though, is hand washing, which is of paramount importance. Most infections are spread through the hands, as most people do not have a very good hand-washing technique. Before preparing bottles for a baby or preparing any food, it is important to wash your hands thoroughly.

Q My feelings about my husband have changed; I feel flat and don't know what to do. Any advice?

Try not to be too hard on yourself if you have only recently given birth. Most women are still trying to cope with their baby's demands and adjust to parenthood in the weeks and first few months after the birth. Tiredness and exhaustion can also make it hard to feel excited about other relationships. Unfortunately, this often leaves very little time to consider your partner and it is not unusual for partners to feel neglected or left out when a baby arrives, as the love and attention that was once shared with their partner has suddenly been transferred to the baby. This can be quite a shock to couples and you may find that you need to make a conscious effort to find time for each other to talk and communicate, as well as allowing yourselves time as a couple to enjoy together (see above).

MIDWIFE WISDOM

You and your partner
nurturing relationships after the birth

The arrival of a baby can put a strain on relationships, as a couple may shower attention on their baby, but neglect each other. It's important therefore to make time for each other too.

✽ Arrange for a babysitter and spend an evening out together to focus on your relationship and to rekindle feelings for each other. Surprise your partner by booking a table at your favourite restaurant.

✽ If you're worried about your relationship, remember that your circumstances aren't unique; keep communicating, finding quiet time to talk when your baby has settled.

Q How soon should I get a babysitter so that we can have a night out?

Having a night out with your partner or friends is a healthy thing to do when you have just become a parent. Coping with a new baby can be stressful and all parents need space to recharge their batteries. There is no rule about how early a babysitter can be used. It depends on how comfortable you feel about leaving your baby with another person, and may also be difficult in the early days of breastfeeding before you start expressing. You may have a family member, friend, or neighbour who you trust to look after your baby; or you could arrange to swap with another parent so that they babysit one night and you return the babysit another night. Or there are professional agencies that provide babysitting services (see p.310). Some services will offer a trial period to see how your baby responds to their minder. If it is successful, you may be able to have the same sitter on each occasion, which gives you peace of mind, and is reassuring for your baby. All babysitters have to be registered with Ofsted Early Years.

ESSENTIAL INFORMATION: A NEW LIFE

Finding a babysitter
Time out with your partner

There are various options for finding a babysitter: advertising locally for a young person, going via an agency, using a registered childminder, joining a babysitting circle with local parents, or asking grandparents to babysit. Any babysitter should have spent some time with your baby so that they feel comfortable with them, understand their routines, likes and dislikes, allergies, and medical conditions. They should always have your contact details, and you should have theirs. As well as personal recommendations, checking references is sensible. Most of all, trust your own instincts.

Enlisting the help of grandparents Asking a grandparent to babysit can be a lovely way for them to build a relationship with grandchildren, and provides you with peace of mind. Bear in mind that today's grandparents have busy lives too!

What other options are there? Babysitting circles are an informal arrangement where parents take it in turn to look after each other's children. Each time you sit for another parent you earn credits, which are then spent when your children are looked after. These sitters tend to be other parents whom your children will know and will have children of their own, which could be an advantage. There are several ways you can find out about babysitting circles, for instance through your local National Childbirth Trust branch, playgroup, or local health clinic.

Your Local Authority will have a list of registered childminders who may offer babysitting services as well. Agencies may charge a fee, but they will provide an enhanced Criminal Records Bureau check that highlights any child protection issues.

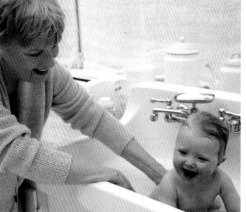

THE HELP OF GRANDPARENTS: Having involved grandparents can be an enormous help, allowing you to take time out knowing that your baby is receiving loving care.

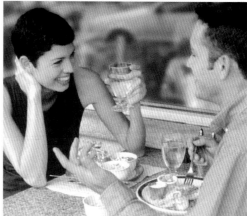

TIME OUT TOGETHER: Getting out as a couple and spending some quality time alone together is important to keep your relationship strong and maintain your identity as a couple.

Q Should I wait until after my postnatal checkup before we have sex again?

This is entirely up to you and your partner! It is perfectly normal to feel like having sex again quite soon after the birth of your baby, but it is also normal not to feel like it for months! Some women prefer to wait until after their postnatal check at around six weeks before resuming their sex life. Your doctor will be able to confirm that an episiotomy wound or tears you had after the birth have healed, and that your body is returning to normal. If all is well, it is likely that sex will not be too uncomfortable, even at first. Other women feel ready to have sex before the postnatal check. As long as you have stopped bleeding, and take things slowly and gently, this is fine. If you do experience any problems, you will be able to discuss them with your doctor at the time of the checkup.

Q I'm the only mum in a group of friends. I can't relate to them as I just want to talk about my baby!

When you become a mother, your life takes on a whole new focus – your baby. Everything about her naturally enthrals and concerns you, so it is to be expected that you will want to talk about her a lot. Unfortunately, you will find that, although your friends will love to hear about your baby, they will not share your intense interest. Being a mum is wonderful and all-consuming, but it is important to take time to focus on other areas of your life, such as socializing with your friends. Talking about other things and other interests will also help you to keep hold of your own identity, as well as that of being a mother.

Q Is it true that I don't need birth control while I'm breastfeeding?

In theory, breastfeeding should be a fairly reliable form of contraception if certain strict criteria are met, because the hormone prolactin, produced by the body to stimulate the production of breast milk, also acts to prevent the release of eggs from the ovaries. However this is not a guaranteed method of

Don't feel rushed into sexual relations. Try to see this as a time when you both need to find other ways to be loving

contraception, and if becoming pregnant again at this stage would be totally unacceptable for you and your partner, it would be best to play safe and use an additional form of contraception while you are breastfeeding your baby. As a general guideline (although as already stated this is not a guarantee), the chances of you conceiving while breastfeeding are extremely small if:

* **You are breastfeeding on demand** night and day without going for more than about six hours maximum without feeding.
* **Your baby has no additional form of nutrition** such as formula or solid food.
* **Your baby is less than six months old**.

Once changes occur, such as your baby sleeping through the night or starting solids, for example, it is possible that your periods, and therefore your fertility, will soon return. Since you will ovulate before your first period after the birth occurs, it is hard to pinpoint the return of fertility.

Q We want our baby to sleep in our room, but how can we have sex when she is so near?

It is currently recommended that your baby shares the same bedroom as you for the first six months as this helps to reduce the risk of cot death (see p.276). Many couples do not mind having sex when their baby is in the same room as long as she is soundly asleep and unlikely to wake up, while other couples do not feel at all comfortable with this idea, and so may need to consider other options if they want to

TIME OUT FOR US: NURTURING RELATIONSHIPS | **301**

continue sexual relations. If you really feel uncomfortable about making love so close to your baby, you may need to consider other places in which to enjoy some intimacy with your partner – it doesn't have to be the bedroom! You could try the sitting room, or a spare bedroom if you like comfort, or even the kitchen or bathroom if you are feeling more adventurous!

Alternatively, you might, in time, settle your baby to sleep in her own room and bring her into your room after the first night waking. This may allow you some private time in your room earlier in the evening.

I want some romance back in our life, but my husband seems to be avoiding sex. What can I do?

You need to talk to your husband about why he is avoiding sex as there may be several reasons for this, all of which can be resolved over time. Perhaps he is simply exhausted, as being a new parent is hard work. If this is the case, trying to find time for extra naps could help, and things should improve over time as the baby sleeps more and for longer. Your husband may be nervous about hurting you, especially if you had any stitches at the time of the birth. If things feel comfortable for you, then reassure him, and just take things slowly. He may be worried about the baby disturbing you during lovemaking. This is completely understandable, and doesn't have an easy solution, although this should hopefully become less of a concern once the baby has a more predictable sleep pattern. In the meantime, perhaps there is a friend or relative who could take the baby out for a while so that you can have some time alone with each other.

Sometimes, it is simply that couples can find it hard to swap roles – being a parent one moment and then being part of a loving couple the next and then back to being a parent again. As you get more used to your roles as parents, it should become easier to swap between the roles. Lastly, trying to make time for each other, to talk, to hold hands, and simply have a cuddle, is so important – if this can be achieved, a sex life will usually follow.

MIDWIFE WISDOM

Rebuilding intimacy
sex after birth

Having sex can be a daunting prospect after giving birth. You may be feeling unsexy, tired, and uncomfortable from stitches, and your partner may be unsure about when to initiate sex. It's best to ease slowly back into lovemaking.

✱ Don't launch straight back into penetrative sex. Spend time first simply caressing and massaging each other.

✱ You may experience more vaginal dryness as a result of hormonal changes, in which case, using a lubricant can help to make lovemaking more comfortable.

✱ Be open with each other about your feelings to avoid resentment and misunderstanding.

We had a baby six weeks ago, but I still don't feel ready for sex – is that normal?

Yes, that is totally normal! Even if you have physically recovered from the birth, you may not feel ready for sex again for quite some time – many couples take quite a few months to get their sex life back on track. If you are breastfeeding, hormones may also be playing a part in reducing your desire for sex. You may also be feeling self-conscious about the changes in your body, and you may just simply feel too tired for sex. This is all totally understandable.

Talk to your partner about the way you are feeling and make sure you have some relaxed time together to chat and simply show affection for each other. The rest will follow with time.

My partner wants me to stop breastfeeding because he is jealous. What should I do?

You need to talk to your partner about what exactly he is feeling jealous of. Perhaps he is jealous that you are the only one who can feed the baby. If this is the case, it may help to suggest other aspects of baby care that he can become involved with, such as winding the baby after a feed, nappy changing, or settling the baby. Once your baby is a few weeks old, you could express some milk for your partner to feed your baby. Once your baby is old enough for solid food, there will be plenty of opportunities for your partner to feed her.

It may be the case that your partner sees your breasts as purely sexual and feels uncomfortable seeing the baby feeding from them. Also, maybe you don't view your breasts in a sexual way so much at the moment, which is totally understandable, and your partner senses this.

Although you can be sympathetic, remind your partner that this phase in your baby's life won't last long, and that things will return to normal after your baby has stopped breastfeeding – maybe even before. Whatever his reasons for feeling jealous, remind him that breastfeeding gives your baby the best possible start in life, which is surely what you both want for your baby. You really need your partner's support in this.

Q Can I express milk so that we can go out?

Yes, you can express milk so that someone else can feed the baby. However, many breastfeeding experts advise waiting for around four to six weeks before doing this to give you and your baby time to get used to and establish breastfeeding, and give your body time to produce milk on a "supply and demand" basis (see p.233). Once you do start expressing, you can do this any time of day, although many women find their supply is greatest in the morning. Expressing milk also gives your partner a chance to become involved in feeding and help him to bond with his baby.

Q Will it harm my two-month-old baby if we leave him with his grandparents for the weekend?

No, it won't harm your small baby to leave her for a couple of days with people who love her. If you are bottlefeeding, this will be fairly straightforward, but if you are breastfeeding, it may be trickier. First, you will need to ensure that your baby is happy to take

Relationships after birth

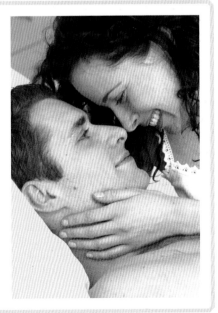

It's common for one or both partners to feel neglected after the birth, and the constant demands of a new baby can put a strain on the best of relationships. For the mother, it's easy to feel unattractive as her body takes time to return to its pre-pregnancy state. Both partners can feel inhibited by the presence of a baby in the house – probably in your own room – and are likely to be exhausted from weeks of broken sleep. Fathers often feel that all the mother's attention is now directed towards the baby, and they can sometimes begin to feel like an onlooker, expected to be supportive throughout. To ensure that your relationship remains strong, communicate constantly. It's vital that you recognize each other's needs and try to spend some time focusing on each other and being attentive to your partner.

TIME ALONE: You may be too exhausted to even contemplate sex, but simply being affectionate towards each other and maintaining a language of intimacy will help your relationship to thrive.

milk from a bottle, which can take some time if she has only had the nipple so far. You will then need to decide whether she will have expressed breast milk or formula milk while you are away. If she is going to have formula, you will have to accustom her to it before you go, and if she is having breast milk, you will need to start expressing well in advance and freeze some supplies so that you can leave milk with her grandparents. In addition, if you intend to continue breastfeeding, you will need to take a breast pump, sterilizing equipment, and storage bottles with you to maintain your milk supply while you are away. If this sounds too complicated, you could take your baby with you on your weekend and wait until your baby is a little older and perhaps no longer breastfeeding before you go away without her.

Q My partner wants us to have a break. I'm not ready to leave my young baby yet. What can I do?

Many mothers don't feel ready to leave their baby for more than a few hours in the first few months, so don't worry, this is normal. However, you need to explain this to your partner and reach a compromise. Perhaps you could take the baby with you for a weekend away? Small babies are fairly portable, especially if you're breastfeeding. Or maybe a friend or relative could babysit while you and your partner go out to dinner. If you did go for a weekend away just to please your partner, you may not feel happy or relaxed, which would surely defeat the object of time away, and affect your partner's enjoyment too.

It's good for you and your partner to take time out as a couple. Just a few hours at your favourite restaurant can make a difference

Q My wife wants to do everything herself – now my mum is offended. How can I help her relax?

Many new mums feel like this, so your situation isn't unusual. Perhaps your wife feels that she should be able to do everything herself and sees accepting help as an admission of defeat and that she is failing to cope with her new role as a mother. Reassure her that she is a great mum, and let her know that people want to help, and that she would also benefit from having some time out to relax. Tell your mum about how your wife is feeling, and reassure her too, as she probably feels that her offers of help aren't appreciated. Perhaps your mum could ask your wife what she would like her to help with. For example, she would probably love someone to help with the washing up, dusting, or ironing. Or she may even be happy for your mum to take the baby out for a walk so that she can have a bath or a rest.

Q Is it OK to leave the baby asleep in the car while I dash into a shop?

Unfortunately, in this day and age this is probably not advisable, although ultimately it is up to you. If you have a portable car seat, it is very easy to take your baby into a shop with you without disturbing her if she is asleep.

Q I feel like we're stepping into a new life. What does the future hold for us?

Embarking on parenthood is one of the most complex but wonderful transitions in life. It is a rollercoaster of change and challenges, and of emotional and physical ups and downs. Your relationship with your baby develops continually and your relationship with your partner may change slightly too. You will also develop a new social network based on life with your baby. You may wish to stay at home with your baby or return to work. The main thing to remember is that life will not be the same again, but it tends to improve in many ways with a child. Enjoy it as much as possible as your baby will grow up all too quickly.

MYTHS AND MISCONCEPTIONS

Is it true that...

* I'll lose all the baby weight if I breastfeed?

It's estimated that breastfeeding burns around 300 calories a day, so it certainly helps, but it's unlikely to make you magically return to your pre-pregnancy weight again! To give your body time to recover from labour and birth, wait six weeks or so before you think about weight loss. Be sure to eat sensibly, take regular exercise, and allow nature to do the rest. If you are still breastfeeding by six months, seek professional advice if you wish to diet.

* I should be able to fit into my old jeans?

Is it safe to lose weight so quickly after giving birth? Extreme dieting isn't healthy for a mum or her baby. If you're nursing, you need to take in a certain amount of vitamins, minerals, fat, and other nutrients to maintain the quality of your breast milk. So when you deprive yourself of nutrients, you're also depriving your baby. Plus, you have to remember that giving birth, while natural, is very traumatic for your body – you need time to heal. You shouldn't be pushing yourself to lose weight.

* Grandparents will babysit for us anytime, right?

Don't forget that grandparents still have their own lives, friends, and activities! Grandparents are usually very happy to babysit, but don't just assume they're always free, and don't use them as a drop-off point at any time of the day or night! Your parents will love looking after your baby when you need a break, but don't take them for granted.

Glossary

Abruption The detachment of part of the placenta from the wall of the uterus during late pregnancy, which may result in bleeding.

Accelerated labour The artificial augmentation of contractions, after the cervix has started to dilate, by the injection of oxytocin through an intravenous drip. Often used to speed up a long labour.

Active birth An approach to childbirth that involves upright positions and movements during labour.

Active management of labour The constant monitoring and technical control of labour to monitor its duration.

Alphafetoprotein (AFP) A substance produced by the embryonic yolk sac, and later by the fetal liver, which enters the mother's bloodstream during pregnancy.

Alveoli Milk glands in the breasts, which produce a flow of milk when they are stimulated by prolactin and the baby's sucking.

Amniocentesis The surgical extraction of a small amount of amniotic fluid through the pregnant woman's abdomen. This procedure is usually carried out as a test for fetal abnormalities.

Amniotic fluid The fluid that surrounds the fetus in the uterus. Ultrasound scans may be done in late pregnancy to ensure that enough is present.

Amniotomy The surgical rupture of the amniotic sac, often done to speed up labour. This is referred to as ARM (artificial rupture of the membranes).

Anaemia A condition in which there is an abnormally low percentage of haemoglobin in the red blood cells; it is treated by iron supplements.

Anaesthetic Medication that produces partial or complete insensibility to pain.

Anaesthetic, general Anaesthetic that affects the whole body, with temporary loss of consciousness.

Anaesthetic, local Anaesthetic that affects a limited part of the body.

Analgesics Painkilling agents not inducing unconsciousness

Antenatal Before the birth

Anterior position See *Occipital anterior*.

Antibiotics Substances capable of destroying or limiting the growth of micro-organisms, especially bacteria.

Antibodies Protein produced naturally by the body to combat any foreign bodies, germs or bacteria.

Anti-D An injection of antibodies given to women who have a Rhesus negative blood group if it is thought they may have been exposed to Rhesus positive fetal blood cells.

Antihistamines Tranquillizers that are used in the treatment of nausea, vomiting, and certain allergies.

Apgar scale A general test of the baby's wellbeing given shortly after the birth to assess the heart rate and tone, respiration, blood circulation, and nerve responses.

Areola The pigmented circle of skin surrounding the nipple.

ARM See *Amniotomy*.

Bile pigment See *Bilirubin*.

Bilirubin Broken-down haemoglobin, normally converted to nontoxic substances by the liver. Some newborn babies have levels of bilirubin too high for their livers to cope with. See also *Jaundice, neonatal*.

Birth canal See *Vagina*.

Blastocyst An early stage of the developing egg when it has divided into a group of cells.

Braxton Hicks contractions Practise contractions of the uterus that occur throughout pregnancy, but which may not be noticed until towards the end.

Breast pump A device for drawing milk from the breasts.

Breech presentation When the position of the baby in the uterus is bottom down rather than head down.

Caesarean section The delivery of the baby through an incision in the abdominal and uterine walls.

Candida See *Thrush*.

Cardiotocograph (CTG) An electronic monitor that is used to measure the progress of the mother's contractions and the baby's heartbeat during labour.

Carpal tunnel syndrome Numbness and tingling of the hands arising from pressure on the nerves of the wrist. In pregnancy it is caused by the body's accumulation of fluids.

Catheter A thin plastic tube that is inserted into the body through a natural channel to withdraw fluid from, or introduce fluid into, a particular part of the body. This can be used to draw off urine from the bladder after an operation, or to maintain a constant input of fluids into a vein, or to introduce anaesthetic into the epidural space.

Cephalic presentation (Vertex presentation) The position of a baby who is head down in the uterus. The most common presentation.

Cephalopelvic disproportion A state in which the head of the fetus is larger than the cavity of the mother's pelvis. Delivery must therefore be by Caesarean section.

Cervical dilatation See *Dilatation*.

Cervical incompetence A disorder of the cervix, usually arising after a previous mid-pregnancy termination or damage to the cervix during a previous labour, in which the cervix opens up too soon, resulting in repeated mid-pregnancy miscarriages. It is sometimes treated by suturing to hold the cervix closed.

Cervix The lower entrance to the uterus, or neck of the womb.

Chloasma Skin discolouration during pregnancy, often facial.

Chorion The outer membranous tissue that envelops the fetus and placenta.

Chorionic gonadotrophin See *Human chorionic gonadotrophin (HCG)*.

Chorionic villus sampling A method of screening for genetic handicap by analysis of tissue from the small protrusions on the outer membrane enveloping the embryo that later form the placenta.

Chromosomes Rod-like structures containing genes occurring in pairs within the nucleus of every cell. Human cells each contain 23 pairs. See also *Gene*.

Cleft palate A congenital abnormality of the roof of the mouth.

Club foot A congenital abnormality in which the foot is painlessly twisted out of shape.

Colostrum A kind of milk, rich in proteins, formed and secreted by the breasts in late pregnancy and gradually changing to mature milk some days after delivery.

Conception The fertilization of the ripened egg by the sperm and its implantation in the uterine wall.

Congenital abnormality An abnormality or deformity existing from birth, usually arising from a damaged gene, the adverse effect of certain drugs, or the effect of some diseases during pregnancy.

Contractions The regular tightening of the uterine muscles as they work to dilate the cervix in labour and press the baby down the birth canal.

Cordocentesis A fine needle is passed through the mother's abdomen into the fetal vein in the umbilical cord. The technique allows fetal blood to be tested, facilitates intra-urine blood transfusions, and enables drugs to be injected directly into the baby.

Corpus luteum A glandular mass that forms in the ovary after fertilization. It produces progesterone, which helps to form the placenta, and is active for the first 14 weeks of pregnancy.

Crowning The moment when the baby's head appears in the vagina and does not slip back again.

CVS See *Chorionic villus sampling*.

D and C The surgical dilatation (opening) of the cervix, and curettage (removal of the contents) of the uterus.

Dehydration A physical condition caused by the loss of an excessive amount of water from the body, often resulting from severe vomiting or diarrohea.

Depression, respiratory Breathing difficulties in the newborn baby.

Diabetes Failure of the system to metabolize glucose, traced by excess sugar in the blood and urine.

Diamorphine A narcotic opium derivative used as an analgesic.

Dilatation The progressive opening of the cervix caused by uterine contractions during labour.

Distress See *Fetal distress*.

Dizygotic See *Twins*.

Domino scheme A scheme operated by some hospitals in which community midwives provide antenatal care and are present at hospital for the delivery.

Doppler A method of using ultrasound vibrations to listen to the fetal heart.

Doula A supportive woman helper who provides physical and emotional support during childbirth.

Down's syndrome A severe congenital abnormality caused by an incorrect number of chromosomes that produces physical abnormalities and reduced intelligence.

Drip See *Intravenous drip*.

Eclampsia The severe form of pre-eclampsia, which is characterized by extremely high blood pressure, headaches, visual distortion, flashes, convulsions and, in the worst cases, coma and death. The condition is now rare since the symptoms of pre-eclampsia are treated immediately. See also *Pre-eclampsia*.

Ectopic (Tubal pregnancy) A pregnancy that develops outside the uterus, usually in one of the Fallopian tubes. The mother has severe pain low down on one side in her abdomen at any time from the 6th to 12th week of pregnancy. The pregnancy must be surgically terminated.

EDD The estimated date of delivery.

Electrode A small electrical conductor used obstetrically for monitoring the fetal heartbeat during labour.

Electronic fetal monitoring The continuous monitoring of the fetal heart by a transducer placed on the mother's abdomen over the area of the fetal heart, or by an electrode inserted through the cervix and clipped to the baby's scalp.

Embryo The developing organism in pregnancy, from about the 10th day after fertilization until about the 12th week of pregnancy, when it is termed a fetus.

Endometrium The inner lining of the uterus.

Engaged (Eng/E) The baby is engaged when it has settled with its presenting part deep in the pelvic cavity. This often happens in the last month of pregnancy.

Engorgement The over-congestion of the breasts with milk. If long periods are left between feeds, or the baby is not well latched on, painful engorgement can occur. This can be relieved by putting the baby to the breast or expressing the excess milk.

Entonox A mixture of 50 per cent oxygen and 50 per cent nitrous oxygen, breathed in through a mask during labour, that gives pain relief as contractions peak.

Epidural (Lumbar epidural block) Regional anaesthesia, used during labour and for Caesarean sections, in which an anaesthetic is injected through a catheter into the epidural space in the lower spine.

Episiotomy A surgical cut in the perineum to enlarge the entrance to the vagina.

External version (External cephalic version, or ECV). The manipulation by gentle pressure of the fetus into the cephalic position. This may be done by an obstetrician at the end of pregnancy if the baby is breech or transverse.

Fallopian tube The tube into which a ripe egg (ovum) is wafted along after its expulsion from the ovary, along which it travels on its way to the uterus.

False labour Braxton Hicks (rehearsal) contractions, which are so strong and regular that they are mistaken for the contractions of the first stage of labour.

Fertilization The meeting of the sperm with the ovum or egg to form a new life. See also *Conception*.

Fetal distress A shortage in the flow of oxygen to the fetus, which can arise from numerous causes.

Fetus The developing child in the uterus, from the end of the embryonic stage at about the 12th week of pregnancy, until birth.

FH Fetal heart.

Fibroid A benign (non-cancerous) muscle growth in the uterus.

Forceps Metal tong-like instruments placed either side of the baby's head during labour to help deliver the baby.

Hormone A chemical messenger in the blood that stimulates various organs to action.

Human chorionic gonadotrophin (HCG) A hormone released into the woman's bloodstream by the developing placenta from about six days after the last period was due. Its presence in the urine means that she is pregnant.

Hyperemesis gravidarum Almost continuous vomiting during pregnancy.

Hypertension (High blood pressure) During pregnancy this can reduce the fetal blood supply.

Hypnosis A state of mental passivity with a special susceptibility to suggestion. This can be used as an anaesthetic, and can be self-induced.

Hypotension Low blood pressure.

Identical twins See *Twins*.

Implantation The embedding of the fertilized ovum or egg within the wall of the uterus.

Induction The process of artificially starting off labour and keeping it going.

Insulin A hormone produced by the pancreas that regulates the level of carbohydrates and amino acids in the system. It may be used as a means of controlling the effects of diabetes. See also *Diabetes*.

Internal monitoring See *Electronic fetal monitoring*.

Intravenous drip The infusion of fluids directly into the bloodstream by means of a fine catheter introduced into a vein.

Intravenous injection An injection into a vein.

Invasive techniques Any medical technique that intrudes into the body.

In vitro fertilization (IVF) A type of assisted conception where fertilization occurs outside of the womb and fertilized embryos are tranferred back into the womb.

Jaundice, neonatal A common complaint in newborn babies, which is caused by the inability of the liver to break down successfully an excess of red blood cells. See also *Bilirubin*.

Lanugo The fine soft body hair of the fetus.

Lateral position Transverse lie or horizontal position of a fetus in the uterus (sometimes occurring if the mother has a large pelvis), where the presenting part is either a shoulder or the side of the head.

Let-down reflex The flow of breast milk into the nipple.

Lie The position of the fetus within the uterus.

Linea nigra A line of dark skin that appears down the centre of the abdomen over the rectus muscle in some women during pregnancy.

Lochia Postnatal vaginal discharge.

Longitudinal lie The position of the fetus in the uterus in which the spines of the fetus and the mother are parallel.

Low-birthweight baby A baby who weighs below 2.5 kg (5½ lb) at birth.

Meconium The first contents of the bowel, present in the fetus before birth and passed during the first few days after birth. The presence of meconium in the amniotic fluid before delivery is usually taken as a sign of fetal distress.

Miscarriage The spontaneous loss of a baby before 24 weeks of pregnancy.

Monitoring See *Electronic fetal monitoring*.

Monozygotic See *Twins*.

Morula A stage in the growth of the fertilized egg when it has developed into 32 cells.

Moulding The shaping of the bones of the baby's skull, which overlap to allow the baby to pass through the birth canal.

Mucus A sticky secretion.

Multigravida A woman in her second or subsequent pregnancy.

Multiple pregnancy The development of two or more babies. See also *Twins*.

Mutation A damaged genetic cell. This can occur naturally or, more commonly, as an effect of outside agents, such as radiation.

Neural tube defects Abnormalities of the central nervous system. See also *Anencephaly; Hydrocephalus; Spina bifida*.

Nicotine A highly poisonous substance that is present in tobacco. During pregnancy this can enter the bloodstream of a woman who smokes and may affect the efficiency of the placenta, which often results in a low-birthweight baby.

Nucleus The central part or core of a cell, containing genetic information.

Occipital anterior The position of the baby in the uterus when the back of its head (the crown or occiput) is towards the mother's front (anterior).

Occipital posterior The position of the baby in the uterus when the back of its head (the crown or occiput) is towards the mother's back (posterior).

Oedema Fluid retention, which causes the body tissues to be puffed out.

Oestriol A form of oestrogen.

Oestrogen A hormone produced by the ovary.

Opioids (Narcotics) Painkilling drugs that induce drowsiness and stupor.

Ovary One of the two female glands, set at the entrance of the Fallopian tubes, which regularly produce eggs until the menopause.

Ovulation The production of a ripe ovum or egg by the ovary.

Oxytocin A hormone secreted by the pituitary gland that stimulates uterine contractions during labour and stimulates milk glands in the breasts to produce milk.

Palpation Feeling the parts of the baby through the mother's abdominal wall.

Pelvic floor The springy muscular structure set within the pelvis that supports the bladder and the uterus, and through which the baby descends during labour.

Pelvis The pelvis is a solid ring of bone at the base of the abdomen; it shields the bladder and portions of the genital tract.

Perinatal The period from the 24th week of gestation to one week following delivery.

Perineum The area of soft tissues surrounding the vagina and between the vagina and the rectum.

Pethidine See *Analgesics*.

Phototherapy Treatment by exposure to light, which may be used when a baby has jaundice.

Pituitary gland A gland set just below the brain that, among other functions, secretes various hormones controlling the menstrual cycle. In late pregnancy it releases a hormone, oxytocin, into the bloodstream, which stimulates uterine contractions and also the milk glands.

Placenta The organ that develops on the inner wall of the uterus and supplies the fetus with all its life-supporting requirements and carries waste products to the mother's system.

Placental insufficiency A condition in which the placenta provides inadequate life support for the fetus, often after 40 weeks, resulting in a baby at special risk.

Placenta praevia A condition in which the placenta lies over the cervix at the end of pregnancy. This part of the uterus stretches in the last few weeks of pregnancy, but the placenta cannot stretch, so it may separate; the result is bleeding during late pregnancy. A woman with a complete placenta praevia is delivered by Caesarean section.

Posterior See *Occipito posterior*.

Postnatal After the birth.

Postpartum After delivery.

Post-traumatic stress disorder Panic and anxiety experienced by some women after traumatic and disempowering childbirth.

Pre-eclampsia (Pre-eclamptic toxaemia or PET) An illness in which a woman has high blood pressure, oedema, protein in the urine, and often sudden excessive weight gain. See also *Eclampsia*.

Premature A baby born before the 37th week of pregnancy and weighing less than 2.5 kg (5 lb).

Presentation The position of the fetus in the uterus before and during labour.

Presenting part The part of the fetus that is

lying directly over the cervix.

Preterm See *Premature*.

Primigravida A woman having her first pregnancy.

Progesterone A hormone produced by the corpus luteum and then by the placenta.

Progestogen A synthetic variety of the hormone progesterone used in oral contraceptives.

Prolactin A hormone that stimulates milk production for breastfeeding.

Prostaglandins Natural substances that stimulate the onset of labour contractions. Prostaglandin gel may be used to soften the cervix and induce labour.

Proteinuria The presence of protein in the urine, which may be a sign of pre-eclampsia. See also *Pre-eclampsia*.

PTSD See Post-traumatic stress disorder

Pubis The bones forming the front of the lower pelvis.

Quickening The first noticeable movements of the fetus felt by the mother.

Respiratory depression See *Depression, respiratory*.

Rhesus factor A distinguishing characteristic of the red blood corpuscles. All human beings have either Rhesus positive or Rhesus negative blood. If the mother is Rhesus negative and the fetus Rhesus positive, severe complications and Rhesus disease (the destruction of the red corpuscles by antibodies) may occur, unless prevented by anti-D gamma globulin.

Rooting The baby's instinctive searching for the breast.

Rubella (German measles) A mild virus that may cause congenital abnormalities in the fetus if it is contracted by a woman during the first 12 weeks of pregnancy.

Scan (Screen) A way of building up a picture of an object by bouncing high-frequency soundwaves off it. The sonar or ultrasound scan is used during pregnancy to show the development of the fetus in the uterus. See also *Transducer*.

Show A vaginal discharge of bloodstained mucus occurring before labour, resulting from the onset of cervical dilatation. A sign that labour is starting.

Small-for-dates Babies who are born at the right time but who for a range of reasons have not flourished in the uterus. See also *Placental insufficiency*.

Sperm (Spermatozoon) The male reproductive cell that fertilizes the female ovum or egg.

Spina bifida A congenital neural tube defect in which the fetal spinal cord forms incorrectly, outside the spinal column.

Spinal anaesthesia An injection of local anaesthetic around the spinal cord.

Steroids Drugs used in the treatment of skin disorders, asthma, hay fever, rheumatism, and arthritis. Because they alter the chemical balance of the metabolism they may, very rarely, cause fetal abnormalities if used extensively during pregnancy.

Stillbirth The delivery of a dead baby after the 24th week of pregnancy.

Streptomycin A broad-spectrum antibiotic that should not be taken in pregnancy. See also *Antibiotics*.

Stretch marks Silvery lines that sometimes appear on the skin after it has been stretched during pregnancy.

Supplementary feeding Additional bottles given to a breastfed baby.

Surfactant A creamy fluid that reduces the surface tension of the lungs so that they do not stick together when deflated. Preterm babies may have breathing difficulties if surfactant has not developed sufficiently.

Suture The stitching together of a tear or a surgical incision.

Syntocinon A synthetic form of oxytocin, which is used to induce or accelerate labour.

TENS machine See *Transcutaneous electronic nerve stimulation*.

Term The end of pregnancy: this is measured at 38–42 weeks from the first day of the last menstrual period.

Tetracycline A wide-spectrum class of antibiotic that should be avoided during pregnancy, because it can affect the development of the fetal teeth and bones. See also *Antibiotics*.

Thrombosis A blood clot in the heart or blood vessels.

Thrush A yeast infection that can form in the mucous membranes of the mouth, genitals, or nipples.

Toxoplasmosis, congenital A parasitic disease that is spread by cat faeces. If it crosses the placenta during pregnancy, it can cause eye or central nervous system damage in the baby.

Transcutaneous electronic nerve stimulation A method of pain relief that uses electrical impulses to block pain messages to the brain.

Transducer An instrument that translates echoes of very high-frequency soundwaves, bounced off the developing fetus in the uterus, to build up an ultrasound image on a monitor. See also *Scan*.

Transition A phase between the first and second stages of labour when the cervix is dilating to between 7 and 10 cm.

Trial of labour A situation in which, although a Caesarean section may be necessary, the mother labours in order to see if a vaginal delivery is possible.

Twins The simultaneous development of two babies in the uterus, either after two eggs are fertilized independently by two sperm – dizygotic or fraternal twins – or, more rarely, after one fertilized egg divides to produce monozygotic or identical twins.

Ultrasound See *Scan; Transducer*.

Umbilical cord The cord connecting the fetus to the placenta.

Uterus (Womb) The hollow muscular organ in which the fertilized egg becomes embedded, where it develops into the embryo and then the fetus.

Vacuum extractor An instrument, used as an alternative to forceps, which adheres to the baby's scalp by suction and, with the help of the mother's bearing down, can be used to guide the baby out of the vagina.

Vagina The canal between the uterus and the external genitals. It receives the penis during intercourse and is the passage through which the baby is delivered.

VE Vaginal examination.

Vernix A creamy substance that often covers the fetus in the uterus.

Vertex presentation (VX) See *Cephalic presentation*.

Vulva The external part of the female reproductive organs, that includes the labia and the clitoris.

Water birth Birth of a baby under water.

Resources

Fertility

www.gettingpregnant.co.uk
Fertility advice

www.hfea.gov.uk
020 7291 8200
Human Fertilisation and Embryology
Authority

www.midwivesonline.com
'Trying for a baby' section

www.surrogacy.org.uk
0844 4140181

Pregnancy

www.bpas.org
0845 730 4030
British Pregnancy Advisory Service

www.fpa.org.uk
0845 310 1334
Family Planning Association

www.maternityalliance.org.uk
020 7490 7638
Advice for pregnant women and new parents

www.midwivesonline.com
Information on pregnancy, birth, and new
babies; includes Ask a Midwife support
service

Labour and birth

www.activebirthcentre.com
020 7281 6760

www.aims.org.uk
Helpline 0870 7651433
Association for Improvements in Maternity
Services

www.birthchoiceuk.com

www.birthtraumaassociation.org.uk

www.caesarean.org.uk

www.doula.org.uk
0871 433 3103
Support for women during labour and birth

www.homebirth.org.uk

www.independentmidwives.org.uk
0845 4600105

www.midwivesonline.com

www.nct.org.uk
Pregnancy and birth 0870 444 8709
National Childbirth Trust

www.rcm.org.uk
020 7312 3535
Royal College of Midwives

Support groups

www.apni.org
020 7386 0868
The Association for Postnatal Illness

www.bliss.org.uk
Helpline 0500 618140
Organisation supporting special-care babies
and their families

www.careconfidential.com
Helpline 0800 028 2228
Support and advice for unplanned
pregnancies

http://caretolearn.lsc.gov.uk
Support for childcare costs for teenage
parents who wish to continue education
or training

www.clapa.com
020 7833 4883
Cleft Lip and Palate Association (CLAPA)

www.connexions-direct.com
Support and advice for 16–19 year-olds in
their education decisions

www.cry-sis.org.uk
Helpline 08451 228669
Advice for parents for dealing with
excessive crying and sleep problems

www.diabetes.co.uk
02476 712712

www.downs-syndrome.org.uk
Helpline 0845 2300372
Downs Syndrome Association

www.drinkaware.co.uk
020 7307 7450
Advice on alcohol and risks

www.gosmokefree.co.uk
NHS helpline 0800 1690169
Support for quitting smoking

www.hyperemesis.org.uk
Advice and information on hyperemesis
gravidarum

www.lupus.org.uk
St Thomas' Lupus trust

www.mind.org.uk
0845 7660163
Support for sufferers of mental illness

www.ocupport.org.uk
The Obstetric Cholestasis Support website

www.pelvicpartnership.org.uk
01235 820921
Support and information for sufferers of
symphysis pubis

www.pni.org.uk
Information and advice on postnatal
depression

www.pre-eclampsia.co.uk

www.steps-charity.org.uk
Helpline 0871717 0044
Information and advice on talipes/club foot

www.talktofrank.com
Helpline 0800 776600
Information and support for drugs
and alcohol addiction

Parent groups

www.healthvisitors.com

www.mama.org.uk
01525 217064
MAMA (Meet-A-Mum Association)

www.multiplebirths.org.uk
020 8383 3519
The Multiple Births Foundation

www.parentlineplus.org.uk
Helpline 0808 800 2222
Support and advice for parents

www.tamba.org.uk
Twinline 0800 138 0509
Twins and Multiple Birth Association

www.twinsuk.co.uk
01670 354463

www.fatherhoodinstitute.org
0845 634 1328
Support for fathers

Breastfeeding

www.abm.me.uk
Helpline 08444 122949
Association of Breastfeeding Mothers

www.babyfriendly.org.uk
0870 606 3377
The Baby Friendly Initiative by Unicef
promoting breastfeeding

www.breastfeedingnetwork.org.uk
Helpline 0844 412 4664

www.laleche.org.uk
Breastfeeding helpline 0845 1202918

www.midwivesonline.com
Breastfeeding advice

www.nct.org.uk
Breastfeeding helpline 0870 444 8708
National Childbirth Trust

Family

www.bestbear.co.uk
08707 201277
Information and advice on childcare

www.grandparents-association.org.uk
Helpline 0845 4349585

www.gingerbread.org.uk
0800 018 4318
Self-help groups for single-parent families

www.healthvisitors.com

www.mynightoff.com
Babysitting circle service

www.raisingkids.co.uk
020 8883 8621/020 8444 4852
Information for families

www.relate.org.uk
0845 4561310
Relationship counselling

www.sitters.co.uk
0800 3890038
Babysitting site

Benefits and rights

www.citizensadvice.org.uk

www.direct.gov.uk
Employment and benefits

www.dwp.gov.uk
Department for work and pensions

www.hse.gov.uk
Health and Safety Executive

www.workingfamilies.org.uk
020 7253 7243
Advice and support for working parents

www.worksmart.org.uk
Information on maternity rights

Bereavement

www.crusebereavementcare.org.uk
Helpline 0870 167 1677
Bereavement counselling

www.fsid.org.uk
Helpline 020 7233 2090
Foundation for the Study of Infant Deaths

www.miscarriageassociation.org.uk
Helpline 01924 200799

www.uk-sands.org
Helpline 020 7436 5881
Stillbirth and Neonatal Death Society

General

www.baaf.org.uk
020 7421 2600
British Association for Adoption and
Fostering

www.eatwell.gov.uk
Food Standards Agency; advice on
healthy eating

www.healthvisitors.com
01274 427132
Information and support for parents

www.iaim.org.uk
020 8989 9597
The International Association of Infant
Massage

www.idfa.org.uk
020 7836 2460
Infant and Dietetic Food Association;
information on specialist nutritional needs

www.nhsdirect.nhs.uk
0845 4647

www.nice.org.uk
0845 003 7780
National Institute for Health and Clinical
Excellence

www.rcog.org.uk
020 7772 6200
Royal College of Obstetricians and
Gynaecologists

www.tommys.org
08707 70 70 70
Tommy's Maternal and Fetal Research Unit

Index

A

abdomen
  flabbiness 266
  measuring 101
abnormalities, fetal 116, 122–3, 125
abortion 40
abuse 115
acupressure 82
acupuncture 144, 176
adoption 71
AFP (alpha-fetoprotein) 117, 119
afterbirth see placenta
afterpains 264
age
  adapting to pregnancy 68
  and fertility problems 19
air travel 46
alcohol
  and breastfeeding 235
  and cot death 235, 276
  in pregnancy 35–7, 53
  preparing for pregnancy 15, 16
allergies 54, 297, 298
alternative therapies, pain relief 175–6
ambulances 159
amniocentesis 123, 125
amniotic fluid
  ARM (artificial rupture of membranes)
    180–81, 191, 192
  "waters breaking" 167–8
amniotic hook 180–81, 192
amniotomy see ARM
anaemia 81, 109–10, 117, 217
anaesthesia
  Caesarean section 207, 208, 210
  epidural 174, 176, 177–8, 271
  episiotomy 205
  forceps delivery 203
anger, grief 260
animals, safety 297
anomaly scan 119, 120, 121
antacids 43
antenatal care 74–80
  booking appointment 41, 74–5, 78
  tests 116–26
  work and 61, 63
antenatal classes 142, 194
anterior position 145
antibiotics 43
antibodies
  in breast milk 237
  in colostrum 227
  Rhesus incompatibility 79
anti-D injections 79

anti-depressants 281, 282, 283–4, 194
antiemetics 43
antihistamine 43, 86
Apgar score 212, 216, 217
aquanatal classes 55, 58–9, 142
areola 228
ARM (artificial rupture of membranes)180–81,
  191, 192
arnica 265
aromatherapy 175–6
artificial insemination by donor (AID) 29, 33
aspirin 43
assisted conception 27
assisted delivery 202–5
asthma 45, 250
Association for the Improvement in Maternity
  Services 310

B

babies see fetus; newborn babies;
  premature babies
"baby blues" 247, 281, 282
baby clothes 138, 254
baby monitors 138–9, 246
babysitters 298, 299, 300, 304
backache 58, 84
bacteria
  baby's exposure to 298–9
  food poisoning 47
  infections 158–9
balls, birthing 175
barrier cream 253
Bart's test 119
baths
  baby baths 139
  in early labour 168
  nappies 244
  newborn baby 248, 250–51
  in pregnancy 44
  "rebirthing" 256
bed sharing 276, 277–8
bedding 138, 254–5, 280
bedrest 88
belly button see navel
benefits 62
bile, obstetric cholestasis 90
bilirubin 164, 203, 222, 223
biological fathers, tracing 33
biparietal diameter 118
birth see delivery; labour
birth certificate 71
birth control see contraception
birth plans 149, 155

birth preparation classes 79–80
birthing balls 175
birthing partners 158, 177, 194–200
birthing pools 156–7
birthing units 154–5
birthmarks 219
blastocysts 21
bleeding
  gums 83
  lochia 224, 264
  miscarriage 22–3
  nosebleeds 84
  in "show" 167
  vaginal 75, 90
blood clots 58, 86, 209, 213, 225, 267
blood flow scans, Doppler 120
blood pressure
  high 83, 87, 89
  low 81
  twin pregnancies 131–2
blood spot test 220–21
blood tests 75, 117–19, 222
"blooming" 108, 110
BMI (Body Mass Index) 18, 126
body
  after birth 264–71
  changes to in pregnancy 105–12
bonding 216, 286–9
  father and 198, 288
  in pregnancy 94–5, 102
  skin-to-skin contact 188
  with special care babies 165
  with twins 130–31
bones, baby's 121
booking visit 75
bottlefeeding 236–42
  bowel movements 252
  and colic 274
  combining with breastfeeding 239
  equipment 139, 236, 237
  establishing a routine 275
  formula milk 166, 227, 236–7, 240
  leaving baby with grandparents 303–4
    and sleep 248–9
  sterilizing equipment 238, 239, 241, 242
bowel movements
  after birth 265
  after episiotomy 270
  bottlefed babies 242
  meconium 252
  passing in labour 186, 188
brain
  development of 94, 95
  premature babies 164–5

Acknowledgments

Author's acknowledgments

Without doubt, it would not have been possible to compile this book without the numerous expectant and new parents entrusting their personal and confidential questions to us in the first place – so a huge thank you to all the expectant and new parents who continue to place such faith in midwives and entrust their very precious cargo to us – without you there would be no midwives. Equally, a book like this could not have been compiled by me alone, and I wish to thank sincerely the great midwives and fellow workers who have made no small and invaluable contribution in terms of their time to research and respond to numerous questions from parents, and for their contribution to special articles. The following midwives contributed to the questions: **Diane Jones RM; Joanne Daubeney RM; Dawn Lewis RM; Julie Scott RM; Emma Whapples RM; Tamsin Oxenham RM; Sarah Fleming RM; Anne Thysse RM;** and **Dr Mary Steen RM**. The consultant midwifery editors were **Peggy Plumbo RN, MS, CNM** and **Dr Mary Steen RM**. For the special articles, thanks to **Anne Thysse RM** and **Joanne Daubeney RM**.

Personal thanks to the following people who tirelessly assist with Midwivesonline.com and in particular our Ask a Midwife service, without whom this book would not have been possible. To my gorgeous husband, who is my number one cheerleader in all my activities on Midwivesonline.com and *Ask a Midwife* – I love you and thank you Chris for your many sacrifices on my behalf xx; to my sister, PA & senior administrator, Teresa Fleming – Teresa, without your dedication, loyalty and hard work, none of this would have ever happened – thank you.

My second team of cheerleaders include my mentor and fellow director John Kirkby; also Robert & Gillian Clarkson and administrator Maureen Terry – for all your hard work and effort in launching our services - thanks. Technical workers: Tim Snell, Georgina Stretch & Syed Zeeshan Ali – gold dust indeed. All the midwives and health visitors who daily contribute to *Ask a Midwife* and *Ask a Health Visitor* services – sincere thanks.

Thanks also to the numerous health professionals who tirelessly respond to parents' questions at all the baby shows we attend, too numerous to mention.

Last but by no means least, I would like to thank the staff at DK for daring to believe in me producing this book. Special thanks to Esther Ripley and Peggy Vance for all your guidance and encouragement; thanks to Claire Cross for all your tireless editing, and to Carole Ash for all your inspiring design work. Thanks, too, to Emma Woolf, Nicola Rodway and Marianne Markham at DK for your contributions and guidance.

Publisher's acknowledgments

Dorling Kindersley would like to thank Alyson Silverwood for proof-reading, Hilary Bird for the index, Jenny Baskaya and Romaine Werblow for assistance with images, and Debbie Maizels and Philip Wilson for the illustrations.

Picture credits

The publisher would like to thank the following for their kind permission to reproduce their photographs:

(Key: a-above; b-below/bottom; c-centre; f-far; l-left; r-right; t-top)

Alamy Images: Angela Hampton Picture Library 68l, 244; Richard Baker 279bl; Bubbles Photolibrary 38br, 82tr; ImageState 46r; Janine Wiedel Photolibrary 176cr, 209r; PHOTOTAKE Inc. 209l; Picture Partners 214tr, 254; Profimedia International s.r.o. 38bl, 56cb, 208; Chris Rout 12bl, 35, 56l; Stockbyte 32; thislifeBaby 262tl; Peter Usbeck 163r; **Bubbles:** Chris Rout 112; Corbis: Cameron 185cb; Pascal Deloche/Godong 165; Annie Engel/zefa 6c, 38tl, 72tr; Rick Gomez 214cl, 262cr; Annie Griffiths Belt 130; Jack Hollingsworth 150cr; Jose Luis Pelaez, Inc. 294; Don Mason 62; David Raymer 300r; H. Schmid/zefa 68r; Holger Winkler/zefa 63bl; **Getty Images:** Chad Ehlers - Stock Connection 97cla; Food Image Source 82ca; William King 63bc; Photodisc 224; Louie Psihoyos 150br; **iStockphoto.com:** Scott Fichter 191r; Nathan Maxfield 213; **Prof. J.E. Jirasek MD, DSc.:** CRC Press/Parthenon 96tr, 97tc, 97tr; **Life Issues Institute:** 98tr; **LOGIQlibrary:** 118bc, 118bl, 118cb; Masterfile: Aluma Images 44r; **Mother & Baby Picture Library:** 3l, 4c, 4t, 6b, 7b, 7t, 12tl, 38cl, 44l, 46l, 72bl, 72br, 72tl, 77l, 85, 89, 103, 111, 115, 117, 149, 150bl, 150cl, 150tl, 150tr, 155tc, 155tr, 156c, 156cl, 156r, 168, 174bl, 174r, 179, 184l, 184r, 185clb, 185crb, 191l, 195, 196bc, 196cb, 214br, 262br, 282, 303; **Photolibrary:** 49; LWA-Dann Tardif 4b, 11; **PunchStock:** 51bc; BananaStock 76, 185t; Blend Images 171, 38cr; Brand X Pictures 225cb; Design Pics 285; Digital Vision 225l, 300l; Image Source 12tr; Photodisc 140, 225bc; Purestock 279tr; zefa 282; **Science Photo Library:** 28cb; Marco Ansaloni / Eurelios 30br; Neil Borden 121cb, 121clb; BSIP, Laurent 192; Mauro Fermariello 12br, 29; Adam Gault 2r, 72cl, 77c; Ian Hooton 2l, 3r, 8, 38tr, 51t, 72cr, 77r, 146; Dr Najeeb Layyous 28bc, 28clb, 97tl, 124bc, 124br, 124fbr; Living Art Enterprises, Llc 121bc, 121bl; Cordelia Molloy 17r; Professors P.M. Motta & J. Van Blerkom 20bl, 21bc; Joseph Nettis 163l; Dr Yorgos Nikas 20br; D. Phillips 20bc, 21bl; Philippe Plailly / Eurelios 31bl; Chris Priest 30bl, 31br; P. Saada / Eurelios 118clb; John Walsh 28bl; Zephyr 25l; **SuperStock:** age fotostock 6t, 12cr; **Wellcome Library, London:** Yorgos Nikas 21br; Anthea Sieveking 153, 219

Jacket images: Front: **PunchStock:** Polka Dot Images br; **Science Photo Library:** Ian Hooton bl, tr; Paul Whitehill bc. Back: **Corbis:** Jack Hollingsworth tr; JLP/Sylvia Torres tl; **Mother & Baby Picture Library:** tc. Spine: **PunchStock:** Blend

All other images © Dorling Kindersley
For further information see: www.dkimages.com

kisses and then again the shutting and
and bureau drawers and both of them,
acking up, preparing to get out.

at that table with all those stacked-up
frozen, paralyzed, wanting, oh desper-
rush through that door and not even
as still standing there behind her. Only
rases and all to be put together, pieced
, 'not paying the old lady,' 'running out
here.' Had she heard something about
e story that had been accepted? Maybe,
up. There she had sat and listened and
e door stealthily opening and then feet
of thieves, the boards creaking in the
opening of the outer door; then faint
g of the area gate behind them.

That music, what was it, she had asked herself, occurring in her heart, feeling it climb, ascending to what celestial heights she did not need to ask, but let it climb, let it continue climbing, let the clouds burst and the effulgence stream behind the breaking clouds while she experienced such joy as never was or could be quite imagined, running as she seemed to be backward into childhood with that music, with those intimations and the remembrance of that day in Siena when she'd found and read the incomparable *Ode*, and being there again in that grove in Brookline picking those spring flowers, being in the summer fields above the ocean, a part of that great dance of life. And from whence came such music, she had asked herself, from what fount of knowledge and intuition, yielding herself up to it, letting the heart climb higher, higher, and saying to Felix yes, it is enough, it is sufficient.

After that was over, the spell had been cast, shed on all the guests, and she had walked through the rest of the party treading it had seemed to her upon celestial clouds, the pleasantest compliments in her ears and that delicious sense that everything was going as she'd planned. She'd had in a man to serve and a caterer had furnished the refreshments and with her own Daphne Jordan assisting everything went on without a hitch. Champagne, she had thought, looking at her guests, at the daffodils, the freesia, the narcissus – the perfect wine for such a night as this and she had lifted her glass to drink, as someone had suggested, to the spring and there at her side the young cellist who had played, it was the only word for it, like an angel, and she had told him that his performance was perfection and he had bowed and said 'My dear lady, it was because you were there with that expression on your face that I performed so well.' A lovely compliment she had thought carrying it with her through the evening while this little tableau melted into the next and the whole airy, fairy dream went floating away from her until the last guest had gone and there she'd been alone in her big room thinking of it all with such extreme delight.

And then because she must find somebody to talk to she'd gone downstairs in search of Daphne Jordan and found her stacking up the dishes on the dining table just as she had ordered, tired, considerate, and more than a trifle tipsy, what with all the glasses she'd emptied. Her lady must sit down and have a cup of coffee for she hadn't, she'd reminded her, had a bite to eat. 'Now there,' she'd said, returning with salad, sandwiches, and coffee, 'eat, my lady, eat them sandwiches,' and back she'd gone into her kitchen to finish with the dishes.

Glad enough she'd been of something to sustain her. Pitching into the sandwiches and salad, trying to gather and assemble the various fragments of that lovely dream her party, which for once in a way had been so completely successful, and becoming suddenly aware that something was going on in the front room she'd felt annoyance, irritation. Why should those two young people disturb this mood of happiness and satisfaction with their ugly quarrels? They were in the midst of a regular fracas. She'd not wanted to listen to them, but as a matter of fact she had done so; she'd listened attentively. She could hear them plainly, for they'd raised their voices and oh, she wished they would not use all those ugly words, throwing them at each other like that, words only associated in her mind with certain passages of the Bible and in the mouths of these young people revolting, revolting. The girl was apparently weeping and what was she telling the young man? That she was going to have a baby. Oh God, oh God, she couldn't bear it, and she'd put her hands before her face. 'All right,' he'd said, 'you're going to have a baby. All right, that's your responsibility. No reason at all for me to believe it's mine.' At this the girl had shrieked hysterically. It seemed that she was on the bed. She could hear her moving about and the springs

creaking. '...
nobody bu...
he had call...
could not ...
aware that...
kitchen do...
how could...
and shutti...
girl contin...
you.' 'Shu...
the girl m...
an actual ...
just pelti...
sound of ...
he was h...
over and ...
listened t...
seemed t...
'All righ...
and the ...
heart to ...
what sh...
she'd ne...
so despe...
love an...
though...
drunke...
to exc...
long, h...
as he'd ...
growin...
hear n...
over, ...
him. '...

and there had beer...
the opening of doo...
it dawned upon her,...

And there she'd s...
dishes round her, b...
ately, to get up an...
knowing if Daphne ...
scraps of words and ...
out by her imaginati...
on her,' 'getting out ...
Europe, Paris, about ...
perhaps she'd made ...
finally she had heard...
as cautious as a pair...
basement hallway, th...
but audible the latch...

TEN

Miss Sylvester regarded her little patch of view. She had never been able to accustom herself to it and tonight it was of such transcendent beauty, the air, the sky so clear and that small slice of a moon sailing past the tower, the stars quivering, this astonishing array of windows building up before her eyes their citadels of crystal light. Strange it should have been her portion to look out on such a spectacle as this. Strange to have lived on earth through these last eighty years. And an altogether extraordinary business writing her book, laying it away unopened and then rereading it today, sitting here turning the pages as one might turn the pages of anybody's novel, all the while reliving it, giving it back to memory, to that stream that still continued flowing. It was, she thought, looking out upon the moon, the stars, and all the glittering windows, as though they challenged her, something of a cheat – a cheat, the cutting her story off, rounding it to a finish with all that tragedy and melodrama in the basement.

Life carried on and that knowledge to which she'd been so brutally exposed became as time went on an item of familiar baggage in her heart. How long had she stayed on in Grove Street, three years or four? She wasn't sure, and the year she'd sold the house and moved to that comfortable place in Eighth Street would probably remain uncertain were it not for the fact that luck had been involved, getting out before the crash, selling the house at a good profit and making all those arrangements about the legacy, the settlement of seventy thousand dollars on the grandchild she'd never seen, completed in the spring of that same year, the funds invested soundly, capital and accruing interest to be paid at his majority and all achieved without so much as breaking that agreement never to reveal herself either to her son or to his issue.

And the years that followed her moving out of Grove Street, goodness gracious, more than twenty of them. What with the world events that rushed upon her out of the headlines, off the celluloid, out of the air, collapsing, colliding, careening madly off into time and space, how could she possibly keep track of them? After the crash that period of depression, queues of the unemployed and that soup kitchen right around the corner on Green Street, never emerging from her door without the sight of hungry men. Then there had been Hitler and all the terrifying rumors (just when had she first heard of Hitler?), then Roosevelt and the moratorium, the first inaugural speech, that voice in which you somehow trusted, then suddenly the rolling of the beer barrels so jolly in the midst of all that apprehension, and behold the bars, the mirrors, bottles, the ladies with their glasses, and all the time the rumors growing louder – youth movements, storm troopers, Jews in liquidation, windows broken in Berlin, shops raided in Vienna, the burning of the Reichstag.

How many years since she'd divested herself of her personal possessions and moved into this singularly impersonal room and here, confronted with her lone estate, resolved to write her little story, to sit down every single day and try to tell the secret she had kept throughout the years? Was it the anonymity of her life against which she'd rebelled? One had a right to one's personal history; if one had experienced strong emotion, endured one's special brand of agony, one was entitled to express it. At any rate with all the *Schrecklichkeit* that marched upon the world – Hitler entering Vienna, rolling across the bridge with all that show of military might, Czechoslovakia, Munich, Berchtesgaden, Chamberlain stepping from his plane carrying his scroll and his umbrella – switching on the radio, sallying forth to see the newsreels, how determined she had been to stick to her resolve. Why, it had obsessed her utterly. All the rumors from the air, that sense that everybody had of waiting on some dread, calamitous, unprecedented moment had not been able to deter her. Desperately she'd stuck right at it, working each and every day. It had, she is free to confess it, almost killed her, but when the spring arrived, exceptionally soft and lovely, she'd felt on certain days a curious joy, as though her heart had been assuaged, her spirit given wings to soar, to mount. There, spread upon the Flushing marshes was the great World's Fair – the fountains and the palaces of peace, and she had walked among them in the warm spring weather, an old, old woman in her declining years with something slowly growing, taking shape within her.

The King and Queen had visited the Fair, had eaten frank-furters with Mrs Roosevelt and returned to England safely. Finally in August that cloud that hung above the world exploded, burst asunder – Poland invaded, England, France at war with Germany, Warsaw bombed, the whole world waiting for Paris and London to be strafed from the air. During the long winter of the phony war with what dogged perseverance she had labored at her task. She could bring no order, no organization to her work, it simply fell to pieces in her mind. Up and down the floor she'd paced telling herself she was the greatest fool alive. Then out of that dead calm, ah God, with what swiftness came those bolts of lighting, Norway invaded, the overrunning of Denmark, the occupation of Belgium, the overrunning of France, Sedan, the fall of France, and the miraculous Dunkirk; then a pause before the crisis and finally, staged forever on the screen of air and sky, the Battle of Britain, all those nightly bombings, conflagrations, the show put on for everyone to see – that English bravery, with Churchill looming like Colossus, and all America invited to stay at home and listen to those cheerful voices of the bombed-out people in their shelters, jovial as though assembled at some pleasant nightclub, London every day in flames at all the movie theaters, and there she'd stayed to watch it, with her novel weaving through the holocaust and the horror.

After that to cap the climax Rudolf Hess flying to Scotland, and then to cap all climaxes and all surprises Hitler invading Russia, nothing to think about but Russia, those place names tolling in the mind like dirges, Kiev, Smolensk, Nizhni Novgorod. Would they hold, had they fallen? That meeting – Churchill shaking hands with Roosevelt aboard the battleship, the Atlantic Charter. And on a Sunday, the seventh of December, breaking through the music. Was it a prank by Orson Welles – a jamming of the radio? Pearl Harbor. Where exactly was it? What did it mean? Were we at war, lined up against the Axis, in it with our allies to the finish?

Disaster falling on disaster, Wake Island, Bataan, the stand at Corregidor, the sinking of the English ships, Hong Kong, Singapore, the Malay Peninsula, the Dutch East Indies; and presently the celluloid offering the eyes the visual images, the far-flung lines of battle, that wilderness of snow in Russia, the armies fighting in the snow, the cities holding – Moscow, Leningrad, and in the spring those corpses on the leafless trees in the demolished hamlets, convoys in the Atlantic, sinkings, aircraft carriers in the Pacific, dogfights in the waste of sky and ocean, landing craft, soldiers disembarking on the lonely beaches, battles in the jungles, flaming tanks, the boys arrayed in leaves and branches, with Mickey Mouse and Donald Duck and Popeye running in and out of Armageddon – sitting in that macabre twilight, wondering if she had the courage to complete her novel, Alamein, Guadalcanal, Roosevelt and Churchill at Casablanca, our landings in North Africa, and Stalingrad, the bleak, the desolated city, Eniwetok, Tarawa, Okinawa, Truk, Stalin under the palms with Roosevelt and Churchill.

And then again the voices, the announcements, sitting beside the radio – the channel safely crossed, the epic beach-heads, Caen and the channel ports. And in the summer, voices that announced the Russian conquests, cities taken back, that gathering sense of safety, victory approaching, the Battle of the Bulge and hopes set back at Christmas, confidence restored, that softening up, the ceaseless strafing of the German cities, our armies on the march, the crossing of the Rhine (victory so close that you could touch it), Stalin, Churchill, Roosevelt at Yalta (the black cape, the skeletal face) – peace and the spring approaching. Suddenly that voice that struck out like a blow – Roosevelt dead at Warm Springs, the funeral train (lilacs in the dooryard blooming), the crowds at stations weeping. Then spring with all the blossoms; peace in Europe long awaited. And summer with the victories in the Pacific, the Philippines regained, the islands hopped. Truman in conference with Attlee. Truman's announcement on the sixth of August, those words reverberating round the world. Alamogordo, Hiroshima.

Nagasaki; peace.

Peace, repeated the old woman, peace, and remembering the news that she had read that morning, said aloud, or thought that she had said it, 'What is man that Thou art mindful of him, and the son of man that Thou visitest him?' and she attempted to get up, for she was late and Adam waiting for her (dear me, dear me, how much money had he said he wanted? She must go to her desk and get it. Fifty dollars was the sum? No, no, she would not leave her manuscript to Adam, she would destroy it when she returned from dining. Plenty of novels in the world already. She had had the experience of writing it – that was sufficient, quite sufficient) and had she risen to her feet, had someone dealt her a stupendous blow and was it Nanny at her elbow urging her, 'Yes, now, take another step, the money's in the desk, go there and get it,' or was it the august angel with his hand upon her shoulder?

She fell, her head escaping by the fraction of an inch the corner of the desk and there she lay stretched out upon the carpet while the telephone upon the table by her bed began to ring, continued ringing.

And Adam who was mad and standing in the booth at the Armenian restaurant cursed roundly. 'Damn the old woman, damn Mol,' he said, banging the receiver onto the hook and then as he heard the coin click in the cup beneath the telephone, he pocketed his last remaining nickel and went back into the dining room to wait for his old lady, under the impression that she was on her way.